ACTS OF CARE

ACTS OF CARE

Recovering Women in Late Medieval Health

SARA RITCHEY

CORNELL UNIVERSITY PRESS
Ithaca and London

First published 2021 by Cornell University Press

Library of Congress Cataloging-in-Publication Data

Names: Ritchey, Sara Margaret, author.
Title: Acts of care : recovering women in late Medieval health / Sara Ritchey.
Description: Ithaca [New York] : Cornell University Press, 2021. | Includes bibliographical references and index.
Identifiers: LCCN 2020022417 (print) | LCCN 2020022418 (ebook) | ISBN 9781501753534 (hardcover) | ISBN 9781501758324 (paperback) | ISBN 9781501753541 (epub) | ISBN 9781501753558 (pdf)
Subjects: LCSH: Women healers, Medieval—Benelux countries. | Medical care—Religious aspects—Christianity. | Medical care—History—To 1500.
Classification: LCC R141 .R563 2021 (print) | LCC R141 (ebook) | DDC 610.9/02—dc23
LC record available at https://lccn.loc.gov/2020022417
LC ebook record available at https://lccn.loc.gov/2020022418

To my parents,
Margaret Maraist Ritchey and Ronald Ritchey

Contents

Abbreviations

AASS	Acta sanctorum, edited by Jean Bolland et al., 68 vols. (Paris: Palmé, 1863–1925)
BHL	Bibliotheca hagiographica Latina antiquae et mediae aetatis, 2 vols. (Brussels: Société des Bollandistes, 1949)
VAS	[Vita] de B. Aleyde Scharembekana
VAV	Vita Arnulfi conversi Villariensis
VBJ	Vita Beatae Juettae reclusae
VBN	Vita Beatricis, priorisse in Nazareth
VCM	Vita Christinae mirabilis
VIC	Vita Ioannis Cantipratensis
VILeau	Vita Idae Lewensis
VILeuv	Vita Idae Lovaniensis
VIN	Vita Idae de Nivellis
VJM	Vita Iulianae de Corelion
VLA	Vita Lutgardis Aquiriensis
VMO	Vita Mariae Oigniacensis
VMY	Vita Margarete de Ypres
VOL	Vita B. Odiliae Viduae Leodiensis

ACKNOWLEDGMENTS

This book seeks to make visible the hidden labor that enabled late medieval European communities to survive and thrive. The author could not have endured its coming into being but for the quiet care acts of so many friends, family members, colleagues, and service workers. I compose these final words from the security of my home during a national lockdown undertaken to limit the spread of the virus known as COVID-19. My writing is thus made possible, as it always was, by service and care laborers who daily risk their own well-being so that others can enjoy the privileges of comfort and connection. Let us sustain the visibility of their labor, and recognize and value it as essential, long after our collective re-emergence.

Throughout the period of this book's research and writing, my colleagues and students at the University of Louisiana at Lafayette and the University of Tennessee, Knoxville have been a source of intellectual generation and solidarity when public support for higher education in the humanities has often devalued our work. Under the leadership of Amy Elias and with the support of Ernie Freeberg, the Humanities Center and the Department of History at the University of Tennessee enabled me to participate in a monthly seminar on the medical humanities that led to many productive insights; they also hosted a workshop of the complete manuscript in which Montserrat Cabré, Susan Lawrence, Jay Rubenstein, and Laura Smoller offered extensive feedback. I am grateful for their perspectives and criticisms, but especially for their friendship. Other chapters or portions of this book have benefited from workshops and talks hosted by various universities and institutions, where a great deal of the organizational labor for my visit was undertaken by graduate students; I thank them for their time and intellectual energy, especially Elizabeth Harper, Mark Lambert, Jacqueline Victor, Anna Weerasinghe, and Sarah Zanolini. My colleagues at the University of Tennessee and the University of Louisiana have become dear friends and have greatly enhanced this project by sharing work and citations, offering feedback, and lifting my spirits. Thank you especially to Ian Beamish, Monica Black, Kristen Block, Manuela Ceballos,

Emily Deal, Nikki Eggers, Rich Frankel, Katie Hodges-Kluck, Chad Parker, Liz Skilton, Tina Shepardson, Lena Suk, Alison Vacca, and Shellen Wu. Other friends and scholars have also answered persistent questions, helped me to acquire resources, invited me to share work, and generally cared for my emotional life; I am especially grateful to Paul Barrette, Winston Black, Jennifer N. Brown, Naama Cohen-Hanegbi, Adam Davis, Daisy Delogu, Jay Diehl, Jen Edwards, Nahyan Fancy, Peggy McCracken, Cathy Mooney, Amy Ogden, Lucy Pick, Jeff Rider, Alan Rutenberg, and Sharon Strocchia. Their patience and kindness, so rare in this field, have allowed me to find a place in medieval studies when once my presence seemed so uncertain. The amount of support and guidance these scholars imparted should have resulted in a more perfect book; its remaining flaws are very much my own.

I remain perpetually grateful to and awed by three women in particular. Monica Green has fundamentally transformed not only my scholarship and career, but that of multiple generations of scholars. In addition to her constant supply of resources and feedback, her efforts to create online and in-person pedagogical and mentoring communities are absolutely unprecedented, such as the MEDMED-L list and the NEH seminar on Health and Disease in the Middle Ages. Without her scholarly generosity, advocacy, and intellectual labor, I simply could not have written this book. Alison Frazier and Martha Newman were my first and most dedicated mentors, making space for me in an academy into which I did not at once comfortably fit, and introducing me to hagiographic sources. Their meticulous scholarship, careful mentoring, and community building is a gift to our field. Words do not adequately capture my gratitude for the work of these three scholars, but my actions, I hope, can recapitulate their generous support by welcoming into the field and providing navigational assistance to those who are finding their way.

In the midst of writing this book, I transitioned to an R1 university and to geographic proximity to the institutional resources and scholarly communities positioned along the eastern seaboard of the United States. That move has brought into sharp relief the cumulative effects on scholars and scholarship of the unequal distribution of our resources and networks among academic geographies of prestige. I wish to acknowledge that much of this book could not have been completed from the margins of those institutional hierarchies, and I pledge to continue the work of building an inclusive academy in which resources are shared more equitably. Such exclusions muffle multitudes of voices, the grand polyphonic harmonies of medieval studies. I also wish to recognize the intellectual and emotional labor of scholars of color in our field, some of whom are involved in the professional collectives known as Medievalists of Color and RaceB4Race. They are doing the constant and uncompensated work of lifting the veil that has for so long attempted to conceal the foundational and structural racism, misogyny, and institutional elitism of our field. I am thankful for their voices, their work, and their presence.

Numerous institutions have made this book possible. I am grateful to them as well as to the people who have enabled me to acquire their resources and participate in their support. Funding for the research and writing of this book was provided by the National Endowment for the Humanities, the American Council of Learned Societies, the Renaissance Society of America, the American Philosophical Society, and the Louisiana Board of Regents. My ability to accept their funding and to present myself as a competitive candidate was entirely contingent on a cadre of caregivers, alternate kinship networks, and taxpayer-funded schools and after-care programs. Thank you especially to Pearson and Lisa Cross, Juliet Guzzetta, Joshua Yumibe, and Alex Zapruder, who provided me and my family with affective care as well as encouraged, prepared meals, organized playdates, and otherwise made my work and life possible. I also wish to thank the librarians and staff at the KBR, the Université de Liège, the Archives de l'État en Belgique, the British Library, and Hodges Library, especially Shaina Destine and Rachel Caldwell, and the administrative staff in my department and in the UT Humanities Center, Mary Beckley, Kim Harrison, Bernie Koprince, and Joan Viola Murray. The ability to access resources requires not only extensive time and funding, but also mobility. During this book's final stages, I was aided immeasurably by my research assistant, the remarkable Bradley Phillis, who helped me sort through sources when I was unable to do so on my own; this book could not have been completed without his efforts. Also at those final stages, the incredible editorial team at Cornell University stepped in with a fresh supply of enthusiasm and rhetorical wizardry. My sincere appreciation goes to Mahinder Kingra, Bethany Wasik, and Karen Hwa for shepherding this book to publication.

I have enjoyed the outstanding unearned privilege of being born into a family that heeds no bounds in matters of love, adventure, support, and good humor. Each one of them has cared for me in ways that have fundamentally enabled this book's existence. Lynne Bauersfeld, Jay Krachmer, Kathryn Maraist Krachmer, Liz Maraist, Christine Ritchey Weber, and my (as of this writing) 103-year-old grandmother, Gertrude Melancon Maraist, have been a constant source of material and emotional support. Malisa Troutman Dorn, Chris Dorn, Kit and Carl Dorn, and Dolores Vaughn make my family complete and help me to cherish the memory and example of Rebekah Vaughn Troutman and John Vaughn, whose absence grips me daily. Every page of this book is a memorial to Rebekah's work, to her capacity to infuse life and dignity into her community through acts of care. Scot Ritchey, Carly Ingvalson, and my beloved William Jude Ritchey supply me with the heartiest love and laughter I have ever known; I am so grateful that they are part of my life. And I cherish the love and partnership of John Troutman, who, in addition to reading drafts and suggesting revisions in all of my writing, maintains the work of our family while I travel every week. He has believed in me, whoever I am, and provided every support for the person I am still becoming; I can think of no greater gift. None of these efforts would be worth expending without the imagination and wit of our son, Jack Florian, who supplies the soundtrack of our days, their rhythm and harmony, and a reason to celebrate. My thanks to all of you for the richness and possibility you have brought into my life.

This book is dedicated to my parents, Ron Ritchey and Margaret Maraist Ritchey. All that I really know about health and care has come from experiencing their love. My father's boundless reserves of creative energy and his will to research and revise his own care practices have taught me how to use art, work, and care of self and others to overcome my isolation. He has been my source of serenity and encouragement when I could not muster the strength to supply my own. My mother is a most rare creature: every person she encounters is transformed by her ability to pierce humanity deep within the layers of pain and performance we all carry. She has given me everything, while staring directly into the eyes of strife, melting it, and radiating joy. It is an honor to call myself theirs.

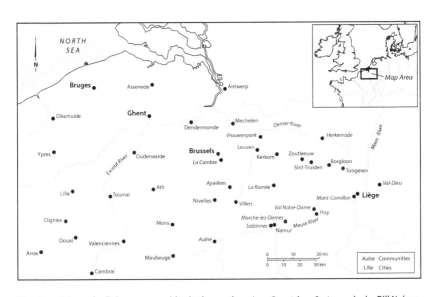

MAP 1. Cities and religious communities in the southern Low Countries. Cartography by Bill Nelson.

ACTS OF CARE

Introduction: To Heed the Trace

A young beguine named Ida, who later joined the Cistercian community of Roosendaal, routinely visited the poor and sick in her hometown of Leuven, providing them with food, clothing, and other bodily comforts.[1] The unnamed Cistercian monk who recorded her *Life* in the later thirteenth century reports that Ida was once called to a nearby home where she found a man in bed (*aegrotus*), nearly dead, and already having received the viaticum. She quickly inquired into the man's illness, eliciting information about the exact site and symptoms he experienced. After inspecting his pestiferous swelling, Ida drained the puss, and oversaw the salubrious results, which included the reduction of pain and swelling. Ida's success in healing the man proved pivotal for her reputation in the larger community:

> Thus the virgin of God, from this day forward and hereafter, is held in
> great esteem, clothed with the ornament of sanctity by all that received
> notice of these events. Indeed all who had seen it for themselves, or had
> heard of it, shared the unwavering conviction that it was through the
> merits of the venerable Ida that the vexation of the harshest pain was
> so dispersed and health, arriving just so suddenly and unexpectedly,

---

1. *Vita Idae de Lovanio* (BHL 4145), in *Acta sanctorum* (*AASS*) April II, 157D–189F; hereafter *VILeuv*.

took new form in the same sick person. Many took to telling the story of it far and wide, which promoted the fame of Ida's virginal holiness throughout the surrounding region.[2]

According to this report, Ida's successful treatment of the patient promoted her reputation for "virginal holiness"; that is, her health-giving intervention cinched her *fama* not as a healthcare practitioner, but as a "virgin of God." As the citizens of Leuven rendered this healing event into story, they crafted Ida's image as a holy woman. A Cistercian monk then recorded this orally circulating story and assembled it, along with other tales of her "virginal holiness," into a narrative of Ida's sanctity. This transmission process points to the ways that religious women's therapeutic authority was encoded, and then eroded, in other social norms in thirteenth-century Europe. Ida's activity as an efficacious bedside healer was subsumed by her gendered reputation for sanctity. Her therapeutic actions were recorded not as demonstrations of medical acumen but as examples of her intense religiosity.

The case of Ida spotlights the kinds of historical trajectories through which the healthcare behaviors she exhibited, behaviors displayed by numerous women in the thirteenth-century southern Low Countries, failed to be translated as "medical" sources and thus as "medical" history.[3] Women living as beguines and Cistercian nuns in this region served as nurses, herbalists, everyday caretakers, and wonder-workers who assisted patients using charms, blessings, relics, meditations, and prayers, in addition to herbs, stones, purgatives, phlebotomy, and maintenance of a daily regimen. Their labor was increasingly necessary as social needs became more visible under the pressure of the region's rapid urbanization, a response to the growth of the textile industries and the associated expansion of overland trade from Bruges to Cologne throughout the course of the thirteenth and fourteenth centuries.[4] Women immigrated

---

2. *VILeuv* 171D: "Ex tunc igitur et deinceps in magna veneratione Dei virgo praetextu suae sanctitatis, apud omnes, ad quorum haec pervenere notitiam, his diebus est habita. Cunctorum quippe, quibus haec videre vel audire permissa sunt, una fuit immutabilisque sententia, quod per venerabilis Idae merita tam acerbissimi doloris fugata molestia tamque repentine et improvise succedens sospitas in eodem esset aegroto procul dubio reformata. Quod cum ex frequenti relatione multorum longe lateque notitiae patuisset, ac virginalis sanctimoniae titulum his temporibus in omni circumjacenti vicinia mirabiliter extulisset."

3. My use of the term "medicine" throughout this book should be distinguished from contemporary Western concepts of "biomedicine." The term "medicine" is more encompassing than biology-based systems of health knowledge because it appreciates various cultures of illness and treatment. On this distinction, see Atwood Gaines and Robbie Davis-Floyd, "Biomedicine," in *Encyclopedia of Medical Anthropology: Health and Illness in the World's Cultures*, ed. Carol Ember and Melvin Ember (New York: Springer, 2004), n.p.

4. On the expansion of trade and urbanization, see Peter Stabel, *Dwarfs among Giants: The Flemish Urban Network in the Late Middle Ages* (Louvain: Garant, 1997). On the connection between

to centers of industry and manufacturing such as Cambrai, Ypres, Bruges, Douai, Leuven, and Brussels, where they found domestic, textile, and hospital work, and regularly engaged in public activities.[5] The women investigated in this book inhabited this urban social scene. They founded, managed, and staffed hospitals, leprosaria, and infirmaries; they cared for the dead and prepared bodies for burial; and they sometimes worked outside of institutional settings, begging for food, medicines, or clothing on behalf of the sick and infirm. They visited the sick and dying at bedsides in private homes, and occasionally the sick would journey from afar to access their healthcare services. This book seeks to reconstruct the therapeutic epistemologies that animated their practices; that is, it looks for the kinds of thinking, the logic or specific rationale, that brought together the variety of caregiving practices religious women used.

Such an endeavor must confront the vexing question of sources, of their supposed scarcity, and of what "counts" as medical history or medical knowledge. It is a lack of sources, scholars have assumed, that makes it difficult if not impossible to write a history of women practitioners in the later Middle Ages. For example, after remarking on the extensive healthcare institutions founded and staffed by beguines, Walter Simons notes that although these women must have received training, "such expertise has unfortunately remained undocumented."[6] And Simons would know. His *Cities of Ladies* is the most comprehensively researched recent account of beguine foundations in this region. At one point, he notes that caregiving was so closely associated with beguine patterns of charity that the terms "beguine convent" and "beguine hospital" were often used synonymously in the sources.[7]

urbanization and the need for hospital work, see Pierre de Spiegeler, *Les hôpitaux et l'assistance à Liège: Aspects institutionnels et sociaux* (Paris: Les Belles Lettres, 1987), 55.

5. On the demographics suggesting that women outnumbered men in the southern Low Countries, see Roger Mols, *Introduction à la démographie historique des villes du Europe du XIVe au XVIIIe siècle* (Gembloux: Duculot, 1954), 2:374–75; and Martha Howell, *Women, Production, and Patriarchy in Late Medieval Cities* (Chicago: University of Chicago Press, 1986). Walter Simons discusses the unequal migration patterns of women and men in "The Beguine Movement in the Southern Low Countries: A Reassessment," *Bulletin de l'Institut Historique Belge de Rome* 59 (1989): 63–105; Henri Pirenne, "Les dénombrements de la population d'Ypres au XVe siècle (1412–1506): Contribution à la statistique sociale du Moyen Âge," *Vierteljahrschrift für Sozial und Wirtschaftsgeschichte* 1 (1903): 1–32 is slightly later but discusses the role of women as domestic servants. On the public visibility of women as stall managers, vendors, teachers, and innkeepers, see Walter Simons, *Cities of Ladies: Beguine Communities in the Medieval Low Countries, 1200–1565* (Philadelphia: University of Pennsylvania Press, 2001), 10; and Jan Van Gerven, "Vrouwen, arbeid en sociale positie: Een voorlopig onderzoek naar de economische rol en maatschappelijke positie van vrouwen in de Brabantse steden in de late Middeleeuwen," *Revue Belge de Philologie et d'Histoire* 73 (1995): 947–66.

6. Simons, *Cities of Ladies*, 77–78.

7. Simons, 77.

It is here that I stake my intervention into the history both of premodern medicine and of medieval religion and gender. The sources for religious women's caregiving exist. Their recovery simply demands a shift in our thinking about how gendered interactions shape the documentary record. For too long, medievalists have read the sources we do have—psalters, prayers, saints' *Lives*, miracles, relics, liturgical rites—as having little to say about health, healing, care work, and medical practice.[8] Indeed, the overdetermination of late medieval holy women as imitating Christ's suffering has masked the historically situated ways that their embodied performances of prayer and penance also carried medical significations that mattered deeply to the communities surrounding them. Their prayers were experienced as efficacious healthcare practices by those who supported them. Any version of medieval medicine that excludes the demand for, and the perceived effects of, prayer and penance, therefore, is incomplete. The sources of women's bodily therapies, I argue, come not in the form of coherent academic treatises, but in "fragile traces" detectable in liturgy, poetry, recipes, meditations, sacred objects, and the everyday behaviors that constituted their world.[9]

The sources I explore in this book are necessarily fragmentary. They are traces of a practice long forgotten as therapeutic.[10] These traces often appear to scholars of medieval history and religion, and are interpreted and perpetuated by them, as "religious" texts or ritualistic behavior, not as medical practices. I refer to these traces of past practices as "therapeutic" in order to frame them as knowledge and behaviors that fall somewhere in between our current conceptualizations of medicine and religion, as "treatments." There is an abundance of scholarly precedence for framing premodern healthcare in this way. For example, the medical historian Vivian Nutton notes that Galen used the term *therapeutes* to indicate a kind of caregiving and body knowledge connected

---

8. This is a point made repeatedly by Monica Green in "Gender, Health, Disease: Recent Work on Medieval Women's Medicine," *Studies in Medieval and Renaissance History*, ser. 3, 5 (2005): 1–46.

9. Informing my approach here is the work of Patricia Hill Collins, who provides a framework for deciphering examples of Black women's knowledge and resistance. She argues that "suppression of Black women's ideas within white male-controlled social institutions led African American women to use music, literature, daily conversations, and everyday behavior as important locations for constructing a Black feminist consciousness." Patricia Hill Collins, *Black Feminist Thought: Knowledge, Consciousness, and the Politics of Empowerment* (New York: Routledge, 2002), 251–52. Nancy Rose Hunt addresses the search for "fragile acoustic traces" in "An Acoustic Register, Tenacious Images, and Congolese Scenes of Rape and Repetition," *Cultural Anthropology* 23.2 (2008): 220–53.

10. On this process of forgetting the original significations of social practices, see Diana Taylor, "Remapping Genre through Performance: From 'American' to 'Hemispheric' Studies," *PMLA* 122.5 (2007): 1416–30.

to "active worship."[11] More recently, the literary historian Daniel McCann has opted for the terminology of "treatment" to encompass the biological, psychological, and social factors pertinent to efficacy.[12] My use of "therapeutic treatments" as a frame for examining premodern healing practices is informed by my experiences growing up in an Acadian bayou town in southern Louisiana, a region to which I returned as an adult professor of medieval history. There, healers known as *traiteurs* and *traiteuses* have for centuries used prayer, herbal remedies, touch, and ligatures to address an array of afflictions ranging from bug bites to angina.[13] They do not accept money as payment, and their *traitements* (treatments), along with the power to wield them efficaciously, are passed down orally. They do not position themselves in competition with professional biomedical practitioners, but they are an essential component of the healthcare landscape of this region (or at least they were until the mid-twentieth century— these practices have slowly begun to fade as the Acadiana region has become more commercialized, medicalized, and suburban).[14] I propose the term "therapeutic treatments" to describe the caregiving work provided by thirteenth-century religious women because it mingles the physical, social, emotional, and spiritual aspects of their approach to health and care. Like *traiteurs*, their treatments included prayer, touch, counsel, and herbal remedies, in addition to feeding, cleaning, and the provision of daily comfort and assurance. If we consider these treatments from within the context of religious women's communal circuits of care, we can begin to restore their therapeutic meanings.

11. Vivan Nutton, "God, Galen, and the Depaganization of Ancient Religion," in *Religion and Medicine in the Middle Ages*, ed. Peter Biller and Joseph Ziegler (York: York Medieval Press, 2001), 25.

12. Daniel McCann, *Soul Health: Therapeutic Reading in Late Medieval England* (Cardiff: University of Wales Press, 2019), 6.

13. This occupational title might best be rendered in English as "treaters." The *Dictionary of Louisiana French* translates *traiteur* as "traditional healer, faith healer." See *Dictionary of Louisiana French: As Spoken in Cajun, Creole, and American Indian Communities*, ed. Albert Valdman et al. (Jackson: University of Mississippi Press, 2009), 628. This rendering, however, does not quite grasp the blended modes of therapy used by *traiteurs*, which involved prayers, incantations, nonsensical secret phrases, touch, *cordons* (ligatures), *benisons* (blessings), and herbal remedies, especially teas, tonics, and *catepans* (poultices). Some basic remedies involved burying a nail after making the sign of the cross on an afflicted body part and applying holy water or wax to an afflicted limb while saying a prayer. These *traitements*, along with the power to wield them efficaciously, are passed down orally. It is for this reason, in part, that very few historians have examined *traiteurs*, although they do have a place in folklore studies. An earlier study, from the perspective of folklore, is Anna Boudreaux, "Les remèdes du vieux temps: Remedies and Cures of the Kaplan Area in Southwest Louisiana," *Southern Folklore Quarterly* 35.2 (1971): 121–40.

14. The legal and professional process of eroding these healthcare practices was underway even earlier. A February 1919 action in the circuit court of appeals sitting at Baton Rouge, for example, made injunction against two "notorious" traiteurs from Lafayette parish, prohibiting them from practicing medicine. *Abbeville Meridional*, 8 Feb. 1919.

Reading "Nonevidence"

Scholars have long noted that the household operated as the first "port of call" for the sick within premodern Europe, where women provided "the basic recourse for medical care."[15] They were primarily responsible for daily "bodywork"—the maintenance of diet, cleanliness, and comfort.[16] As Mary Fissell has noted, women were central to the practice of everyday healthcare: "Almost everyone in early modern Europe was brought into the world by women and ushered out of it by women. Women's hands birthed babies, cut umbilical cords, and swaddled newborns. Women's hands treated the sick, comforted the dying, and laid out bodies, readying them for burial."[17] Peter Pormann and Emilie Savage-Smith have made similar observations about the omnipresence of women practitioners in Islamicate societies, noting that they were responsible for the medical needs of children, husbands, and other members of the extended family and "contributed fundamentally to the health of the wider society."[18] Anthropological and sociological analysis confirms the picture of woman-dominated caregiving within the domestic sphere.[19] In other words, we *know* that the daily healthcare needs of medieval

15. Margaret Pelling, "Thoroughly Resented? Older Women and the Medical Role in Early Modern London," in *Women, Science, and Medicine, 1500–1700*, ed. Lynette Hunter and Sarah Hutton (Gloucestershire: Sutton, 1997), 70; Alicia Rankin, *Panaceia's Daughters: Noblewomen as Healers in Early Modern Germany* (Chicago: University of Chicago Press, 2013), 3. In this book, I will use Monica Green's definition of "female medical practitioners" as "women who at some point in their lives would have either identified themselves in terms of their medical practice or been so identified by their communities." Monica Green, "Documenting Medieval Women's Medical Practice," in *Practical Medicine from Salerno to the Black Death*, ed. Luis García-Ballester, Jon French, Jon Arrizabalaga, and Andrew Cunningham (Cambridge: Cambridge University Press, 1994), 335–36. Green's definition is an adaptation of Margaret Pelling and Charles Webster's notion of medical practitioner as "anyone whose occupation is basically concerned with care of the sick." See Margaret Pelling and Charles Webster, "Medical Practitioners," in *Health, Medicine, and Mortality in the Sixteenth Century*, ed. Charles Webster (Cambridge: Cambridge University Press, 1979), 165–235.

16. Mary Fissell developed the concept of "bodywork" to grasp the range of caregiving approaches to suffering bodies. Fissell writes, "I am not proposing that we replace the category 'medicine' with bodywork; rather, that we investigate the relationship between the work we consider medicine and the broader category of attending to the human body, and perhaps place medicine and its learned traditions within or next to the larger category of bodywork or body technologies." Mary Fissell, "Introduction: Women, Health, and Healing in Early Modern Europe," *Bulletin of the History of Medicine* 82.1 (2008): 11. Fissell builds on previous scholarship, such as Sandra Cavallo's notion of "artisans of the body," in *Artisans of the Body in Early Modern Italy: Identities, Families, and Masculinities* (Manchester: Manchester University Press, 2007); Montserrat Cabré's notion of modification of body surfaces, in "From a Master to a Laywoman: A Feminine Manual of Self-Help," *Dynamis* 20 (2000): 371–93; and Monica Green's term "technologies of the body" in "Gender, Health, Disease."

17. Fissell, "Introduction," 1.

18. Peter Pormann and Emilie Savage-Smith, *Medieval Islamic Medicine* (Washington, DC: Georgetown University Press, 2007), 103.

19. For caregiving statistics, see Nicholas T. Bott, Clifford Sheckter, and Arnold Milstein, "Dementia Care, Women's Health, and Gender Equity: The Value of Well-Timed Caregiver Support," *JAMA*

communities were numerically dominated by women, the vast majority of whom did not develop reputations as saints. And yet, as Monica Green has noted, scholars are confronted by the abiding problem of "nonevidence"; that is, women rarely appear in documents of medical practice or in our resulting historical narratives of premodern medicine.[20]

Where professional records do exist, they scarcely capture the presence of women healthcare practitioners. For example, Danielle Jacquart's 1981 study of three centuries of medical practitioners in France, which included midwives, turned up just 127 women, or 1.5 percent of the total recorded practitioners.[21] In England, women made up 1.2 percent of the total, and in the Kingdom of Aragon three women out of five hundred (or 0.6 percent) appear to have held titles as practitioners of healthcare.[22] Turning from archival sources to medical treatises, we find that, on the rare occasions that practitioners identified as women do appear in academic medical literature, it is only to denounce their foolishness in matters of the body that should be left to trained—that is, to literate male—physicians. For example, when Teodorico Borgognoni, the thirteenth-century Dominican bishop of Bitonto and later of Cervia and sometime master of medicine and surgery at the University of Bologna, transmitted a small sample of verbal remedies in his Latin *Chirurgia*, he professed deep hesitation, stating that they struck him as "more the concoction[s] of old women than the prescriptions of a prudent man."[23] Gendered comparatives such as Teodorico's, which distinguish women's verbal remedies from men's learned prescriptions, are found throughout later medieval European texts of scholastic medicine and surgery.[24] In order to legitimize the transmission of

---

Neurology 74.7 (2017): 757–58; on gender, caregiving, and emotional labor, see Arlie Russell Hochschild, *The Commercialization of Intimate Life: Notes from Home and Work* (Berkeley: University of California Press, 2003); and Amy Wharton, "The Sociology of Emotional Labor," *American Review of Sociology* 35 (2009): 147–65; for a historical approach in the US context, see Susan Reverby, *Ordered to Care: The Dilemma of American Nursing, 1850–1945* (Cambridge: Cambridge University Press, 1987).

20. Green, "Gender, Health, Disease," 18.

21. Danielle Jacquart, *Le milieu médical en France du XIIe au XVe siècle* (Geneva: Droz, 1981), 47–55; Monica Green supplemented Jacquart's list with an additional six healers in "Documenting Medieval Women's Medical Practice." On the English sources, see Stuart Jenks, "Medizinische Fachkräfte in England zur Zeit Heinrichs VI (1428/9–1460/61)," *Sudhoffs Archiv* 69.2 (1985): 214–27.

22. For England, see Monica Green, "Women's Medical Practice and Health Care in Medieval Europe," *Signs* 14 (1989): 434–73; for Aragon, see Carmel Ferrargud Domingo, *Medicina i promoció social a la baixa edat mitjana: Corona d'Aragó 1350–1410* (Madrid: Consejo Superior de Investigaciones Científicas, 2005), 76.

23. Teodorico Borgognoni, *Chirurgia*, in *Ars chirurgia Guidonis Cauliaci* (Venice, 1546), fol. 158v: "quia magis videntur nobis vetularum esse quam prudentis viri"; trans. E. Campbell and J. Colton, *The Surgery of Theodoric* (New York: 1960), 2:17.

24. On denunciations of women's remedies in scholastic medical treatises, see Jole Agrimi and Chiara Crisciani, "Savoir médical et anthropologie religieuse: Les représentations et fonctions de la *vetula* (XIIIe–XVe siècle)," *Annales: Économies, Société, Civilisations* 48.5 (1993): 1281–1308.

remedies culturally associated with women practitioners, Teodorico and other scholastic physicians had to obscure any suggestion of feminine origin to assert that *theirs* were affirmed by learned men.

Our current historical narrative of the emergence of medicine in western Europe is progressive; it depends upon an intellectual posture that reaches back in search of familiar professional markers and diagnostic habits, the antecedents of present practice.[25] Such a posture reifies categories of knowledge production separating medicine and religion that were by no means stable or universally embraced in the thirteenth century.[26] For instance, Naama Cohen-Hanegbi has shown that the construction of medicine as a distinct field of investigation in medieval Europe was penetrated by Christian concepts, as scholastic physicians sought to determine how to approach an ensouled body that was premised on its susceptibility to immaterial forces. In those moments of elaborating a medicine that addressed the soul in order to shape the body, practitioners were concerned with a medicine of self, with the continuities of body and spirit. For example, the Italian physician Giovanni Matteo Ferrari da Grado (d. 1472) prescribed the experience of joy to counteract the melancholic fevers of a young patient.[27] While thirteenth-century practitioners and theologians clearly recognized distinctions between medicine of the body and medicine of the soul, the phenomenological experience of embodiment was expressed in mutual terms.

Although an elite minority of educated men known as *physici* attempted to articulate medicine according to natural and rational principles of matter, a vast array of other practitioners understood and deployed the language of medicine and health (*salus*) in far more fluid and unbounded ways. While those medical others were not exclusively women, their vilification and erasure in the learned treatises of medieval medicine resulted in an explicit gendering of certain forms of healthcare practice. When physici chose to distinguish their remedies from those of practitioners unschooled in Galenic principles of medicine, they relied upon the image of the loathsome *vetula*, or "old woman."[28] For instance, Arnald

---

25. Fissell, "Introduction."

26. Iona McCleery, "Christ More Powerful than Galen: The Relationship between Medicine and Miracles," in *Contextualizing Miracles in the Medieval West*, ed. M. M. Mesley and Louise Wilson (Leeds: Medium Aevum, 2014), 127–54.

27. Giovanni Matteo Ferrari da Grado, *Consilia* (Lyon, 1535), fol. 7v, in Naama Cohen-Hanegbi, *Caring for the Living Soul: Emotions, Medicine, and Penance in the Late Medieval Mediterranean* (Leuven: Brill, 2017), 74.

28. Jole Agrimi and Chiara Crisciani chronicled the increasing suspicion on the part of learned medical practitioners and clerics, who from the thirteenth century onward cast *vetulae* as deviant and untrustworthy in their "Savoir médical et anthropologie religieuse." See also Karen Pratt, "*De vetula*: The Figure of the Old Woman in Medieval French Literature," in *Old Age in the Middle Ages*

of Villanova, seeking to establish the superior knowledge of physicians, referred to *vetulae* as the very incarnation of neglect of reason and natural causes of disease.[29] Guy of Chauliac thought that "women and idiots" were most interested in using herbal charms and incantations.[30] And the French surgeon Henri de Mondeville reported that simple patients (*vulgi*) rejected learned physicians and sought instead "divine surgeons" (*divini cyrugici*) such as the anchorites and "old harlots" (*antiqui meretrices et metatrices*) who, they believed, gained medical knowledge directly from God and the saints.[31] Henri feminized categories of healer other than the scholastic physician when he associated barbers, fortune-tellers, alchemists, midwives, Jewish converts, and Muslims with the ignorance and religiosity of *vetulae*.[32] In order to emerge as distinct, as professional, proponents of academic medicine explicitly lambasted certain practices that they associated with women. These practices included charms, prayers, poetry, liturgical rituals, and meditations. To be sure, many varieties of practitioner, women and men, dabbled in these kinds of affective, performative remedies. But scholastic physicians characterized those remedies as feminine and hence as irrational, unlearned, sometimes even as wicked. As Peregrine Horden has lamented, women healthcare practitioners were the "first and largest casualty of scholasticism triumphant."[33]

The presences and practices of women's caregiving have thus been erased by historical trajectories premised on recorded professional and genre-defined documents, that is, on mechanisms of power from which women

---

and the Renaissance: Interdisciplinary Approaches to a Neglected Topic, ed. Albrecht Classen (Berlin: De Gruyter, 2007), 321–42. It was hardly physicians alone who cast suspicion on old women using herbs and charms to care for their neighbors. Theologians engaged in similar maneuvers in which they theorized certain ritual actions, like blessings and charms, as permissible among trained clerics but dangerous when used by the uneducated, especially by old women. See Michael Bailey, "The Disenchantment of Magic: Spells, Charms, and Superstition in Early European Witchcraft Literature," *American Historical Review* 111.2 (2006): 383–404. As Agrimi and Crisciani have shown, clerics and physicians shared biases about *vetulae*, leading to even greater suppression.

29. Joseph Ziegler, *Medicine and Religion, c. 1300: The Case of Arnau de Vilanova* (Oxford: Clarendon Press, 1998), 123. See, for example, Arnald of Villanova's *De cautelis medicorum*, trans. Henry Sigerist, in "Bedside Manners in the Middle Ages: The Treatise *De cautelis medicorum* Attributed to Arnald of Villanova," in *Henry Sigerist on the History of Medicine*, ed. Felix Marti-Ibañez (New York: MD Publications, 1960), 132–40.

30. Don Skemer, *Binding Words: Textual Amulets in the Middle Ages* (University Park, PA: Pennsylvania State University Press, 2006), 235n1.

31. *Die Chirurgie des Heinrich von Mondeville (1306–1320)*, ed. J. Pagel (Berlin: Hirschwald, 1892), 68.

32. *Die Chirurgie*, 661: "sicut barberii, sortilegi, locatores, insidiatores, falsarii, alchemistae, meretrices, metatrices, obstetrices, vetulae, Iudaei conversi, Sarraceni."

33. Peregrine Horden, "Religion as Medicine: Music in Medieval Hospitals," in *Religion and Medicine in the Middle Ages*, ed. Peter Biller and Joseph Ziegler (York: York University Press, 2001), 137; Monica Green's *Making Women's Medicine Masculine* shows that it was women's estrangement from Latin medical texts and university centers of medical learning that phased out their participation.

were eclipsed. Because women's practices were not preserved as "legitimate" medical knowledge, their voices were not recorded as medical authorities. Women-identified practitioners, in other words, were socially alienated from professional markers and from the production of generic textual sources, the commentaries and *consilia* (medical case histories) produced by academic or licensed physicians. Therefore, neither occupational markers nor formal medical treatises convey the full range of women's healthcare activities.[34] Recognizing this disjunction between women's daily healthcare practice in medieval Europe and their lack of archival substantiation raises questions about the validity of historical methods that rely on the very media from which women were estranged.[35] Given women's vexed relationship to what was recorded as authoritative medical knowledge and practice, the goal of locating them and their constructions of therapeutic knowledge might behoove us to critically stretch our understanding of the kinds of reading, writing, and performance that inform medical history. By continuing to construct our histories of medicine on these genre-defined sources and technologies of power from which women were socially, culturally, and sometimes legally distanced, we only reproduce feminine erasure and silence.[36]

Rather than searching for women's presence among professional markers in diplomatic or scholastic medical sources, I consider how women's healthcare practices were translated into textual representations. As Montserrat Cabré has shown, women's healthcare roles were subsumed under the semantic domain of *mother*, *woman*, and other categories of feminine life stages.[37] To ascertain women's roles in the medieval health economy, we must desist from imposing "categories clearly alien to women's work."[38] Women's positions in caring for and curing sick and dying bodies in hospitals,

---

34. That occupational markers were the exception, not the rule, for female healthcare practitioners is a foundational argument of Monica Green's "Documenting Medieval Women's Medical Practice."

35. This point about historical practice and the process of uncovering silenced and estranged voices is derived from Marissa J. Fuentes, *Dispossessed Lives: Enslaved Women, Violence, and the Archive* (Philadelphia: University of Pennsylvania Press, 2016).

36. Laws limiting women's medical practice appear in Valencia in the fourteenth century and in England in the fifteenth. Licensing regulations affected women as early as the thirteenth century, but only insofar as they were uneducated, not *as* women. On Valencia, see Luis García-Ballester, Michael McVaugh, and Augustin Rubio Vela, *Medical Licensing and Learning in Fourteenth-Century Valencia* (Philadelphia: Transactions of the American Philosophical Society, 1989); on England, see Eileen Power, "Some Women Practitioners of Medicine in the Middle Ages," *Proceedings of the Royal Society of Medicine* 15.6 (1922): 20–23.

37. Montserrat Cabré, "Women or Healers? Household Practices and the Categories of Healthcare in Late Medieval Iberia," *Bulletin of the History of Medicine* 82.1 (2008): 23.

38. Cabré, 23.

leprosaria, and private homes reflected their social roles as caretakers of children, preparers of food, attendants at childbirth, and custodians of the dead.[39] This healthcare work failed to be translated textually as medical labor. Instead, as in the case of Ida, communities expressed their gratitude for religious women's care and cure through attributions of sanctity and holiness.

While many different kinds of women in medieval societies cared for the infirm, not all of them developed reputations for sanctity. In this book, I use the records of those that did garner such standing in order to piece together a coherent impression of the array of therapeutic practices and concepts available to women—particularly religious women—in the thirteenth-century southern Low Countries. These sources demonstrate that several communities of religious women in the southern Low Countries were able to position themselves at the center of phenomenological descriptions of health events in their region.[40] In other words, the women who gained reputations for sanctity left behind the kinds of records we can use to better understand women's roles more generally as charitable caregivers in the later Middle Ages. These women were not exceptional; my interest is not in the "saints," but rather in how we can use the stories of saints—and saints identified as women in particular—to learn more about feminine caregiving roles and therapeutic knowledge, forms of care that have been devalued and underrecognized in our historical records and in our resulting historical narratives.

I show that religious women's social association with penitential prayer placed them in proximity to the sick and dying, where they performed a wholly integrated spiritual and corporeal therapeutics that blended prayer with bodily and emotional care and cure. They offered both a conceptualization of the body that was tied cosmically to a community of the dead and living and a therapeutic practice that linked body and soul with individual and communal health. In a culture where death was immanent and among people who earnestly believed that to die unconfessed would lead to eternal misery for their souls and the resulting anguish of their dearest loved ones, certain assemblages of religious women were able to console and care as an efficacious form of therapy.[41] They, and those they treated, were bound

---

39. Carol Hill, *Women and Religion in Late Medieval Norwich* (Woodbridge: Boydell and Brewer, 2010), 134.

40. On similar positionings, but in the Caribbean, see Pablo Gómez, *The Experiential Caribbean: Creating Knowledge and Healing in the Early Modern Atlantic* (Chapel Hill: University of North Carolina Press, 2017), 106.

41. Stacey Langwick, *Bodies, Politics, and African Healing: A Matter of Maladies in Tanzania* (Bloomington: Indiana University Press, 2011), 6.

together through social obligations of caring and curing, relationships that were perpetuated and strengthened in the form of stories of sanctity.

"Religious Women" and Their Stories

Stories of sanctity form a starting point for this book. I investigate how tales of women's holiness conveyed information about therapeutic resources. The stories of sanctity I explore comprise a unique corpus of *Lives* of so-called living saints written and transmitted in the thirteenth-century southern Low Countries.[42] The saints' *Lives* from the thirteenth-century Low Countries have been variously described as a "corpus," a "canon," and a "dossier."[43] In an effort to recognize the flourishing in this region of stories of meritorious people living in the thirteenth century, I use the terminology of "corpus," but I am intentionally open-ended with regard to the texts and other content that constitute this corpus because I wish to be expansive about who was deemed a "saint" in the thirteenth-century lowlands.[44] The "saints" whose *Lives* appear in this book, for example, were never canonized.[45] But they left

---

42. On living saints, see Aviad Kleinberg, *Prophets in Their Own Country: Living Saints and the Making of Sainthood in the Late Middle Ages* (Chicago: University of Chicago Press, 1992); Gabriella Zarri, *Le sante vive: Cultura e religiosità femminile nella prima età moderna* (Turin: Rosenberg & Sellier, 1990); C. Ruhrberg, *Der literarische Körper der heiligen Leben und Viten der Christina Stommeln* (Tubingen: Bibliotecha Germanica, 1995).

43. The "canon" of thirteenth-century southern Netherlandish saints' lives can be found in Barbara Newman, preface to *Send Me God*, trans. Martinus Cawley (University Park: Pennsylvania State University Press, 2011), xlviii-xlix. Newman describes the canon as "probably unique in the annals of hagiography" (xxx). A slightly expanded enumeration of the canon can be found in Anneke Mulder-Bakker, *Living Saints of the Thirteenth Century* (Turnhout: Brepols, 2011). Although not all of the lives of mulieres religiosae in this corpus contain information about caregiving, they have all been critical to my understanding of the process of translation of care into textual representations of women's sanctity. As discussed in chapter 2, I also consider the male lives in the larger corpus, though they exhibit far fewer examples of caregiving.

44. On this approach to expanding who we identify as "saints," see Anneke Mulder-Bakker, "The Invention of Saintliness: Texts and Contexts," in *The Invention of Saintliness*, ed. Anneke Mulder-Bakker and Han J. W. Drijvers (London: Routledge, 2002), 3–23; and Julia Smith, "Oral and Written: Saints, Miracles, and Relics in Britany, c. 850–1250," *Speculum* 65 (1990): 309–43. According to Barbara Newman's canon, there were twenty-five total saints' *Lives* (fourteen women and eleven men) produced "around" the thirteenth century in the southern Low Countries. This number does not include the many brief anecdotes and summarized *Lives* that appear in collections such as Caesarius of Heisterbach's *Dialogue on Miracles* (*Dialogus miraculorum*), Thomas of Cantimpré's *Book of Bees* (*Bonum universale de apibus*), the *History of the Monastery of Villers* (*Chronica Villariensis monasterii*), and the *Deeds of the Saints of Villers* (*Gesta sanctorum Villariensium*).

45. The Bollandists' enterprise of editing saints' *Lives* originated among the Jesuits of Antwerp, particularly Heribert Rosweyde, who conceived to publish the *Lives* of the saints of the Catholic Church in an eighteen-volume collection that assembled "authentic" documents, dispensing of legend. Rosweyde's idea was brought to fruition by his pupil, Jean Bolland, who commenced the production as the *Acta sanctorum*, or *AASS*. While irrefutably useful, the *AASS* is still a political product. Decisions about truth and legend and the canon law concept of sainthood determined its contents. On the

enough of an impression on their neighbors that those neighbors shared stories of wonder and merit about them, and in some cases, those stories were written down in note form or compiled from notes into life narratives. Saintliness is the chance detail that has enabled the survival of a record of the medical services provided by thirteenth-century women. I contextualize these details of sanctity among an array of other manuscript and archival sources circulating in women's religious communities, such as regimens, prayer books, charms, meditations, testaments, songs, images, relics, and liturgical practices. In reading saints' *Lives* in this context, I seek to peel back the layers of the textual codification of sanctity, to consider why stories of sanctity began circulating in the first place.

Thus far I have described the subjects of this book as "religious women." This is a fraught term, and yet it is one that I am not prepared to discard. The sources used in this book employ a variety of labels to identify women, including nuns (*moniales*), handmaidens (*ancillae*), holy virgins (*sanctae virgines*), and beguines (*beghinae*); but the vocabulary appearing most commonly in the sources is *mulieres religiosae*, "religious women." What this phrase meant in the thirteenth century is not always clear, though it is important to note that *religio* had a meaning rather different from the way we currently tend to conceptualize it in the twenty-first-century North America in which I am writing.[46] To Christians in medieval Europe, *religio* referred to the bond between a devout human and their God, a bond commonly formalized in monastic vows.[47] In the thirteenth-century lowlands, however, it could also be applied to women who were not legally recognized as nuns, but were nevertheless described as "religious."

Who were these mulieres religiosae? Scholars have long struggled to answer this question, to sort the sources of thirteenth-century European women's lives into the appropriate categories of religious life.[48] Jennifer Kolpacoff Deane,

---

enterprise, see David Knowles, "The Bollandists," in *Great Historical Enterprises: Problems in Monastic History* (Edinburgh: Nelson and Sons, 1963). On this critical process, see Jan Machielsen, "Heretical Saints and Textual Discernment: The Polemical Origins of the *Acta sanctorum* (1643–1940)," in *Angels of Light? Sanctity and the Discernment of Spirits in the Early Modern Period*, ed. Clare Copeland and Jan Machielsen (Leiden: Brill, 2012), 103–41.

46. Jonathan Z. Smith, "Religion, Religions, Religious," in *Critical Terms for Religious Studies*, ed. Mark Taylor (Chicago: University of Chicago Press, 1988), 269–84. As Smith notes of sixteenth-century attributions of this term by Europeans attempting to describe the indigenous cosmologies they encountered in Peru, "Religion is not a native category. It is not a first-person term of self-characterization. It is a category imposed from the outside on some aspect of native culture. It is the other, in these instances colonialists, who are solely responsible for the content of the term."

47. See Peter Biller, "Words and the Medieval Notion of Religion," *Journal of Ecclesiastical History* 36.3 (1985): 351–69.

48. Alison More uses the term "rubric" to explain how clerics sought to slot religiously inclined women into clear-cut categories. See More, *Fictive Orders and Feminine Religious Identities, 1200–1600*

Michel Lauwers, Elizabeth Makowski, Alison More, Tanya Stabler Miller, and so many other scholars have illuminated the rich and complex individual communities and larger "movements" of women in late medieval northern Europe, raising important questions about the ways that we draw lines around religious identities that defined women as nuns, beguines, penitents, tertiaries, or laywomen.[49] The patient and diligent work of these scholars has exposed the limitations of our language as well as our binary and often teleological thinking when attempting to describe the world in which these women attempted to express their devotion.

Some of the mulieres religiosae discussed in this book lived at least part of their lives as Cistercian nuns. They often appear in the sources as nuns (*moniales*), sisters (*sorores*), or religious women (*mulieres religiosae, religiosae feminae, devotes mulieres*), and they usually took formal, canonical vows; but their status as "cloistered" and even as "Cistercian" was hardly stable in this period.[50] In the early thirteenth century, they often behaved more like lay religious women by involving themselves in various forms of active charity in hospitals, leprosaria, and homes on their diverse granges, outside of or adjacent to their cloister; moreover, in the thirteenth-century lowlands, they often lived as lay religious women or canonesses attached to other independent houses or hospitals before formal incorporation as Cistercian nuns. The hagiographic sources used in this book to examine the charitable caregiving offered by Cistercian nuns are shaped by clerical interests that often projected a stable Cistercian identity on religious women

---

(Oxford: Oxford University Press, 2019), 2. She asserts that men "who were charged with providing [women's] spiritual care (*cura*) struggled to find a rubric that would both explain the existence of these women and place them in a recognizable category under canon law" (2).

49. Jennifer Kolpacoff Deane, "Beguines Reconsidered: Historiographical Problems and New Directions," *Commentaria* 34.61 (2008), n.p.; Sean Field, "On Being Beguine in France, c. 1300," in *Labels and Libels: Naming Beguines in Northern Medieval Europe*, ed. Letha Böhringer, Jennifer Kolpacoff Deane, and Hildo van Engen (Turnhout: Brepols, 2014), 117–33; Michel Lauwers, "L'expérience béguinale et récit hagiographique à propos de la *Vita Mariae Oigniacensis* de Jacques de Vitry," *Journal des Savants* 11 (1989): 61–103; Elizabeth Makowski, "Mulieres Religiosae, Strictly Speaking: Some Fourteenth-Century Canonical Opinions," *Catholic Historical Review* 85 (1999): 1–14; Tanya Stabler Miller, *Beguines of Medieval Paris: Gender, Patronage, and Spiritual Authority* (Philadelphia: University of Pennsylvania Press, 2014); More, *Fictive Orders*; Anneke Mulder-Bakker, *Lives of the Anchoresses: The Rise of the Urban Recluse* (Philadelphia: University of Pennsylvania Press, 2005).

50. On the evolution of Cistercian nuns in Liège and Cambrai, see Sara Moens, "Beatrice's World: The Rise of Cistercian Nunneries in the Bishoprics of Liège and Cambrai," *Ons Geestelijk Erf* 89.3–4 (2018): 225–74; on their development more broadly in France and the Low Countries, see Constance Berman, *The White Nuns: Cistercian Abbeys for Women in Medieval France* (Philadelphia: University of Pennsylvania Press, 2018); Erin Jordan, *Women, Power, and Religious Patronage in the Middle Ages* (New York: Palgrave, 2006); Anne Lester, *Creating Cistercian Nuns: The Women's Religious Movement and Its Reform in Thirteenth-Century Champagne* (Ithaca: Cornell University Press, 2011).

prior to their own formal affiliation with or identification as Cistercian. Those sources thus reflect practices that would fit within the parameters of proper behavior for what a cleric might consider a "good" Cistercian nun; this clerical investment in Cistercian women's propriety, in the promotion of "virgins of God," served to mediate and translate these women's lives. Religious women's healthcare acts are thus depicted in these sources as taking place either prior to the time when their saintly subjects entered the cloister or as part of their attendance to the sick within the cloister. But when read alongside the resistance of some communities of Cistercian nuns to strict enclosure, these hagiographic portraits suggest multiple dimensions of their active charity. For instance, from 1229 to 1233, as the abbot of the Cistercian monastery of Savigny in Normandy, Stephen of Lexington visited a number of women's abbeys in northern France. At Blanches-Abbaye and Villers-Canivet, he forbid the nuns to provide "care" to secular women, and he advised the nuns to be highly cautious when determining who, among the sick and pregnant, would be allowed to enter; at Moncey, he ordered the porteress to allow only women and children under the age of four to enter the hospice, and he entirely forbid the entrance of women nearing childbirth.[51] That nuns protested this kind of abbatial visitation and enforcement throughout the 1240s suggests that we should question claims to strict, rigid enclosure, at least prior to the 1249 agreement between Pope Innocent IV and the abbots of the Cistercian order, which legislated that women's houses would be visited by abbots rather than bishops.[52] Even as late as 1257, Cistercian codifications of legislation were reiterating that secular women should not be permitted to stay overnight in the infirmary, an indication that this practice may have occurred with some regularity.[53] Turning from these centrally enforced sources to more local and unofficial documents provides an entirely different picture of Cistercian women's active charity, as Anne Lester has shown

---

51. Berman discusses these examples of visitation in *The White Nuns*, 23. Stephen of Lexington, "Registrum epistolarum," in *Analecta Sacri Ordinis Cisterciensis* 13 (1232): 241–42.

52. Constance Berman notes that the Cistercian *Statuta* for 1243 record nuns' upheavals in protest of abbatial visitation (regulation and control) at Droiteval, Saint-Antoine-des-Champs, Beaufays, Goujon, Salzinnes, Hocht, Tarrant-Keynes, Notre-Dame de l'Isle at Auxerre, Moncey, Marquette, Heiligenkreuz, Parc-aux-Dames (Vrouwenpark), and Lieu-Notre-Dame at Romorantin. Berman writes, "The nuns were described as insubordinate: some for having locked out their newly appointed visitors and denying their authority, others for shouting and clapping their hands to drown out the new visitors' decrees." Berman, *The White Nuns*, 21.

53. *Les codifications cisterciennes de 1237 et de 1257*, ed. Bernard Lucet (Paris: Centre National de la Recherche Scientifique, 1977), no. 4: mulieres autem seculares in claustris ipsarum vel in infirmitoriis non pernoctent.

with regard to small women's communities in Champagne that cared for the sick and leprous.[54] For much of the thirteenth century, some Cistercian women, like beguines, found ways to exercise an interest in charitable care.

Indeed, there was quite a bit of overlap and contact among Cistercian nuns and beguines and, as we will see, among both of them and anchoresses, hospital sisters, Augustinian canonesses, and recluses. The struggle to define categories of religious women is not unique to our contemporary disciplinary practice. Devout women confounded preexisting categories in the thirteenth century as well. The Franciscan Guibert of Tournai (d. 1288) famously bemoaned that "there are among us women whom we have no idea what to call, ordinary women or nuns, because they live neither in the world or out of it."[55] The Cistercian miracle collector, Caesarius of Heisterbach, referred to uncloistered religious women as "holy women," who "live among people wearing lay clothes [yet] still they surpass many in the cloister for the love of God."[56] And the preacher, hagiographer, and cardinal Jacques de Vitry (d. 1240) used the term "beguine" in a generic sense when he referred to women who lived piously outside of recognized canonical orders. But, as Alison More points out, Jacques also used other terms to describe religious women who chose not to live as nuns: "In France they are known as 'papelardae,' in Lombardy, 'humilitatae,' 'bizoke' (bizzoche) in other parts of Italy, and 'coquennunne' in the German lands."[57] We can add to this list of terms to describe women who lived religious lives outside of formal orders "anchorites," "recluses," "tertiaries," and "penitents."[58]

---

54. Lester, *Creating Cistercian Nuns*, 117–46. Sherri Franks Johnson also demonstrates the benefit of nuance that comes from questioning the affiliation of women's religious communities. See her *Monastic Women and Religious Orders in Late Medieval Bologna* (Cambridge: Cambridge University Press, 2014). In the case of Cistercian abbeys in German lands, as Lucy Barnhouse has shown among the hospital sisters of St. Agnes in Mainz, small communities of women could use Cistercian customs and share pastoral staff while maintaining their independence. Lucy Barnhouse, "Disordered Women? The Hospital Sisters of Mainz and Their Late Medieval Identities," *Medieval Feminist Forum* 3 (2020): 60–97.

55. Guibert of Tournai, "Collectio de scandalis ecclesiae," *Archivum Franciscanum Historicum* 24 (1931): 58: "Et apud nos mulieres aliae, de quibus nescimus utrum debeamus eas vel saeculares vel moniales appellare. Partim enim utuntur ritu saeculari, partim etiam regulari."

56. *Dialogus miraculorum*, VIII.

57. More, *Fictive Orders*, 5; Jacques de Vitry's second sermon to the virgins, *Secundus sermo ad virgines*, trans. Carolyn Muessig, *The Faces of Women in the Sermons of Jacques de Vitry* (Toronto: Peregrina Press, 1999), 89, 140–41, 218–20.

58. Catherine Mooney, "The 'lesser sisters' in Jacques de Vitry's 1216 Letter," *Franciscan Studies* 69 (2011): 1–29; Brenda Bolton, "Some Thirteenth-Century Women in the Low Countries: A Special Case?," *Nederlands Archief voor Kerkgeschiedenis/Dutch Review of Church History* 61.1 (1981): 7–29. Bolton demonstrates that there was a great deal of similarity between the women who lived as "anchorites" in Britain and those called "beguines" in the Low Countries.

The terminological indeterminacy that troubles both past and present attempts to identify religious women (or "quasi-religious" or "lay religious women") points to an important aspect of the lives they led.[59] What we can say about these women is that they strove *not* to fit into accepted and clear categories of religious and social life.[60] They sought to live outside of the regulations of canonically sanctioned religious life as nuns, and away from the expectations of patriarchally sanctioned marital life in a family.[61] It was precisely this twinned rejection of existing gender paradigms that enabled these women to practice charitable caregiving, to fulfill a niche in the landscape of thirteenth-century healthcare options.[62] Their efforts at charitable caregiving were clearly appreciated, and much needed. Individuals of varying ranks became their clients and patients, supporting their caregiving practices and sharing stories of their efficacy. But it was the very slipperiness of categories that also led to difficulties and distortions in reporting those stories, in creating textual records of their care. Because their care was valued, institutions emerged to sustain their efforts and to "protect" their chaste bodies, which were seen as a source of their healing as well as a requirement for the intimate forms of contact that their caregiving demanded. Because they were so successful, clerical overseers became increasingly invested in explaining their lives, representing their practices in acceptable terms, thus imposing what Dyan Elliott has called the "frame" of female spirituality.[63] The *Lives*, miracles, and *exempla* that transmit their stories, often our only evidence of their existence, reflect a clerical effort to fashion their activities in acceptable terms. It was through this process of protection and promotion that religious women's roles as medical service providers were distorted in narrative sources. As I will show, at precisely the same moment that scholastic physicians were defining their practices as a distinct category based on a privileged

---

59. This point is also made by Field, "On Being a Beguine in France."

60. On this negative terminology, see Jennifer Kolpacoff Deane, "Beguines Reconsidered"; and Carol Neel, "The Origins of the Beguines," *Signs* 14.2 (1989): 321–41.

61. As we will see, some of the women were widows, but also appear to have vehemently rejected second marriages and went to great lengths to extricate themselves from obligations to their children.

62. On the rejection of preexisting paradigms, see More, *Fictive Orders*, 7. She uses the term "extra-regular" to describe their rejection in the technical sense, arguing that this extra-regular way of life was characterized by reaching out "to the poor, the destitute, lepers, and those outside of society."

63. Dyan Elliott has figured the representation of female spirituality as a "frame," referring to the factors that played a role in how female spirituality was presented, allowing it to flourish but also repressing certain features that struck clerical promoters of women as unsavory. See her *Proving Woman: Female Spirituality and Inquisitional Culture in the Later Middle Ages* (Princeton: Princeton University Press, 2004), 6.

learning to which women had little to no access, ecclesiastical authorities were invested in translating religious women's healthcare activities into spiritual ideals. Women who had built vibrant reputations serving a loyal clientele as caretakers of the leprous and managers of hospices—women like Elizabeth of Thuringia, Marie of Oignies, Juliana of Mont-Cornillon, Lutgard of Aywières, and Yvette of Huy—underwent a process of hagiographic transformation in which their treatments appear so totally spiritualized that they strike us as no more than literary craft, the tired trappings of Christic mimesis or hagiographic topoi. The hagiographic "frame" that was imposed on these women cast their dedication to confession, penance, and the Eucharist as exemplars of righteous feminine spirituality; but their penitential practices, their visions and other communions with the dead, their foreknowledge of death, and their advocacy of confession and communion were also tools of their trade, extensions of the broader caritative outreach that placed them in proximity to the sick and dying.

As Walter Simons has shown, from roughly 1190 to 1230, pious laywomen commonly called "beguines" in the Low Countries began to gather and live in informal communities dedicated to charitable service and prayer.[64] These small communities of laywomen were regulated and enjoyed papal privileges: they had to wear distinguishing clothing, share property, and observe certain liturgical rites, and following these customs, they were allowed to engage in active service. But they were not nuns according to canon law.[65] For example, by 1190 in the town of Huy there were gatherings of devout women around the widow Yvette, who served a leprosarium before taking up a cell as an anchoress inside the building's chapel. Around 1191, a married woman named Marie left her home in Nivelles to serve with her husband in a leprosarium in Willambroux. She later became a recluse in an Augustinian priory in Oignies, and a cluster of women began to form around her as well. By about 1208 a group of beguines had begun to gather in Nivelles, around the church of St. Sépulchre and the leper hospice of Willambroux. In

---

64. Simons describes the gatherings of the first beguine communities in the Low Countries in *Cities of Ladies*, 36–48. The first communities of lay religious women to receive formal regulation in the Low Countries begin to appear in ecclesiastical records around 1216, when Jacques de Vitry was traveling in Italy. At that time, Jacques sought papal approval for a rule governing the mulieres religiosae who were already flourishing in Liège. Approval eventually came from Pope Honorius III (r. 1216–27), who issued *Litterae tuae nobis* in August of 1218, which permitted preexisting little dwellings (*domicilia*) of unmarried "women" or "virgins" (*virgines et aliae mulieres*) to continue as long as they received appropriate and regular pastoral care. Honorius did not address this decree specifically to the Low Countries beguines; in fact, it was a response to the movement of poor laywomen in Italy.

65. Makowski, "Mulieres Religiosae, Strictly Speaking"; James Brundage, *Medieval Canon Law* (New York: Longman, 1995), 215.

Liège in the first quarter of the thirteenth century a group of women began to congregate at the leprosarium of Mont-Cornillon, and at the same time another band of women were amassing at the parish church of St. Christopher in the heart of the city, where they also served and attended services at the hospital. Around 1259, a number of religious laywomen began to assemble near the hospital of Gratem just outside of the town of Borgloon, where the laywomen Jutta and Christina (later known as Christina Mirabilis ["the Astonishing"]) lived as recluses. Such thirteenth-century urban hospitals welcomed parishioners who were not patients: vagabonds, pilgrims, and other residents attended Mass in their chapels.[66] Archival and hagiographic sources depict religious women not only gathering around such hospitals and attending services there, but deliberately building communities around hospices and leprosaria so that they could serve patients—an expression of active charity. The care that they provided in these small-scale hospitals and leprosaria was largely palliative and regimental. They made patients comfortable by changing linens, dressing wounds, offering an appropriate diet, preparing simple herbal remedies from the hospital garden, and ensuring that they had access to salubrious prayers, liturgy, and sacraments.[67] While the hagiographic sources that document their emergence depict them as ecstatics and visionaries—and there is little reason to doubt that they indeed engaged in contemplative practice—the foundational interest among these women, around which they began to organize themselves, was caritative. Caregiving was part of their group identity as mulieres religiosae, even if each individual beguine did not engage in caregiving.

The mulieres religiosae of the southern Low Countries were frequently in contact with one another, traveling roads that connected the cities and towns of the Sambre-Meuse valley, Brabant, and Loon.[68] They sought refuge and protection from one another, they appear in one another's *Lives*, *exempla*, and visionary accounts, and they learned from one another. It was not just beguines, anchoresses, and other pious laywomen who participated

---

66. James Brodman, *Charity and Religion in Medieval Europe* (Baltimore: Johns Hopkins University Press, 2009), 262.

67. The physical and spiritual approaches to caregiving, as we will see, were always intertwined. I make every effort throughout this book not to separate them anachronistically unless analytically necessary or explicitly separated in the sources. On the hospital as a locus of care for body and soul, see John Henderson, *The Renaissance Hospital: Healing the Body and Healing the Soul* (New Haven: Yale University Press, 2006); Carole Rawcliffe, *Medicine for the Soul: The Life, Death, and Resurrection of an English Medieval Hospital; St. Giles's Norwich, 1249–1550* (Stroud: Sutton, 1999); Jessalyn Bird, "Medicine for Body and Soul: Jacques de Vitry's Sermons to Hospitallers and Their Charges," in Biller and Ziegler, *Religion and Medicine in the Middle Ages*, 91–108.

68. Simons, *Cities of Ladies*, 45.

in these feminine communications and affiliations. Cistercian and Benedictine nuns and Augustinian canonesses also demonstrate accommodation of and cooperation with other mulieres religiosae in the region. For example, in 1241, John, the chaplain of St. Gilles in Liège, left his home to the Cistercians at Val-Benoît so that they could offer hospitality to twenty-four beguines, a legal act that founded the beguine convent of la Madeleine.[69] Val-Benoît also offered refuge to Juliana of Mont-Cornillon and her companions when property disputes at the leprosarium she oversaw left the women homeless after the year 1247; Juliana would find asylum in two additional Cistercian women's abbeys as well. At Lille, the hospital sisters who accepted the Rule of Augustine were continually referred to as beguines in the archival records, and possibly represented the female staff who departed from the Hôpital Comtesse to found a beguinage after 1239.[70] And several *Lives* of mulieres religiosae in this region depict their heroines living as beguines, at least temporarily, before transitioning into what they portrayed as a "more perfect" state of Cistercian observance; Lutgard of Aywières, Ida of Nivelles, Ida of Leuven, and Beatrice of Nazareth were among this group.[71] Thus, in both the institutional and the narrative documentation on mulieres religiosae in the thirteenth-century southern Low Countries, there is a great deal of intersection and overlap in identities and categories of religious life available to women.

These affinities are reflected in the manuscript transmission of the corpus of saints' *Lives*, which provide some of the earliest historical sources for the caregiving work of the mulieres religiosae in this region. Although the narrative *Lives* in the corpus fall under the genre now called "hagiography," none of

---

69. This was the same John who was known as "the abbot" and, as I discuss in chapter 2, was the son of Odilia of Liège, for whom we have a *Life*. The abbess and nuns of Val-Benoît would supervise the beguine hospital of la Madeleine. See entry for 28 August 1241 in *Cartulaire de l'abbaye du Val-Benoît*, ed. Joseph Cuvelier (Brussels: Kiessling, Ibreghts, 1906), no. 80, 93–94.

70. Aubertus Miraeus and Joannes Foppens, eds., *Opera diplomatica et historica* (Leuven: Denique, 1723), 3:594. The suggestion of the possible splitting off of the beguines from the Hôpital Comtesse comes from Simons, *Cities of Ladies*, 285–86n63; he acknowledges that this interpretation differs from Bernard Delmaire, "Les béguines dans le nord de la France au premier siècle de leur histoire (vers 1230–1350)," in *Les religieuses en France au XIIIe siècle*, ed. Michel Parisse (Nancy: Presses Universitaires de Nancy, 1985), 158–59.

71. Their association with Cistercian abbeys stems in part from the efforts of clerical promoters to render their way of life as saintly, hence, as falling within the recognizable confines of monastic life. There is also a lingering historiographical impression, left by Herbert Grundmann's classic *Religious Movements in the Middle Ages*, that all quasi-religious or lay religious movements found their fulfillment in monastic orders. Scholars have had to work through these mediations to situate the sources in their original contexts. Herbert Grundmann, *Religious Movements in the Middle Ages* (South Bend: University of Notre Dame Press, 1999).

these women were ever canonized.[72] The *Lives* were written partly in an effort to manage the reputations these women had already developed. They are depicted as having accrued local followings when they were still alive; that is, they garnered reputations for holiness during their lives, a phenomenon that some historians have called "living sanctity."[73] What distinguished the "living saints" from other women in the surge of thirteenth-century religious activity was the public attribution to them of a perceived infusion of grace. For example, Jacques de Vitry's prologue to the *Life* of Marie of Oignies opens by praising the throngs of women, "many holy virgins," who served the city of Liège in prayer, manual labor, and vigils.[74] Yet when he proceeds to describe not the mulieres religiosae as a group, but the individual holy women among them, he fixates on their reception of grace: "I call your holiness as my witness, for you have seen with your own eyes the wondrous workings of God and the distribution of graces in different people."[75] Observers witnessed the distribution of grace working within and through these women, the spectacle of their sanctity. If the dispersal of grace was involved in this performance, however, a prudent cleric was needed to manage matters. The *Lives* served as a means of clerical control of the image, reputation, and access to the "distribution of grace" among the saintly mulieres religiosae.

Although I rely on hagiographic narratives, I am less interested in the exceptional saintly heroines than in how we can use these narratives to understand the practices, body knowledge, and caritative mission shared by the many anonymous women that made up the social network of mulieres religiosae in the thirteenth- and early fourteenth-century lowlands. Those few exceptional *Lives*, keep in mind, were persuasions, promotions. They safeguarded and protected the work of the many, the unnamed. As the story of Ida of Leuven's treatment of a tumor illustrates, the healthcare interactions and healing relationships established by some of the mulieres religiosae could be experienced or reported as miraculous, grace-filled, or holy. Their

---

72. A liturgical office for Marie of Oignies was composed for celebration at Villers by Goswin of Bossut, around 1250; her relics had been translated about a quarter century prior to this composition. She is the most likely to have received any sort of official veneration in the thirteenth century, though she was not canonized.

73. Gabor Klaniczay provides a description of the external signs of living sanctity in "Using Saints: Intercession, Healing, Sanctity," in *The Oxford Handbook of Medieval Christianity*, ed. John Arnold (Oxford: Oxford University Press, 2014), 227–28.

74. *Vita Mariae Oigniacensis* (*BHL* 5516–17), ed. Daniel Papebroche, in *AASS* 23 June XXV, 542–72; the modern edition is edited by R. B. C. Huygens in Corpus Christianorum, vol. 252 (Turnhout: Brepols, 2012); hereafter *VMO* refers to this edition. A translation by Margot King can be found in *Mary of Oignies: Mother of Salvation*, ed. Anneke Mulder-Bakker (Turnhout: Brepols, 2006), 37.

75. *VMO*, prol., 49; trans., 45: "Testem invoco sanctitatem tuam: oculis enim tuis vidisti mirabilem dei operationem et in diversis personis divisiones gratiarum."

behavior—visiting the sick, caring for bodies, encouraging and sometimes hearing confession, their proximity to the dead and dying, their frequent, vehement prayer and contemplative ecstasies—was susceptible to suspicion, to condemnation. Living as *non*-nuns, *non*-wives, *non*-daughters in the homes of their fathers, the mulieres religiosae needed the protection of clerical promoters and the safety of their hagiographic tropes. It was far too easy for skeptics to deem their behavior offensive, demonic, unorthodox.[76] Hagiography was only one of many clerical methods of controlling and reforming women's religious life in the region. Oversight was another. For example, Jacques Pantaleon (d. 1264), who was archdeacon of Liège before becoming pope (1261–64), promulgated in 1245 statutes for the life of beguines in the bishopric of Liège.[77] According to principles of reform, episcopal supervisors were also appointed to check in on beguines and "other religious women, ailing and well, living in reclusaria, hospitals, or leprosaria."[78] The hagiographic

---

76. Rachel Smith, *Excessive Saints: Gender, Narrative, and Theological Invention in Thomas of Cantimpré* (New York: Columbia University Press, 2019), 66. Grundmann's model of the women's religious movement understood the proliferation of independent women's communities as a response to the refusal of male clerics to accommodate women in religious orders. Grundmann fashioned all religious movements in a teleological development as "achiev[ing] realization in religious orders or in heretical sects" (*Religious Movements*, 1). Scholars no longer see mulieres regliosae as a reactionary movement, or as entirely distasteful in the eyes of male clerics. See John Freed, "Urban Development and the 'Cura monialium' in Thirteenth-Century Germany," *Viator* 3 (1972): 311–28.

77. Ecclesiastical regulation and suspicion of lay religious women would persist, and increase, throughout the thirteenth and fourteenth centuries. But this intensifying regulation should not be confused for complete resistance, persecution, or repression. In 1298, Pope Boniface VIII issued the decretal *Periculoso*, which appears to have been aimed at women, like the Cistercians I examine in this book, who may have been involved in caritative work in hospitals and leprosaria near their abbeys or visiting the sick in their granges. *Periculoso* was aimed at "certain nuns" (*quarundam monialium*) who "sometimes go outside their monasteries in the dwellings of secular persons." Boniface VIII, "Periculoso," in *Corpus iuris canonici*, ed. Aemilius Richter and Emile Friedberg (Leipzig: Bernhard Tauchnitz, 1829), vol. 1, c. 119. The 1311 Council of Vienne then addressed beguines and other lay religious women involved in "detestable practices," but absolved the pious beguines among them: "We do not intend to prevent those pious women who live honorably in their hospices, with or without a vow of chastity, from doing penance and serving the Lord with the spirit of humility. They will be allowed to do that." *Decrees of the Ecumenical Councils*, ed. and trans. Norman Tanner (London: Sheed and Ward, 1999), 1.374. As Jennifer Kolpacoff Deane has pointed out, the decrees of Vienne highlight the problem of labels—there was no single canonical category to talk about beguines or religious women who were not nuns. Vienne's decrees thus made all lay religious women seem suspect. But even despite these decrees, lay religious communities of women flourished in the Low Countries and Germany throughout the fourteenth century and beyond. There were occasional local persecutions, but on the whole, houses of lay religious women continued to thrive. See Deane, "From Case Studies to Comparative Models: Würzburg Beguines and the Vienne Decrees," in Böhringer, Deane, and Van Engen, *Labels and Libels*, 53–82.

78. See Mulder-Bakker, *Lives of the Anchoresses*, 131. The original document no longer exists, but a reconstruction based on a charter of 1 August 1266 from Henry of Guelders, bishop of Liège, to his diocesan administrator, Renier of Tongres, can be found in Jean Paquay, "L'archidiaconat liégeois d'Urbain IV," *Leodium* 2 (1903): 61: "aliarum religiosarum personarum infirmarum et sanarum,

promotions of the few local "living saints" as chaste, prayerful, and so closely associated with clerics or with specific abbeys facilitated the many nameless mulieres religiosae to carry on with their caregiving work.

Although I focus on the Low Countries as a case study of the caregiving that religious women provided in later medieval Europe, the mulieres religiosae from this region were no geographic exception. Mary Doyno and Janine Peterson have recently published monographs exploring the late medieval Italian phenomenon of laypeople living religious lives, some of whom became recognized locally as saints.[79] Among these saints a number of women were noted for their charitable activities, including the Italian penitent Umiliana of Cerchi (d. 1246), who fed and clothed the poor. After becoming a widow, Margaret of Cortona (d. 1297) founded the hospital of Santa Maria dalla Misericordia. Another widow named Aldobrandesca (d. 1309) worked in the hospital Saint'Andrea in Siena; and a single woman named Ubaldesca (d. 1206) served the hospital of St. John of Jerusalem in Pisa.[80] A community of women who provided charitable healthcare was approved in 1254 by the bishop of Spoleto, Bartolomeo Accoramboni, who regulated their care according to the Augustinian Rule in the Ospedale Nuovo.[81] And in 1216, when Jacques de Vitry wrote to an interlocutor in Liège from his travels in Perugia, he commented on the habits of the religious laywomen whom he observed. Jacques asserted that these *sorores minores* "abide together in various hospices near the city."[82] The many varieties of religious women in northern Italy who lived outside of regular orders thus

---

in reclusoriis, hospitalibus ac leprosorum domibus degentium." The bishop affirms the presence of holy women in the region known as beguines and orders that Jacques Pantaleon's statute (*libellum*), confirmed by Robert de Thourotte, be enforced.

79. Mary Harvey Doyno, *The Lay Saint: Charity and Charismatic Authority in Medieval Italy, 1150–1350* (Ithaca: Cornell University Press, 2019); Janine Peterson, *Suspect Saints and Holy Heretics: Disputed Sanctity and Communal Identity in Late Medieval Italy* (Ithaca: Cornell University Press, 2019). James Palmer has uncovered testamentary evidence of a "medica," Alegranza di Rogerio Anici, who was revered as a local saint in Rome; see his *Virtues of Economy: Governance, Power, and Piety in Late Medieval Rome* (Ithaca: Cornell University Press, 2019), 141–47.

80. André Vauchez, *Sainthood in the Later Middle Ages* (Cambridge: Cambridge University Press, 1997), 200–201. A number of Italian laymen also worked in hospitals and earned the aura of sanctity, including textual representation in *Lives*. As I will show, although plenty of religious men in the Low Countries worked in hospitals, none of them received *Lives*. The Italian lay saints would make an interesting case study on gender and caregiving because there appear to have been more caregiving saints identified as men.

81. Sandro Ceccaroni, *La storia millenaria degli ospedali della città e della diocesi di Spoleto* (Spoleto: Ente Rocca di Spoleto, 1978).

82. Catherine Mooney, *Clare of Assisi and the Thirteenth-Century Church: Religious Women, Rules, and Resistance* (Philadelphia: University of Pennsylvania Press, 2016), 43. The letter is in Jacques de Vitry, *Lettres de Jacques de Vitry, 1160/70–1240 évêque de Saint-Jean d'Acre*, ed. R. B. C. Huygens (Leiden: Brill, 1960), 71–78: "Mulieres vero iuxta civitates in diversis hospitiis simul commorantur."

also demonstrated a predilection for charitable caregiving. There is certainly merit to investigating a broader Pan-European caregiving phenomenon among pious women, but here I limit my sources to those produced in and around the lowlands so that I can weave together a vast array of documents and other forms of witness to religious women's caregiving, thereby supplementing the picture offered by clerics concerned with orthodox appearances. By reading saints' *Lives* alongside miracles, charters, theology, images, medical writing, regimens, prayer books, and archaeological findings, I am able to focus on the tiny details, the fragments that together built a world of knowledge transmission and caregiving communities. This attention to the processes of feminine caregiving and knowledge production has yet to sufficiently inform either our understanding of women's religious life or our reckoning of healthcare in the Middle Ages.

Medical Trajectories

The traditional narrative of medieval European medical history tells the story of the emergence of *physici* who professionalized healthcare. Practitioners known as *physici* arose, this narrative states, after a period of stagnancy or "lack" in medical theory and practice that lasted from roughly 550 to 1050 in western Europe.[83] Although the Christian Roman Empire in the West had translated and absorbed a small portion of Greek medical learning, such as Soranus, Oribasius's synopsis of Galen and Hippocrates, and Dioscorides, this medical knowledge was confined to monasteries, where it was infused with notions of Christian charity and the supernatural healing acuity of the saints and their relics.[84] By contrast, in the urban centers of the Abbasid Caliphate, numerous physicians and philosophers were digesting and building upon Greek medical learning to create encyclopedias of medical knowledge, in addition to developing methods for clinical training and establishing hospitals.

In this narrative trajectory, books drove the progress and proliferation of medical learning. By around 1150 Europeans began to develop a formal,

---

83. In terms of medical knowledge, the West "came to life again" around 1050, in the words of Roy Porter, *The Greatest Benefit to Mankind: A Medical History of Humanity from Antiquity to the Present* (New York: Norton, 1999), 106. On the traditional narrative and methods for dismantling it, see also Vivian Nutton, "Medicine in Medieval Western Europe, 1000–1500," in *The Western Medical Tradition, 800 BC to 1800 AD*, ed. W. F. Bynum (Cambridge: Cambridge University Press, 1995); and Peregrine Horden, "What's Wrong with Early Medieval Medicine?," *Social History of Medicine* 24.1 (2011): 5–25.

84. Nancy Siraisi, *Medieval and Early Renaissance Medicine: An Introduction to Knowledge and Practice* (Chicago: University of Chicago Press, 1990), 10–11.

theoretical interest in medicine because, by then, Western readers had access to Latin translations of Hippocrates and Galen, as well as the Arabic encyclopedists, many versions of which were made by Constantine the African, Gerard of Cremona, and Burgundio of Pisa. Salerno and Montpellier emerged as centers of medical knowledge and practice.[85] Book learning, and thus schooling and literacy, came to symbolize the successful healer.[86] Individual questions about natural and biological phenomena were isolated and examined by means of *quaestiones*, and medical learning was broadened and disseminated via the commentary tradition.[87] By 1300, a new form of medical knowledge had been fully introduced to western Europe. In this model, universities adopted the medical curriculum, first at Bologna, Paris, and Montpellier, then civic bodies sought to provide technically trained medical practitioners to serve the health problems of their communities.[88] It was at Salerno that medical practitioners began to distinguish themselves from other varieties of healer (*medici*) that had included a number of women (the *mulieres salernitanae*) in addition to the famed Trota of Salerno.[89] These new healers preferred the moniker *physici* to denote their possession of a certain kind of specialized knowledge about the natural world and the constitution of matter and the cosmos that they used to explain the relationship between the components of living matter (the elements, qualities, and humors) and the processes of illness and health.[90] Because this knowledge was communicated through texts, and increasingly in university settings, non-Latin literate women were excluded from the development of professional medicine.[91]

Over the last few decades the picture of healthcare in medieval Europe has begun to expand. Spearheaded by discussions in the social history of

---

85. Monica Green, "Salerno," in *Medieval Science, Technology, and Medicine: An Encyclopedia*, ed. Thomas Glick, Steven Livesey, and Faith Wallis (New York: Routledge, 2005), 452–53; see also Danielle Jacquart, ed., *La scuola medica salernitana: Gli autori e i testi* (Florence: SISMEL, 2007).

86. See Vern Bullough, *The Development of Medicine as a Profession: The Contribution of the Medieval University to Modern Medicine* (New York: Karger, 1966).

87. Luis García-Ballester, "Construction of a New Form of Learning and Practicing Medicine in Medieval Latin Europe," *Science in Context* 8.1 (1995): 79–85.

88. García-Ballester, 76; Danielle Jacquart and Françoise Micheau, *La médecine arabe et l'Occident médiévale* (Paris: Maisonneuve et Larose, 1990).

89. Maaike Van Der Lugt, "The Learned Physician as Charismatic Healer: Urso of Salerno on Incantations in Medicine, Magic, and Religion," *Bulletin of the History of Medicine* 87.3 (2013): 307–46. On the *mulieres salerniternae* and Trota of Salerno, see Monica Green, ed. and trans., *The Trotula: A Medieval Compendium of Women's Medicine* (Philadelphia: University of Pennsylvania Press, 2001).

90. Luke Demaitre, *Medieval Medicine: The Art of Healing from Head to Toe* (Santa Barbara: ABC Clio, 2013), 3. See also Jerome Bylebyl, "The Medical Meaning of *Physica*," *Osiris* 6 (1990): 16–41.

91. On women practitioners and the rise of book-based medical practice, see Monica Green, *Making Women's Medicine Masculine: The Rise of Male Authority in Pre-modern Gynaecology* (Oxford: Oxford University Press, 2008).

medicine, scholars have begun to attend to the so-called margins, the local healers, barbers, empirics, herbalists, and saints who populated the majority of daily healthcare interactions in this period, and thus were hardly marginal. Monica Green has developed an interpretive framework for locating women healthcare practitioners in western Europe by incorporating analyses of power into the investigation of medieval medical history. Her attention to the workings of power has brought greater visibility to the variety and complexity of the medieval medical marketplace.[92] Following Green's lead, scholars have begun to supplement the picture of medical care as narrowly represented by university medical treatises and licensed professionals.[93]

This recognition of multiplicity has illuminated many of the lived, embodied practices that regulated what Peregrine Horden has called "the non-natural environment."[94] The non-natural environment refers to the six external factors (the so-called non-naturals) that were understood to influence bodily health in humoral medicine.[95] The Islamicate physician Hunayn ibn Ishaq delineated these factors as air, food and drink, diet and rest, sleeping and waking, evacuation and retention, and the passions of the soul.[96] The primary mode of medical treatment involved what we tend to consider now as preventative care: maintaining a regimen, diet, and the proper functioning of the non-naturals. By emphasizing that the maintenance of the non-natural environment was a *medical* activity in later medieval and Renaissance Europe and the Mediterranean, many recent scholars have begun to broaden the kinds of behaviors that constituted medical care.[97] This amplified view

---

92. Monica H. Green, "Women's Medical Practice and Healthcare in Medieval Europe," *Signs* 14 (1989): 343–73.

93. Michael McVaugh, *Medicine before the Plague: Practitioners and Their Patients in the Crown of Aragon, 1285–1345* (Cambridge: Cambridge University Press, 1993); Rawcliffe, *Medicine for the Soul*; Peregrine Horden, *Hospitals and Healing from Late Antiquity to the Later Middle Ages* (Aldershot: Ashgate, 2008).

94. Peregrine Horden, "A Non-natural Environment: Medicine without Doctors and the Medieval European Hospital," in *The Medieval Hospital and Medical Practice*, ed. Barbara Bowers (Aldershot: Ashgate, 2007), 133–45.

95. The non-naturals (*res non naturales*) stood in distinction from the *res naturales*, which were internal, such as the humors, elements, and complexion. A third category, the *contra naturales*, were pathological conditions, harmful to health. Most physicians first counseled an adjustment of the non-naturals in order to restore humoral balance.

96. Hunayn's work was translated from Arabic into Latin by Constantine the African as the *Isagoge* of Johannitius. In this latinized version it would enter Western medical training.

97. Cohen-Hanegbi, *Caring for the Living Soul*; Nicole Archambeau, "Healing Options during the Plague: Survivor Stories from a Fourteenth-Century Canonization Inquest," *Bulletin of the History of Medicine* 85.4 (2011): 531–59; Daniel McCann, "Medicine of Words: Purgative Reading in Richard Rolle's Meditations on the Passion," *Medieval Journal* 5.2 (2015): 53–83.

has enabled scholars to recognize how everyday embodied activities, such as prayer, pilgrimage, cooking, cleaning, and bathing, participated in a larger care economy. These practices of care garnered little discursive commentary. Instead, they were performatively elaborated by habituated practices, transmitted as craft or know-how.[98] These kinds of treatments were learned through observation, repeated practice, and informal learning arrangements as a kinesthetic form of embodied knowledge.[99]

Scholars such as Carole Rawcliffe, Montserrat Cabré, Naama Cohen-Hanegbi, and Peregrine Horden have worked to contribute a particularly expansive picture of the range of therapeutic technologies in use in medieval western Europe.[100] They have focused on the non-natural environment and particularly on the passions of the soul in medical practice as a way to make visible the varied ways that practitioners deployed meditation, music, and literature as a means to stimulate the health of the body.[101] The passions of the soul constituted one of the six non-natural factors determining health or sickness. As defined by Hunayn ibn Ishaq, they were "incidental states of the soul [that] have an effect on the body, such as those which bring the natural heat from the interior of the body to the surface of the skin."[102] Certain emotions, such as delight or hope, were considered as potentially curative; whereas others, like grief and anger, were deleterious. Depending on context, a meditation or an illustration, a song or a relic, might have operated with medical valence as a means of triggering salubrious passions or dispelling toxic ones. Seen from the perspective of the passions of the soul, many texts, images, rituals, and social roles bore expressly salutary functions.

---

98. Kathryn Linn Guerts, *Culture and the Senses: Bodily Ways of Knowing in an African Community* (Berkeley: University of California Press, 2002). On embodied knowledge and women's therapeutic practices, see the essays in Sara Ritchey and Sharon Strocchia, eds., *Gender, Health, and Healing, 1250–1550* (Amsterdam: Amsterdam University Press, 2020).

99. Susan Broomhall, *Women's Medical Work in Early Modern France* (Manchester: Manchester University Press, 2004), 2. On embodied knowledge, see also Pamela H. Smith, *The Body of the Artisan: Art and Experience in the Scientific Revolution* (Chicago: University of Chicago Press, 2004); and Pamela Long, *Artisan Practitioners and the Rise of the New Sciences* (Corvalis: Portland State University Press, 2011).

100. Rawcliffe, *Medicine for the Soul*; Cohen-Hanegbi, *Caring for the Living Soul*; Ziegler, *Medicine and Religion*; Horden, *Hospitals and Healing*.

101. Glending Olson and Simo Knuttila were among the first anglophone scholars to elaborate on the therapeutic uses of the passions of the soul in medieval society. See Glending Olson, "The Hygienic Justification," in *Literature as Recreation in the Middle Ages* (Ithaca: Cornell University Press, 1982), 39 ff.; and Simo Knuttila, *Emotions in Ancient and Medieval Philosophy* (Oxford: Clarendon Press, 2006).

102. Gregor Maurach, "Johannicius: Isagoge ad Techni Galieni," *Sudhoffs Archiv* 62 (1978): 160: "Sunt quaedam accidentia animae quae faciunt intra corpus, sicut ea, quae commovent calorem ab interiori parte ad superficiem cutis."

Historians have often coded these cultural artifacts, however, in categorically bounded ways as "religious," thus distorting their therapeutic uses.[103]

This book participates in ongoing efforts to build an explanatory framework for the history of late medieval medicine that includes the therapeutic knowledge and practices of the nonelite. It represents an exercise in imagining how people sought care and reported cure in thirteenth-century northwestern Europe. In communities in this region, individuals from across the social spectrum could rely on assistance from religious women. These women cared for the sick and indigent with prayers, penitential exercises, and other bodily comforts. Although hundreds of them engaged in charitable caregiving, only a few narrative examples, in the form of hagiographic *Lives* and miracles, describe the character of their care. Supplemented by other sources used in their therapeutic interactions, such as prayers, poetry, liturgy, images, objects, and regimens, this concatenation of source material indicates that religiously affiliated Christian women in the late medieval southern Low Countries formed vital microcommunities of care, local economies of salvation.[104] They were the linchpin in establishing and sustaining salubrious relations within and across their community, the community of the living, the dead, and the divine. In other words, they consolidated the relations that constituted remedy. Within the limited healthcare infrastructures of late medieval cities and towns, it was often religiously affiliated women who mediated relationships, offered care, and prepared the sick and their loved ones for bodily transitions.

Expansive Methodologies

This book seeks to recuperate the feminine therapeutic epistemologies that guided religious women's caregiving practices. This work would be impossible to achieve, however, without turning to the guidance of scholars working beyond the traditional boundaries of medieval European history— particularly those working in performance studies, Native American and Indigenous studies (NAIS), the history of enslaved communities in North America and the Caribbean, and the medical anthropology of sub-Saharan Africa. These scholars have developed methods for making visible voices and

---

103. Religion was *absent* as a category from medieval thinking. It invites a process of distortion to use it analytically in our process of thinking about the cultural products of the period. On the postmedieval genealogical formation of the Western category of religion, see Smith, "Religion, Religions, Religious."

104. On the formation of microcommunities of salvation, see João Biehl, *Will to Live: AIDS Policies and the Politics of Survival* (Princeton: Princeton University Press, 2007), 48.

presences that have been suppressed by technologies of power maintained by white, elite, colonial, and settler archives and historical narratives.[105] Medievalists, I hope to demonstrate, have much to learn from them about how to hear and to incorporate those voices. Moreover, as Sarah Ahmed has insisted, by naming these scholars and citing them, I acknowledge my debts and I bring them into the space of the medieval, as a necessary part of the intellectual constructions built here.[106]

In performance studies, Diana Taylor has urged scholars to stretch beyond the archive to the repertoire. By "repertoire," Taylor signals the embodied forms of knowledge and memory, conveyed in gestures, orality, song, and dance.[107] Performance, she asserts, is a key means of transmitting and storing knowledge. The search for feminine therapeutic epistemologies, which are not recorded in medieval "medical" sources, requires an interrogation of late medieval women's repertoire. My interrogation has also been guided by the insights of NAIS scholars such as Jean M. O'Brien, Lisa Brooks, Alyssa Mt. Pleasant, and Robert Warrior, who have exemplified how scholars in all historical disciplines can make use of archival and genre-specific materials without replicating their conceptual categories or retransmitting their assumptions about what counts as knowledge; they have also insisted on centering spoken, material, and image-based sources, privileging "what many do not know," questioning the process of knowledge formation, and embracing community-engaged historical work.[108] From these

---

105. Foundational studies that have guided my thought in this book include Saidiya Hartman, *Scenes of Subjection: Terror, Slavery, and Self-Making in Nineteenth-Century America* (Oxford: Oxford University Press, 1997); J. Kēhualani Kauanui, *Hawaiian Blood: Colonialism and the Politics of Sovereignty and Indigeneity* (Durham: Duke University Press, 2008); the essays in Aileen Moreton-Robinson, ed., *Sovereign Subjects: Indigenous Sovereignty Matters* (Crows Nest, Australia: Allen & Unwin, 2008); bell hooks, *Feminist Theory: From Margins to Center* (Boston: South End Press, 2007); Hortense Spillers, "Mamas Baby, Papas Maybe: An American Grammar Book," *Diacritics* 17 (1987): 64–81; Patricia Williams, *Seeing a Color-blind Future: The Paradox of Race*, Reith Lectures, 1997 (New York: Farrar, Straus and Giroux, 1998).

106. Sarah Ahmed, *Living a Feminist Life* (Durham: Duke University Press, 2017), 148–58.

107. Diana Taylor, "Remapping Genre through Performance: From 'American' to 'Hemispheric' Studies," *PMLA* 122.5 (2007): 1416–30.

108. Jean M. O'Brien and Robert Warrior, "Building a Professional Infrastructure for Critical Indigenous Studies: A(n Intellectual) History of and Prospectus for the Native American and Indigenous Studies Association," in *Critical Indigenous Studies: Engagements in First World Locations*, ed. Aileen Moreton-Robinson (Tucson: University of Arizona Press, 2016), 33–48; Lisa Brooks, *Our Beloved Kin: A New History of King Philip's War* (New Haven: Yale University Press, 2018); Alyssa Mt. Pleasant, Caroline Wigginton, and Kelly Wisecup, "Materials and Methods in Native American and Indigenous Studies: Completing the Turn," *William and Mary Quarterly* 75 (April 2018): 207–36. Bitterroot Salish scholar Tarren Andrews has worked to build a constructive space for the collaboration of Indigenous scholars, Indigenous studies scholars, and medievalists; see the collected articles in "Indigenous Futures and Medieval Pasts," edited by Tarren Andrews and Tiffany Beechy, *English*

scholars, I have learned to expand my source base in order to imagine how women living in and alongside religious communities in the thirteenth-century southern Low Countries brokered in a politics of everyday behavior that positioned them at the center of stories about health events when the health of the body included that of the soul, and when the significance of life extended beyond bodily death.[109]

Examining the record of healthcare practices in the Caribbean, Pablo Gómez has worked to uncover "localized circumstances" of knowledge that did not lay claim to grand, universal principles or reduce the human body to an "inert, knowable, regular, predictable entity."[110] Black healers in the Caribbean generated body knowledge in localized circumstances that have often been obscured from traditional histories of medicine because they took place in a social and intellectual atmosphere distant from university-generated medical categories and texts.[111] Gómez's work offers a model for integrating into the history of medicine seemingly incommensurable narratives about traditional healers and formal physicians. In another part of the Caribbean, Marissa Fuentes has opened up the possibility of historicizing the experiences of enslaved women by providing a fresh reading of the archival record of eighteenth-century Barbados. Rather than assenting to a practice of reading around silences and erasures in the archival record, Fuentes probes the very circumstances of archival power, questioning historical methodologies that rely on sources that favor power, that demand statistical verification, and that record a superabundance of white European men's voices and perspectives.[112] By attending to silence, Fuentes offers a method for subverting archival erasure, one that reverses the perspective privileged by white, masculine power.[113]

Language Notes 58.2 (2020), especially Tarren Andrews, "Indigenous Futures and Medieval Pasts: An Introduction," 1–17.

109. Gómez, *The Experiential Caribbean*, 106; Langwick, *Bodies, Politics, and African Healing*, 6.

110. Gómez, *The Experiential Caribbean*, 5. See also his "Incommensurable Epistemologies? The Atlantic Geography of Healing in the Early Modern Caribbean," *Small Axe* (2014): 95–107.

111. Gómez, *The Experiential Caribbean*, 3. On Gómez's choice of "Black" as opposed to African, see his "The Circumstances of Body Knowledge in the Seventeenth-Century Black Spanish Caribbean," *Social History of Medicine* 26.3 (2013): 383–402.

112. Fuentes, *Dispossessed Lives*, 5–6. My thinking here is also influenced by the work of Thavolia Glymph, who has innovated registers for hearing marginalized women's voices and for appreciating the enormous weight of everyday acts of resistance. See her *Out of the House of Bondage: The Transformation of the Plantation Household* (Cambridge: Cambridge University Press, 2008).

113. On the operation of power in the production of history, my thinking is informed by Michel-Rolph Trouillot, *Silencing the Past: Power and the Production of History* (New York: Beacon, 1997). On confronting invisibility and silence in the historical record, see also Hartman, *Scenes of Subjection*. On efforts to expose the manner in which dominant narratives work to suppress certain voices, see

From the standpoint of medical anthropology, Stacey Langwick's work among healers practicing today in southeastern Tanzania has demonstrated methods for reading past biomedical categories, revealing the various ways that experiential circumstances participate in the generation of therapeutic objects and practices, that is, in the delineation of bodies and bodily threats.[114] Practice, she shows, brings into being the matter of bodies, bodily dangers, and bodily experts, even when their generative forces remain invisible, immaterial, unseen. Everyday healthcare practices, which we have often considered as traditional or folk medicine, are coproductive of, and interdependent with, those categories of professional (learned or "modern") medicine.[115] Much of my work in this book is indebted to such observations about category formation, about who has the power to define therapeutic success, and about epistemological violence in the competition over experiential knowledge or whose experiential knowledge is worthy of trust, transmission, and record.[116] At the same time, I recognize that the subjects of my book—Christian European women—benefited from many social privileges and often participated in the oppression and marginalization of other peoples in their communities, particularly Jewish people. While the methodological and theoretical models offered by these scholars have been fruitful for detecting marginalized epistemologies and for recognizing performative modes of caregiving, I attempt throughout the book to articulate the ways that the subjects of this book also benefited from structural regimes that enabled them to develop their therapeutic tools, for them to gain currency in certain settings.

By incorporating these methods, I am able to construct a case study of the caregiving practiced by religious women in the late medieval lowlands. Even though they were often ad hoc and informal, and thus produced fewer official records, these women formed essential communities of care. That is, they formed locally recognized communities of therapeutic expertise;

Gayatri Spivak's notion of "the itinerary of the silencing" in Gayatri Chakravorty Spivak, *The Post-Colonial Critic: Interviews, Strategies, Dialogues* (New York: Routledge, 1990), 31.

114. Langwick, *Bodies, Politics, and African Healing.*

115. On a similar process of fabrication and implantation of traditional or folk medicine in colonial India, see Shinjini Das, *Vernacular Medicine in Colonial India: Family, Market, and Homeopathy* (Cambridge: Cambridge University Press, 2019).

116. Other anthropological works that have been fruitful for approaching the sources used in this book were Nancy Rose Hunt, *A Nervous State: Violence, Remedies, and Reverie in Colonial Congo* (Durham: Duke University Press, 2016); Ann Laura Stoler, *Along the Archival Grain: Epistemic Anxieties and Colonial Common Sense* (Princeton: Princeton University Press, 2009); Byron Good, *Medicine, Rationality, and Experience: An Anthropological Perspective* (Cambridge: Cambridge University Press, 1993); Carolyn Sargent, *The Cultural Context of Therapeutic Choice: Obstetrical Care Decisions among the Beriba of Benin* (Dordrecht: D. Reidel, 1982).

their treatments were culturally valued as healthcare by their neighbors and other observers. These treatments, and the communities in which they were embedded and in which they gained meaning, have remained historically invisible as healthcare practices in part because they often appear as indistinguishable from the expected behaviors of "religious women." These treatments include prayer, the performance of poetry and liturgical rites, passionate meditative reading, in addition to wound care, maintenance of regimen, the provision of bodily comfort, obstetric care, herbal preparations, and all manner of preventative medicine. By centering these treatments within medieval understandings of the word *salus*, which meant both "health" and "salvation," this book reintegrates spiritual and material approaches to healthcare that have become conceptually disentangled by our tendency to view them from the perspective of modern biomedicine. *Salus* was polyvalent and broader in scope than any contemporary verbal or conceptual equivalent; neither "medicine" nor "healthcare," nor even "caregiving," captures the full semantic range that included body and soul, the individual and community, the temporal fluidity of cosmic past, present, and future, and the whole spread of healing technologies used in the treatment of these varied aspects of self.[117] Distinguishing between various elements of *salus*—disentangling medicine from religion—is untenable; instead, I consider the biocultural system forged by the coexisting state of actions, objects, practices, and articulations aimed at *salus*.[118]

Mapping Healthcare in the Late Middle Ages

This book moves from the most outerbound forms of healing captured in the oral circulation of miracle stories to their intimate, tactile embodiment and use in manuscripts housed in individual abbeys. It is divided into three parts, based on the kinds of sources and questions that drive the analysis. The first part relies heavily on narrative hagiographic sources, *Lives* and miracles.

Part 1 asks, What are the stories that contemporaries and near contemporaries told about religious women's acts of care, about their methods of treatment, and the power and authority they held over sick bodies? It begins,

---

117. On this scope, see Miranda Brown, "'Medicine' in Early China," in *Routledge Handbook of Early Chinese History*, ed. Paul Goldin (New York: Routledge, 2018), 465–78. Brown shows that our term "medicine" simply fails to grasp the overlapping systems and contexts of healthcare in ancient China.

118. Patrick Geary, *Living with the Dead in the Middle Ages* (Ithaca: Cornell University Press, 1994), 33. Geary argues that meaning must be sought "in the structure of relationships uniting these elements."

in chapter 1, with an examination of the communal practices of memorialization of beguine and Cistercian women, the so-called living saints of Brabant-Liège, found in recorded storytelling about miraculous healing that took place after their deaths. These narrative sources reveal communications between the living and the dead, and, although clerically mediated, they often provide the only surviving textual witness to a community's memory of the care received at the hands of women. Chapter 2 transitions from posthumous healing miracles to the lived caregiving actions attributed to religious women during their lives, lives lived in part or whole in the service of patients in hospitals, leprosaria, and sickbeds in private homes or monastic infirmaries. This chapter also examines the *Lives* of male living saints in the thirteenth-century southern Netherlandish corpus to show that healthcare practice does not appear as a central component of their stories of sanctity. In addition, it incorporates nonnarrative sources: charters and testaments from the thirteenth-century southern Low Countries that demonstrate the presence of Cistercian and beguine women in hospitals, leprosaria, and infirmaries.

Part 2 (chapter 3) then asks, How did medical and clerical authorities rationalize the kinds of therapeutic treatments used by religious women? How do their rationalizations help us to understand the process through which physicians differentiated their medical authority from that of religious women, and the process through which clerical authors translated religious women's therapeutic power into stories of spiritual merit, stories of grace? Here, I explore a matrix of authoritative discourses—medical, theological, and hagiographic—to imagine how these religious women and their caregiving communities were situated in a broader intellectual and cultural context. Physicians, theologians, and pastors all pondered the role of the soul and its accidents in driving bodily transformation, and their discussions provide insight into claims about authority over certain categories of knowledge and practice and the constitutional interdependence of medicine and religion.

Part 3 asks, What did medieval religious women know about the body and its care? How did they act on that knowledge? How did they transmit it? To answer these questions, Part 3 features the kinds of books to which religious women in this region had access. In chapter 4, I explore several examples from a corpus of Mosan (from the Meuse River Valley) psalters belonging to thirteenth-century beguines, which show that beguines used prayers, liturgy, regimens, images, and poetry as tools in their combined prayer-making and caregiving. Reading these psalters through the lens of performance allows us to detect traces of feminine health knowledge and practice that failed to be recorded as medical acts. In chapter 5 I examine codices that bound together the *Lives* of mulieres religiosae from this region with healing prayers and meditations, blessings, curses, childbirth instructions, and medical charms. I argue that the text of a *Life*, its manuscript materialization, channeled the presence of the saint and became a therapeutic tool, just like her tomb or relics. Finally, the afterword looks forward in time in order to question how the repeatability of habituated caregiving practices generates exclusion from authoritative healthcare knowledge production.

While *physica* brought into being a learned, rational system of body knowledge and its transmission, its success and authority also suppressed social, practical, and tacit ways of identifying health and its threats.[119] Late medieval urban communities in the southern Low Countries clung to a basic perception of the body as dependent on divine and supranatural forces, and they rendered their stories of healing in terms of intimate relationships with those forces. Their stories help us to capture the historical diversity of embodied experience and reveal the extraordinary depths of the medieval medical imagination. This book, finally, is an exploration of those healing stories and of the feminine salutary emblems at their core.

---

119. On the emergence of systems of knowledge classification, see Geoffrey Bowker and Susan Leigh Star, eds., *Sorting Things Out: Classification and Its Consequences* (Boston: MIT Press, 1999); and Simone Lässig, "The History of Knowledge and the Expansion of the Historical Research Agenda," *German Historical Institute Bulletin* 59 (Fall 2016): 38.

PART I

Therapeutic Narratives

CHAPTER 1

Translating Care

The Circulation of Healing Stories

Shortly after Lutgard of Aywières died on 16 June 1246, amid her communal sisters' chanting of the Psalms, the nuns began to care for her corpse, preparing it for burial. During these ministrations, a sister who had long lived with one paralyzed hand began to wash Lutgard's body. Upon a single touch, the sister's hand immediately mended, restored to its full capacity of movement and function. In reporting this occurrence, Thomas of Cantimpré recalled the prophetic words of Marie of Oignies, who had stated of Lutgard, "While she lives, she now performs spiritual miracles; after death she will work bodily ones."[1] Thomas repeated this quip about Marie's prediction three times throughout the *Life* of Lutgard.[2]

Why was her therapeutic competence so important to him and to other authors in the hagiographic corpus? Why did Thomas exert textual control over the bodily miracles that people reported about Lutgard? And what does the textual production of healing miracles communicate about the therapeutic experiences available to residents of the thirteenth-century southern Low

---

1. *De vita S. Lutgardis* (BHL 4950), in *AASS* June III, 237–63; hereafter *VLA*; *Life of Lutgard of Aywières*, trans. Margot King and Barbara Newman, in *Thomas of Cantimpré: The Collected Lives*, ed. Barbara Newman (Turnhout: Brepols, 2008), 211–96. *VLA* III.18, 245; trans., 289: "spiritualia miracula in vita sua nunc facit; corporalia post mortem efficiet."

2. *VLA* III.8 and II.9.

Countries? This chapter pursues answers to these questions by investigating the presentation of the saintly mulieres religiosae as therapeutic agents after their deaths. It explores the handful of posthumous healing miracles in the liégeois corpus, and shows how they served a broader hagiographic agenda in the thirteenth century, a time when the healing miracles of saints were considered by many educated authorities as quite passé.[3]

Thomas of Cantimpré was a well-educated Dominican theologian and hagiographer who, in addition to his hagiographies, compiled a massive encyclopedia of natural history, the Liber de natura rerum.[4] After completing his Life of Lutgard, he embarked in 1248 on a scholastic education at the studium generale in Cologne, where he studied under the natural philosopher and "doctor universalis" Albertus Magnus. Even prior to his studies with Albertus, though, Thomas had exhibited a keen interest in scientific and medical texts.[5] His Liber de natura rerum cites, in addition to biblical, philosophical, and even musical treatises, such medical authorities as Michael Scot's Quaestiones Nicolai, the book of simple remedies known as Circa instans, the Pseudo-Cleopatran Gynaecia, the Metaphysica of Ibn Sīnā (Avicenna), and the Salernitan questions.[6] Thomas likely imbibed this knowledge of natural philosophy in Paris, where, beginning in 1238, he studied among the mendicants at St. Jacques. The mendicants of northern France in the thirteenth century were actively procuring books and assembling libraries that would include the building blocks of "the New Galen," that is, the texts on medical theory, diagnosis, and therapy that would, by the end of the century, constitute the curriculum of advanced study in medicine. This transformation of medical and scientific study took place not in Bologna or Montpellier, but in

---

3. For example, the Cistercian hagiographer of Beatrice of Nazareth commented that her miracles were not wonders of the old style, "the miracles worked by signs and acts of power so copiously and superabundantly by the saints of old." Vita Beatricis is edited and translated by Roger de Ganck in The Life of Beatrice of Nazareth (Kalamazoo, MI: Cistercian Publications, 1991), 285. There is here a sense of temporality, that the miracles of the living saints of Liège are of a different kind.

4. Thomas claims to have completed the Liber while Jacques de Vitry was a cardinal in Rome, thus prior to 1240. British Library, Harley 3717 presents a heavily annotated version of what is possibly an autograph copy of the Liber de natura rerum from the Augustinian priory of Val-Saint-Martin in Louvain.

5. On Thomas's scientific reading, see Mattea Cipriani, "Questio satis iocunda est: Analisi delle fonti di questiones et responsiones del Liber de natura rerum di Tommaso di Cantimpré," Rursus Spicae 11 (2017): 1–58. Cipriani shows that Thomas had access to Arabic translations, perhaps of an intermediary type. For example, she notes that while he may not have had an exact copy of Ibn Sīnā's Canon, he uses a lexicon that demonstrates access to the new medical learning (i.e., "triplex est enim motus rerum: naturalis, violentus et voluntarius").

6. On his auctoritates, see Cipriani, "Questio satis iocunda est."

northern France, facilitated by Dominican scholars.[7] Thomas's exposure to this knowledge lingers in the background of his choice to fashion Lutgard as an agent of bodily healing. It prompts the question, Why would Thomas, who had access to the most sophisticated medical knowledge of the time, position Lutgard as an authority in matters of healing?[8] Why would these traditional healing miracles appeal to him as a way of spotlighting her capacity to recover bodily health?

Two frames of analysis guide my reading of the posthumous healing miracles in the *liégeois* corpus. First, I ask how the posthumous miracles constructed feminine therapeutic authority. In thinking about this question, I consider the hagiographic goals in producing a textual account of miraculous behavior. Like Thomas, many of the hagiographers who recorded the posthumous healing miracles of religious women in this region enjoyed a basic understanding of natural philosophy. Their investment in producing a textual record of women's therapeutic agency suggests something of their need to explain, to control the circulation of stories. As I will discuss momentarily, the sample size of posthumous miracles they transmitted in writing is rather small; thus, even when the number of healing stories in circulation were relatively few and local, these men still felt a sense of urgency to preserve them in writing in a manner that would extend their reach beyond the immediate community from which they were generated.

The second frame of analysis in this chapter is ethnographic. It relies on acts of historical imagination to consider how these posthumous healing miracles would have worked as orally circulating healing stories. How would a person be affected by the sharing of these stories about meritorious women of recent memory who had lived among their community as sisters, neighbors, and religious women? How did these stories shape their listeners' understanding of therapeutic options and the practical realities of relief-seeking? How did they help their listeners to identify healthcare resources,

---

7. On the transmission of medical books to northern France, see Vivian Nutton, *Galen: On Problematical Movements* (Cambridge: Cambridge University Press, 2011), 65. Monica Green has shown that Richard de Fournival was likely the essential key to assembling and promoting medical literature in Paris in the thirteenth century. See her "Richard de Fournival and the Reconfiguration of Learned Medicine in the Mid-Thirteenth Century," in *Richard de Fournival et les sciences au XIIIe siècle*, ed. Joelle Ducos and Christopher Luclean (Florence: SISMEL, 2018), 179–206.

8. Thomas uses the terms *rustica*, *idiota*, and *laica* to describe Lutgard's relationship to language. These terms are not unambiguous, particularly as he also contends that she knew the Bible and meditated on biblical texts. Scholars have discussed Lutgard's illiteracy at length. See Alexandra Barrat, "Language and the Body in Thomas of Cantimpré's *Life of Lutgard of Aywières*," *Cistercian Studies Quarterly* 30.3 (1995): 339–47; and Rachel Smith, "Language, Literacy, and the Saintly Body: Cistercian Reading Practices and the *Life of Lutgard of Aywières*," *Harvard Theological Review* 109.4 (2016): 586–610.

and to regard certain women as capable of providing suitable care? When people went in search of cure at the tombs and with the relics of the saintly mulieres religiosae, what were they looking for? How did they describe their anguish and its relief? I explore the stories from the vantage of one who might be hearing them, who is searching for healthcare resources within what I call a "healing community." These two frames of analysis are intersecting and mutually informing because only the text of the healing miracle supplies the material available to gain insight into the community that shared it orally.

Two technical matters of clarification are in order before exploring the construction of the posthumous miracles. First is the issue of textual design. The protagonists of the posthumous miracle stories in the liégeois corpus were "new" saints, meaning that they had no liturgical celebrations of their own at the time their miracles were recorded.[9] Their Lives and their posthumous healing miracles were composed at the same time, often as part of a single compilation, a single "work," within a few years of their deaths. They were not subject to an authentication process, a canonization inquest, and they were scrutinized by no higher authority than the hagiographer who chose to include them in his Life. In their thirteenth-century Latin iterations, they are local stories, the products of microcommunities whose experience of certain proximate individuals as sources of healing led to the generation of tales about their power and agency that spread no more than a few dozen miles before they were recorded in writing.[10] They represent stories about the behavior of women who were locally and unofficially regarded as saints; at the time of their inscription in the Lives, these posthumous healing stories were circulating orally alongside memories of their actions, behavior, and character during their lifetimes.[11] This timing is critical: the posthumous

---

9. In her section on the miracles of "new" saints, Benedicta Ward covers William of Norwich, Godric of Finchale, and Frideswide (who was only "new" in the twelfth century in the sense that her relics were transferred, inspiring a host of fresh miracle tales).

10. Later vernacular translations of some of the Lives and healing miracles represent a very different tradition; as translations, they were new compositions, produced for new audiences, with new purposes. Jennifer Brown has explored the circulation and community uses of these vernacular translations. See Jennifer N. Brown, Three Women of Liège: A Critical Edition and Commentary on the Middle English Lives of Elizabeth of Spalbeek, Christina Mirabilis, and Marie d'Oignies (Turnhout: Brepols, 2008). Rachel Koopmans notes that the miracles that are extant and preserved in text represent a mere fraction of the tales of miracle cure that actually circulated in saints' cults. See her Wonderful to Relate: Miracle Stories and Miracle Collecting in High Medieval England (Philadelphia: University of Pennsylvania Press, 2011), 5.

11. In many cases, the hagiographer simply continued his narrative after the death of the saint to include her posthumous healing miracles as part of the Life; in some instances, however, such as the Life of Ida of Nivelles by Goswin of Bossut, the hagiographer paused to provide a preface to the

healing miracles recorded in the *liégeois* corpus represent in text some of the earliest murmurings about the mulieres religiosae. Before their fixture in text, those miracle stories were transmitted orally as information about healthcare acquisition.

The second, and related, technical matter concerns gender. Only the shrines of saints identified as women developed thirteenth-century posthumous healing cults. No posthumous healing miracles were recorded as occurring at the tombs of the *viri religiosi* (religious men) in the corpus.[12] Why did the inhabitants of the cities and towns of Brabant-Liège encounter the mulieres religiosae so often as healing saints? The miracles help to explain why the experience of them as religious *women* earned them reputations as meritorious "holy virgins" and, in turn, enabled them to continue that health work, at least for a time. Both of these technical observations about the posthumous miracles point to a distinct dynamic surrounding gender and healing. They raise questions about how the mulieres religiosae were encountered, remembered, and refashioned in hagiographic texts in this place and time. The posthumous miracles are not numerous, nor are they hagiographically unique, nor, even, are they attributed to all of the women in the corpus. But they are uniform in their construction of gender and healing, in their insistence on cultivating a particular affective style among those seeking cure, and in their persuasions of faith in the therapeutic competence of these religious women.

The posthumous miracles represent a first attribution of sanctity, the communal conferral of a distinct power to heal. They provide some indication of how the reputations of saintly religious women served the broader communities in which they were embedded. The posthumous healing miracles gathered in the thirteenth-century *liégeois* corpus have as their source orally circulating stories the hagiographer would have encountered when planning his text. In most cases, the hagiographer gathered these stories from within the monastic complex, from sisters, chaplains, conversi, and staff. The textually fixed healing tales point, however indirectly through the "formaldehyde" of their mediation, to a bustling world of storytelling, a chattering

---

healing miracles. For example, Goswin explained that he had intended to terminate the *Life* of Ida with the details of her death; however, "spontaneously, some miracles have presented themselves for me to write up as well." This preface indicates a recognition that his account of Ida's miracles was distinct from the recorded stories gathered at traditional shrines or prepared by professional miracle collectors in formal compilations.

12. While no miracles occurred at the tombs of the viri religiosi, Walter of Bierbeek is recorded as performing two posthumous healing miracles through the medium of his relics. See *De B. Waltero de Birbeke* (BHL 8794), in *AASS* January II, V.16–17, 450.

chorus convinced that certain saintly persons of recent memory could be trusted to deliver comfort and cure.[13] Miracle stories were told, and retold, and recorded because they retained, for the decades they remained in active circulation, a generative potential. They worked. The posthumous healing miracles worked as persuasions; they convinced their audience of a certain gift, a certain grace, to be found among the mulieres religiosae. I slowly unravel this politics of persuasion in this chapter and the next.

In reading the posthumous miracles in this corpus, I develop the concept of the healing community. I recognize that this concept is not, in fact, a medieval one. Like gender, it is an interpretive lens that makes visible certain patterns of behavior. In this case, it brings into focus healthcare relationships, positioning saints' shrines, relics, and their narrative productions in the continuum of healthcare resources available in the thirteenth-century Low Countries. I incorporate the phrase "healing community" to assist with describing, imagining, and theorizing how stories were shared alongside other healing technologies, like relics, herbal remedies, and methods of wound repair. Healing communities consisted of the informal interpersonal caring relationships that constituted an important form of thirteenth-century healthcare.[14] As I will demonstrate in the following chapter, formal institutional caregiving settings, such as hospitals, monastic infirmaries, and leprosaria, are visible (if often still hazy) in surviving statutes and charters; late medieval healing communities, however, are more difficult to grasp because of their informality, which left little in the way of records. Posthumous healing miracles are one way to begin to decipher how individuals cooperated to assist sufferers in the acquisition of comfort and cure, whether at the hands of a physician, an herbalist, a wise woman, or at a shrine or with the relics of a saint. Unlike *fama sanctitatis* or "cult," the idea of a healing community foregrounds movement, network, and cooperation in the process of accessing healthcare resources. The idea of a "healing community" highlights the fact that healthcare was indeed a communal enterprise in this period. Most preventative and regular sick care took place within the home. The healing community outside the home came into play when sickness

---

13. On the preservative effects of writing down miracles, see Koopmans, *Wonderful to Relate*, 5; on the chattering quality of their oral circulation, see Richard Southern, *Saint Anselm and His Biographer* (Cambridge: Cambridge University Press, 1963), 278.

14. On communities as interpersonal caring relations that constitute some of the most critical aspects of healthcare, see Charlene Galarneau, *Communities of Health Care Justice* (Newark: Rutgers University Press, 2016), esp. ch. 1, where Galarneau argues for the process of making visible the community's role in caregiving, defining community by those who are bound together through race, gender, religion, and culture.

or impairment pressed beyond the abilities of household medicine, when travelers experienced affliction, difficult labors were prolonged, or those suffering from chronic conditions sought greater resolution. No single form of healer yet held a professional monopoly, and thus individuals relied on their neighbors for assistance, and for learning whom to trust, for gathering information about the best resources for care and cure. The concept of a healing community, then, enables me to focus on the site rather than the saint, on the knowledge transmissions and healthcare practices surrounding sick people seeking healthcare resources at tombs and with relics.

"Healing community" is an adaptation of those other useful communities, the textual community and the emotional community, whose ingress into medieval studies has generated such a wealth of insight.[15] Like textual communities, healing communities facilitated a sense of shared purpose and identity. Healing communities embraced and maneuvered between oral and written forms of knowledge about health, knowledge that included an assessment of the saint's healing power and how to access it. Like emotional communities, they valued affective style. They informed sick petitioners about not only the presence and power of a certain saint, but how appropriately to present oneself to her. By attending to the role of the healing community in stories of miraculous healing we can make visible the ways that healthcare knowledge circulated in the form of healing stories, stories of therapeutic options that worked.

The healing community transmitted posthumous miracle stories to potential devotees who had not known a living saint directly or personally, convincing them of her holiness and healing power. They advanced the production of knowledge about a saint as an option for cure. The tombs and relics of local saints feature as loci at which thirteenth-century patrons would gather in search of cure, and from which additional healing stories were generated. For example, when a conversus from the Cistercian women's abbey of Herkenrode came to Villers, to the tomb of Juliana of Mont-Cornillon, he prayed for her intercession "if she had as much merit before God *as she was said to have.*"[16] The conversus traveled to her tomb expecting cure because he was escorted there by people who shared stories of Juliana's merit, people

15. Brian Stock, *The Implications of Literacy: Written Language and Models of Interpretation in the Eleventh and Twelfth Centuries* (Princeton: Princeton University Press, 1983); Barbara Rosenwein, *Emotional Communities in the Early Middle Ages* (Ithaca: Cornell University Press, 2006).

16. *Iuliana virgo* (BHL 4521), in *AASS* April I, 443–77; hereafter *VJM*; translated by Barbara Newman as "The Life of Juliana of Mont Cornillon," in *Living Saints of the Thirteenth Century,* ed. Anneke Mulder-Bakker (Turnhout: Brepols, 2011), 143–302. *VJM* IX, 477; trans., 296 (emphasis added): "si tanti esset, quanti dicebatur, meriti apud Deum."

who conditioned him to believe that her tomb might provide a source of cure. These were the very people who acknowledged his suffering and assisted him in its relief by leading him to a potential source of remediation, one they trusted, one they knew from stories "worked." Another example, from the *Life* of Ida of Nivelles, reports that a Dominican friar who had suffered for many days with a toothache so debilitating that he could neither eat nor sleep apparently came into knowledge (*agnoscens*) of a potential cure from a lay brother of La Ramée, the Cistercian abbey where Ida had lived and was buried. The lay brother traveled nearly fifty kilometers from La Ramée to Liège, carrying Ida's tooth with him. We cannot know specific details about the network bringing together the Cistercian lay brother and the Dominican friar, but we can employ the concept of a healing community to recognize as a healthcare agent the lay brother carrying Ida's tooth on his travels, relaying information about this therapeutic technology, and perhaps repeating the story of this miraculous intervention to his friends back on the grange. Ida's tooth went on to generate additional miracle cures. In this way, the miracle stories not only reflect a single personal experience and interpretation; they also shaped whole communities' experiences of illness, suffering, and healing. Those stories circulated alongside the material manifestations of successful cure—in votives, relics, and texts.

The stories of cure generated by healing communities dedicated to the living saints of the southern Low Countries share structural similarities with the recommendations of academic physicians who counseled medical practitioners on bedside manner. They both centered on the role of the affects and imagination in the therapeutic process. As Fernando Salmón has shown, scholastic physicians theorized the central role of hope for recovery of health. A standard twelfth-century grammatical teaching from Aesop's fables held that sick patients with hope survived, but when hope died, so too did the patient.[17] Both medical prescriptions and the healing communities of saints urged this principle and counseled their adherents to cultivate hope as a salubrious passion. Peter of Spain (d. 1277), for example, argued for the physiological effects of instilling hope for recovery in the patient. Citing Galen and Ibn Sīnā (Avicenna), Peter taught that the imaginative power of

---

17. On this fable, see Fernando Salmón, "The Physician as Cure," in *Ritual Healing: Magic, Ritual, and Medical Therapy from Antiquity until the Early Modern Period*, ed. Ildikó Csepregi and Charles Burnett (Florence: SISMEL, 2012), 206; in Aesopus, *Anonymus Neveleti*, ed. Wendelin Foerster (Heilbronn: Henninger, 1882), XXVIII, "De leporibus et ranis," pp. 111–112: "Speret qui metuit. Morituros vivere vidi, spe duce victuros, spe moriente mori."

the soul affected the health of the body.[18] If the patient had full confidence in the remedies offered by their physician, then the patient's imagination would compel hope and invite salubrious affects. Taddeo Alderoti (d. 1295) added to this explanation, suggesting that confidence and hope facilitated nature in fighting disease just as despair fueled its ravages.[19] The author of the *De cautelis medicorum* made similar claims, extending the effects of the passions of the soul to the patient's social setting. He discussed various rhetorical means of persuading the patient and their company of the physician's competence, advising that physicians must "obtain the favor of the people who are around the sick" because this favor will lead to salubrious hope and confidence.[20] Put another way, hope and confidence in a practitioner's power to heal were contagious. I will return to medical discussions of the passions in chapter 3, but for now I wish to note the magnitude of conviction for the community surrounding the sick.

Just as medical practitioners cultivated hope in their patients in order to see better results, so also did hagiographers portray sick petitioners as requiring hope and confidence in the saint's power to relieve their anguish and facilitate their healing. In these tales, cure was often achieved through the patient's success in dispelling injurious passions such as anger, grief, and aversion, and conjuring salubrious ones such as love, joy, and courage. The healing community was central to this exchange. The healing community assisted the sick in working through their passions, first instructing them on how to relate their story of illness in the presence of the saint, and then promulgating the whole narrative in the form of a miracle story. In both saintly and scholastic medicine, the community surrounding the sick was vital to developing the appropriate passions in the patient, without which the prognosis was grim. The social matrix conferred legitimacy on certain forms of healing, shared knowledge about therapeutic resources and models of sickness, and licensed the patient to expect cure.

Neither in the thirteenth century nor today are healing miracles considered a genre of medical literature; nevertheless, stories of miracle cures form

---

18. Salmón, "The Physician as Cure," 204. Petrus Hispanus (Peter of Spain), *Super Prognostica Hippocratis*, in Madrid, Biblioteca Nacional de España, MS 1877, fols. 124–141; 124v: "Quod fortis ymaginatio est causa salutis et confidentia infirmi de medico est ymaginatio quedam; ergo confidentia est causa salutis."

19. Salmón, "The Physician as Cure," 205.

20. Arnald of Villanova, *De cautelis medicorum*, in *Henry Sigerist on the History of Medicine*, ed. Felix Marti-Ibañez (New York: MD Publications, 1960), 137. Although this treatise circulated under the name of Arnald of Villanova and gained authority through it, McVaugh argues, based on inconsistent phrasing, that there were numerous authors. See his "Bedside Manners in the Middle Ages," *Bulletin of the History of Medicine* 71.2 (1997): 201–23.

an important discourse on medicine and healing. They represent the many ways that individuals reckoned illness and organized their approach to remedy. They reveal how patients explained their symptoms, causes of disease, and rationale for cure. The visit to a saint's tomb or relics was a fundamental means of experiencing and rationalizing illness and its potential for remedy. The stories generated there were cast in what Charlotte Furth has dubbed "the phenomenological plane of medical discourse."[21] This deployment of medical discourse foregrounds sensation, detailing the corporeal and social experience of infirmity. All stories of medical success are based on plausible explanation.[22] In the thirteenth-century southern Low Countries, the women who had lived their lives serving the sick in religious and semireligious communities, who had assisted in the penitential relief of sin, were considered plausible sources of bodily remedy. Some of them were seen this way even after their deaths. Those women were thought of as "saints."

Patterns of the Miraculous

As a means of interpreting personal experiences, miracles had a long history in Latin Christianity. Augustine had explained that visible wonders were affirmations of invisible transformations within the interior self, a way of seeing the world.[23] The miracles of the Gospels, according to Augustine, were designed to convince Christian converts of their new truth. Augustine understood all of creation as radically and miraculously dependent on the incarnate and resurrected God. In his formulation, *all* of the natural world was itself a miracle so that a miracle such as Jesus changing water to wine at Cana was not in fact *against* nature because God was the maker and sustainer of nature. Rather, such liquid transformation was an extension of human perception into the miraculous workings of divine creation. God had created the world with *seminales rationes*, hidden causes within the objects of creation.[24] Their startling eruptions sparked wonder, reverence, and faith. In miracles, it was *human* nature that was temporarily altered by grace, able to

---

21. Charlotte Furth, *A Flourishing Yin: Gender in China's Medical History, 960–1665* (Los Angeles: University of California Press, 1999), 15.

22. Arthur Kleinman, *Patients and Healers in the Context of Culture: An Exploration of the Borderland between Anthropology, Medicine, and Psychology* (Berkeley: University of California Press, 1980).

23. On Augustine's conceptualization of miracle, see Giselle de Nie, *Poetics of Wonder: Testimonies of the New Christian Miracles in the Late Antique Latin World* (Leiden: Brill, 2011).

24. On Augustine and the *seminales rationes* of miracles, see Benedicta Ward, *Miracles and the Medieval Mind: Theory, Record, and Event, 1000–1215* (Philadelphia: University of Pennsylvania Press, 1987), 3.

detect what is usually imperceptible to humanity's fallen senses.[25] Humanity required a sign, a goad to envision the natural world as divinely significant, a physical pressure to conversion. "Why," he asked, "are those miracles, which you affirm were wrought formerly, wrought no longer? I would reply that miracles were necessary before the world believed, in order that it might believe. How is it that everywhere Christ is celebrated with such firm belief in His resurrection and ascension? How is it that in enlightened times, in which every impossibility is rejected, the world has, without any miracles, believed things marvelously incredible? . . . We cannot deny that many miracles were wrought to confirm that one grand and health-giving miracle (*salubrique miraculo*) of Christ's ascension to heaven with the flesh in which He rose."[26] For Augustine, miracles were necessary to convince people of the *greatest* miracle—the resurrection and bodily ascension of Christ. Miracles produced faith; they produced a lived truth. Anchoring the very possibility of miracle was a Christian truth about the body—that Christ's resurrection and ascension in the flesh were "health-giving." It rendered new possibilities, new truths about human corporeality and the means to restore human health.

But Augustine was writing at a time when, he deemed, the grand miracles of the Gospels—the multiplication of loaves and calming of storms— were no longer necessary and no longer occurred. They had performed their work of converting a people to Christianity.[27] Still, he insisted, miracles did continue in his own time, though they were more subtle and thus did not generate grand textual narratives. They did not require scripture. When the relics of the martyr Stephen were transferred from Jerusalem in the year 416, Augustine found an opportunity to record the miracle stories that occurred in the presence of his bones. *"Now,"* he asserted, "miracles are wrought in the name of Christ, whether by His sacraments or by the prayers or relics of His saints; but they are not so brilliant and conspicuous as to cause them to be published with such glory as accompanied the former miracles."[28] Although Augustine declared that miracles were no longer necessary for faith, that they no longer required "publication," he nevertheless proceeded to record narratives of the healing miracles that he had witnessed or that were reported to him. That is, he provided a script to substantiate

---

25. Augustine, *The City of God against the Pagans*, ed. R. W. Dyson (Cambridge: Cambridge University Press, 1998), 22.8–10.

26. *City of God*, 1117.

27. Simon Yarrow, *Saints and Their Communities: Miracle Stories in Twelfth-Century England* (Oxford: Clarendon Press, 2006), 1.

28. *City of God*, 1117 (emphasis added).

the everyday healing miracles that, he claimed, did not warrant scripture. In other words, Augustine fixed in writing healing miracles not because of the wonder of the miracle but because of the power of the story. Miraculous healing narratives had the power to convince their listeners and readers that Christ's salutary resurrection had secured their own avenue to health, both in this lifetime and after their bodily deaths.

By the thirteenth century, when healing miracles about the saintly mulieres religiosae were circulating orally among liégeois healing communities, Thomas Aquinas's definition of miracle was largely accepted, at least by the hagiographers who encountered, interpreted, and recorded these tales. Aquinas distinguished between miracles and wonders, positing that "things that are at times divinely accomplished, apart from the established order of things, are customarily called miracle; for we observe the effect but do not know its cause. And since one and the same cause is at times known to some people and unknown to others, the result is that, of several who see an effect at the same time, some wonder, while others do not. For instance, an astronomer does not wonder when he sees an eclipse of the sun, for he knows its cause, but the person who is ignorant of this science must wonder, for he ignores the cause."[29] As with Augustine, perspective was crucial. Some people, when witnessing powerful transformations in the natural order, experienced wonder, whereas others (studious natural philosophers like himself) knew the natural cause. In miracles, *everyone* experienced wonder because the hidden cause was God. Aquinas's formulation captures a larger thirteenth-century interest in developing rational explanations for material transformation. This interest in natural order explains why the vast majority of miracles that were actually recorded during this time were *not* grand spectacles of nature, but healing miracles.[30] Aquinas reasoned that healing miracles belonged to an entirely separate category. They

---

29. Thomas Aquinas, *Summa contra Gentiles: Book III, Providence, Part Two*, trans. Vernon J. Bourke (South Bend: University of Notre Dame Press, 1975). ch. 101. On thirteenth-century changes in the conceptualization of miracle, see Lorraine Daston and Katherine Park, *Wonders and the Order of Nature, 1150–1750* (Boston: Zone Books, 1998); and Michael Goodich, *Miracles and Wonders: The Development of the Concept of Miracle, 1150–1350* (New York: Routledge, 2007).

30. Caroline Bynum, *Christian Materiality: An Essay on Religion in Late Medieval Europe* (Boston: MIT Press, 2011), 227–30. Benedicta Ward also tracks this change in the pattern of miracle stories. She notes that earlier miracle collections were often recorded anonymously and somewhat haphazardly by guardians at "traditional shrines," that is, the shrines of long-dead saints with an established place in the liturgical life of a church. Those early miracles were attributed to cures or proprietorial claims, in which the saint protected or restored monastery lands, goods, or personnel. Beginning in the twelfth century, however, healing miracles began to dominate and were attached to "new" saints. See Ward, *Miracles and the Medieval Mind*, chs. 3 and 4.

were engineered through grace to provide material benefits on account of faith.[31] His Dominican contemporaries shared Aquinas's understanding of the grace of healing as a separate category of miracle merited by faith and conferred by saints. In the *Life* of Christina Mirabilis, for example, Thomas of Cantimpré reports on the moment when her bodily remains were transferred from the monastery of St. Catherine. He relates that the nuns and clerics who observed the translation were overcome with "sweetness" (*dulcedinis*) and "no one doubted the grace of healing which had been bestowed on those who had come to her tomb in due faith."[32] Those who received healing, he assured readers, were the ones who approached the tomb *in due faith*, linking the reception of healing to conviction in the saint's power, in her divine merit.

While Thomas of Cantimpré delivered no sustained discussion of miracles in his hagiographic or encyclopedic treatises, he did include a number of incidental remarks worthy of deeper scrutiny. His *Life* of Lutgard exemplifies Thomas's approach to the miraculous. As he luxuriated in rich descriptions of Lutgard's seemingly uncanny abilities—her levitations, secretions, prophecies, and other paramystical phenomena—Thomas repeatedly undercut the miraculous, insisting that there was nothing terribly wondrous in Lutgard's bodily transformations.[33] They all fell within the expected natural order. For example, when her fingertips dripped oil in prayer, Thomas insisted that this manifestation was no miracle. Rather, the oil was a natural overflow, a result of her body's condition "so filled up inwardly by superabundant grace."[34] When describing the flame of fire that emitted from Lutgard's mouth as she chanted the Psalms, he paused, "Note, reader," the flame merely signified her "desire of fervid prayer."[35] This pattern is evident again when Lutgard began to levitate in the audience of the entire monastic community. "It is no wonder," Thomas explained; her prayer was enveloped in heaven so that "it

---

31. Thomas Aquinas, *Summa Theologica*, ii.178.

32. *De S. Christina Mirabili virgine* (*BHL* 1746, 1747), in *AASS* July V, 637–60; hereafter *VCM*; *Life of Christina the Astonishing*, trans. Margot King and Barbara Newman, in Newman, *Thomas of Cantimpré*, 127–60. *VCM* V.54, 650; trans., 154: "Nec enim ullus ambigit, gratiam sanitatum collatam esse his, qui cum fide debita ad ejus tumulum accesserunt."

33. Rachel Smith considers Thomas's habit of undercutting his own descriptive efforts as part of an experimental apophatic theology in which he "presses against the possibility of teaching or transmitting such an experience." Smith, *Excessive Saints: Gender, Narrative, and Theological Invention in Thomas of Cantimpré's Mystical Hagiographies* (New York: Columbia University Press, 2019), 178.

34. *VLA* I.16, 194; trans., 231: "quia ex superabundanti gratia repleor interius." He similarly naturalizes the oil that dripped from Christina's breasts and fingers as a normal product of her interior grace.

35. *VLA* II.18, 200; trans., 253: "Nota ergo, lector. . . . Fervidae orationis desiderium figurasse."

was given to her to manifest even through the disposition of her body."[36] And when she tasted a sweet honey in her mouth after a visionary experience of sucking from Christ's wound, he asked: "What is there to wonder in this?"[37]

"Why marvel at this?" he repeatedly demands. "What is wonderful about this? What is new?"[38] Thomas issued these queries at each turn of spectacle, only to cast aside the notion that Lutgard's manifestations were fundamentally "miraculous." Instead, he insisted on an expansion of the natural order to include her manifestations of grace. Appealing to seminal reasons as divine implantations of possible transformation in each created thing, Thomas explained that, "in the creation of heaven and earth, God merely spoke the word and they were created."[39] For each astonishing story he divulged, he provided an exegetical coda in perceiving the seeds of divine grace that took effect within the material world. Lutgard's body, as Rachel Smith has argued, was for Thomas a sacramental sign that manifested the divine "res"; it was less a miracle than a textually mediated sacrament.[40]

I will explore Thomas's physiology of the saintly body in greater detail in chapter 3; for now, I note that it was only when reporting on Lutgard's cures, those undertaken during her life as well as those attributed to her postmortem intercession, that Thomas clearly marked the miraculous. For example, a "most unexpected miracle" occurred when Lutgard cured a sick sister in the infirmary.[41] She accomplished "so great a miracle" when she inserted her finger into the ear of a deaf woman, restoring her audition.[42] And he pronounced that a "wondrous and breath-taking miracle" was secured when Lutgard saved a young nun from debilitating temptation.[43] Just like Augustine before him, Thomas could not resist the compulsion to render healing events in the form of miracle stories. These events were no mere wonders, a matter of perception. For thirteenth-century clerics and hagiographers, healing miracles were real events. They required faith and a mode of understanding possibilities that placed confidence in the healer, the saint who intervened with Christ on behalf of humanity. The posthumous miracles recorded by Thomas and other authors in the liégeois corpus served to promote that faith,

36. VLA I.10, 192; trans., 225: "etiam corporis gestu pro sua possibilitate suscepti."
37. VLA I.13, 193; trans., 228–29: "Quid miri?"
38. VLA II.37, II.42, III.10.
39. VLA III.10, 206; trans., 283: "in creatione enim caeli et terrae, verbo tantum dixit, et facta sunt." Thomas cites Augustine in this discussion, De genesi ad litteram XII.34.67.
40. Smith, Excessive Saints, 7.
41. VLA II.20, 200; trans., 254: "inopinabile multum miraculum."
42. VLA II.22, 200; trans., 257: "tanto miraculo."
43. VLA II.25, 201; trans., 259: "Mirum vere et stupendum miraculum."

to convince various audiences of the reality of their subject's true sanctity and thus her ability to heal not naturally, but supernaturally.

The textual record of the posthumous miracles provides details of how these persuasive tales circulated orally as information about local healing resources, as when the conversus from Herkenrode was recorded as traveling to Juliana's tomb because he had heard stories of her "divine merit." This "divine merit" signified to him a potential therapeutic skill, a health resource available at her tomb. These stories of merit spread as information, as health knowledge, to those who may have been searching for a remedy and did not yet know of the powers of a certain saint or, as we will see, were doubtful of one with whom they were already familiar.

While the textual production of the miracle story emphasized the sanctity of the miracle worker, we can also imagine how the story itself, as *story*, affected listeners. The proliferation of such stories shaped how people thought of their own bodies, illnesses, health options, and potential for recovery. The plotlines, metaphors, and rhetorical devices that characterized healing miracles represent what Arthur Kleinman has called "explanatory models" for illness and healing.[44] Miracles provided an interpretive category— an explanatory model—through which Christians understood that spiritual forces could affect their physical bodies. Without harnessing a precise vocabulary to explain physiological change, they rationalized a real, transformational role for their affective lives in the healing process. Miracle stories from the thirteenth-century canon of living saints emphasize the transformation of person that took place in the presence of a saint, a result of renewed faith.[45] The "abundance" of the saintly encounter meant that sites associated with the saint—her tomb, her relics, the manuscript copy of her *Life*—were coded with significance, with expectation.[46] Through these specific and highly local encounters, individuals reimagined their selves, their bodies, their relationships. The encounter with the saint at her tomb or in her relics, or in the sharing of stories of her healing powers, often represented the beginning of a process of altered perception, seeing the self as whole, completed, or healed. The experience of journeying to the tomb, of seeing and touching

44. Kleinman, *Patients and Healers*, 49.

45. On the transformation of person in the healing encounter, see Thomas Csordas, *Body/Meaning/Healing* (New York: Palgrave, 2002).

46. On the "abundance" of religious events, see Robert Orsi, *History and Presence* (Cambridge, MA: Harvard University Press, 2016), 66–67. Examining the "abundant event" precipitated by the encounter with a saint's tomb or relics emphasizes "the intricacies of relationships in a particular area at a particular time, [and provides] meaning for all the hopes, desires, and fears circulating among a group of people as these were taking shape at a certain place and at a certain time." See his "Abundant History: Marian Apparitions as Alternative Modernity," *Historically Speaking* 9.7 (2008): 14–15.

the saint's relics, of hearing her stories conveyed with conviction, ignited hope and conferred power and authority on the saint. The pilgrimage, the waxen effigy, the petition: these were external models of patients' internal faith, which they placed in the saint's ability to intercede with the divine on their behalf. The petitioner's choice to surrender doubt and visit the tomb, to act upon the possibility of a saint's efficacy, was a choice to live in a world where the possibility of cure was real.[47]

It was a choice with important implications for the thirteenth-century landscape of healthcare. Not only did it mean that there were multiple, overlapping options for seeking cure, a range of therapeutic technologies that included relics, pharmaceuticals, devotional pictures, physicians, liturgy, saints' shrines, barbers, regular confession, empirics, manuscripts, and contemplative gardens.[48] It also meant that practices of the living reached beyond this temporal realm, intersected with the dead, with other bodies, and with other noncorporeal agents. The posthumous miracle stories from the *liégeois* corpus convey those intersections, revealing how residents came to place faith in the power of certain religious women who had lived among them, how well-crafted stories convinced them to access therapy in spaces marked by the material memories of those women.

An Illness Profile

The posthumous healing miracles recorded in the *liégeois* corpus feature small religious communities like Aywières and La Ramée and their environs.[49] They capture local details that stress the ties linking nuns, novices, beguines, lay brothers, chaplains, and other attendants, as well as proximate

47. Godfrey Lienhardt, *Divinity and Experience: The Religion of the Dinka* (Oxford: Clarendon Paperbacks, 1988).

48. For other scholars who emphasize variety in the medical marketplace, see Michael McVaugh, *Medicine before the Plague: Practitioners and Their Patients in the Crown of Aragon, 1285–1345* (Cambridge: Cambridge University Press, 2002); Carole Rawcliffe, "Hospital Nurses and Their Work," in *Daily Life in the Late Middle Ages*, ed. Richard Britnell (London: Stroud, 1998), 43–64; and Rawcliffe, *Medicine for the Soul: The Life, Death, and Resurrection of an English Medieval Hospital; St. Giles's Norwich, 1249–1550* (Stroud: Sutton, 1999); John Henderson, *The Renaissance Hospital: Healing the Body and Healing the Soul* (New Haven: Yale University Press, 2006); Peregrine Horden, *Hospitals and Healing from Late Antiquity to the Later Middle Ages* (Aldershot: Ashgate, 2008).

49. Twenty-nine posthumous healing miracles occur throughout the entire corpus; twenty-seven of them are attributed to female saints. All of the posthumous healing miracles that occurred at tombs were achieved through female saints. On small sample sizes, see Iona McCleery, "Christ More Powerful than Galen: The Relationship between Medicine and Miracles," in *Contextualizing Miracles in the Medieval West*, ed. M. M. Mesley and Louise Wilson (Leeds: Medium Aevum, 2014), 127–54.

neighbors and occasional travelers. Because the saint was in most cases a member of the religious community and had only died very recently, the stories signal how members of the community and their neighbors became convinced that she possessed a genuine option for cure, how they cooperated to share information and convince others of her therapeutic power.

To reiterate the gendered presentation of these healing miracles: there are no posthumous tombside healing miracles that circulated with the *Lives* of male-identified saints in the canon. There are only two relic-related posthumous healing miracles attributed to viri religiosi in the canon. They both occur in the *Life* of Walter of Bierbeek, in both cases an effect of touching his footwear, and in both cases the miracles were granted to knights. While they may have had cults, viri religiosi from this region were not included in stories of cure, as healthcare resources that were shared in healing communities.[50] The healing miracles that circulated in the region thus tell us about the healthcare attributions projected onto local religious women, about the processes through which religious women became centered in these stories.

Even the tiniest sample size of miracles calls out for statistical analysis. As Iona McCleery has remarked, "There is something inherently countable about miracles."[51] Among the twenty-nine miracles in the corpus, twenty-seven were attributed to mulieres religiosae. Of those miracles attributed to the intervention of women, 67 percent represent cures offered to other women. This majority is partly explained by the fact that Ida of Nivelles, Lutgard, and Christina were buried on the grounds of women's communities, which would have made their tombs more accessible to women inhabitants.[52] Yet, tombs were not the main site of miraculous action: twelve of the miracles occurred at tombs, thirteen with relics, and two miracles took

---

50. Walter of Bierbeek's two miracles involved his footwear, and the status of both recipients was that of knight. One had a "dangerous apostema" that was healed by one of Walter's sandals, and the other involved a wealthy knight, Winemarus of Aldendorp, who was paralyzed and requested Walter's socks or leggings (*boti*). He reported that he felt immediate benefit (*beneficium protinus*). *AASS* January II, 447–50, V.16–17, 450. I will discuss Walter's *Life* in the following chapter. Here, I note that Walter's brief *Life*, the only one among the *Lives* of men in the corpus to include healing miracles, circulated in a manuscript with the *Lives* of mulieres religiosae, Brussels, KBR, MS 4459–70. For discussion of this manuscript, see chapter 5.

51. McCleery, "Christ More Powerful than Galen," 140.

52. Christina was buried at St. Catherine's in 1224, then transferred to Nonnemielen in 1231, and then from a grave to a revered place next to the altar in 1249. Lutgard was buried in the church of Aywières in 1246 (elevated in 1616). Ida of Nivelles was buried in La Ramée in 1231. Beatrice of Nazareth was buried in the ambulatory of her community, between the church and the chapter, but her *Life* records no posthumous miracles. Alice of Schaerbeek was likely also buried in her community of La Cambre, though her *Life* records only a series of posthumous visions her devotees experienced shortly after her death.

effect in visions, though both within the confines of a women's abbey. Social status is not indicated in four of the miracles, but in the remaining miracles, recipients included nine nuns, four children or babies, two lay brothers, two beguines, one Dominican friar, one monastic chaplain, one Cistercian monk, one male associate of a women's abbey, and two matrons. While the four unknown statuses remain a mystery, the miracle stories demonstrate that the other characters involved were affiliated with the saint's community, either as a neighbor, benefactor, confessor, or other intermediary such as a servant or beguine. This limited social range suggests intimacy and proximity. Occasionally, as in the example of the lay brother from Herkenrode, a traveler would journey several miles in search of the saint; in most cases, however, these stories circulated in a tight radius around a religious community. They were shared by affiliates of the community, and they reflect how knowledge of therapeutic options might travel in these intimate settings.

The two most common ailments cured by the *liégeois* saints were unspecified illnesses and fevers. Seven cases, 30 percent, fall into the category of unspecified illness, which are described vaguely as *infirmitate grave* or *infirmitate diutina*.[53] The unspecified nature of these illnesses suggests chronic symptoms. For example, one of the patients with unspecified illness was said to be in "continual distress" and unable to sleep or to rise to perform his devotions as a lay brother at La Ramée.[54] Having endured this illness for three years, he visited Ida's tomb and found complete recovery, never again experiencing the languor that had so debilitated him. Unspecified fevers and other head-related woes, such as severe headache, were also common among the healing miracles, and are described in a similar fashion as having an enduring languishing effect.[55] The fevers mentioned are uncategorized, and modified only by descriptions such as "laboring with" or "suffering from."[56]

---

53. *Vita beatae Idae de Nivella sanctimonialis in Monasterio de Rameya* in *Quinque prudentes virgines* (*BHL* 4146–47), ed. Chrysostomo Henriquez (Antwerp: Cnobbaert, 1630), 199–297; hereafter *VIN.* See *VIN* XXXV; *VJM* II.IX.

54. *VIN* XXXV: "continuam infirmitatis molestiam."

55. *VLA* III.iii.27: "gravissimo dolore capitis."

56. Such depictions suggest ephemeral fevers, which Galen often attributed to the overheating of the heart, which then carried inflamed *spirits* throughout the body. Galen, *On the Differences of Fevers* 1.1; Luke Demaitre, *Medieval Medicine: The Art of Healing from Head to Toe* (Santa Barbara: ABC Clio, 2013), 39–42. In the thirteenth century, such fevers would have been treated through a vast range of remedies, including palliation, contraries, massages, cupping, phlebotomy, empirical cures, and saints' interventions.

The sample of miracles also includes four cases of toothaches and three incidents of swellings, some of the most common afflictions in medieval society. In medical practice, toothaches were usually left to empirics; Michelle Savonarola commented that dental problems were "considered to have become a barber's affair and [are] treated mostly by vulgar entrepreneurs on street corners."[57] We can imagine, from this portrait of vernacular medicine, that healing communities might advertise a certain saint's tooth as the most efficacious remedy for pain. As the healing narratives demonstrate, teeth were rather portable relics.[58] Tales of their efficacy, and thus of the saint's healing vigor, could spread quickly in the hands of a lay brother, pilgrim, or merchant, transforming them into itinerant healers.

Additionally, swellings of various limbs featured prominently in the posthumous miracles, where they were reported as having a deleterious effect on patients' mobility.[59] In the three miracles that cure swellings, the term *inflata* is used to describe their patients' afflictions, indicating that they were likely the kind of inflammations that medical writers would have associated with excesses of phlegm or black bile.[60] Another surface disorder, a fistular ulcer, appears as a diagnosis in the posthumous miracles. Fistula was notoriously difficult to cure, and for that reason there were several remedies among the *experimenta* of empirics.[61] As with headaches, fevers, and toothaches, there was no single uniform method of treatment for fistula, so that visiting a saint's shrine or relics was just as hopeful a remedy as many other options, such as herbal treatments or surgery.

Other maladies that received narrative elaboration in the miraculous healing stories are mental illness, catarrh, deafness, wounds, paralysis, ulcers, difficult labor, and hernia. This range of most commonly cured illnesses in the miracle stories allows us to postulate that patients were turning to the saintly mulieres of the southern Low Countries for common, persistent problems that affected every status in medieval society. None of them acted

---

57. Quoted in Demaitre, *Medieval Medicine*, 193. The miracles of toothaches reported intense oral pain and inability to eat.

58. Two of the healings are prompted by contact with teeth from Ida of Nivelles, and two are accomplished by contact with a linen kerchief owned by Juliana of Mont-Cornillon.

59. Galen's *On Unnatural Tumors* (or *On Abnormal Swellings*) treated swellings, which consisted of a general category that Avicenna later refined to specify the various kinds of swellings, including tumors, edema, phlegmon, scrofula, and basic swelling (*inflatio*). This treatise is translated into English by D. G. Lytton and L. M. Resuhr in *Journal of the History of Medicine and the Allied Sciences* 33.4 (1978): 531–49.

60. Demaitre, *Medieval Medicine*, 95.

61. Demaitre, 96.

as a specialist for any one kind of affliction. Rather, they were consulted as general practitioners, available to ease any affliction.

The posthumous healing miracles in the thirteenth-century corpus blend traditional healing tropes with more au courant charitable practices and hagiographic designs. Many of them exhume and repackage healing topoi from the Gospels or from later but equally riveting tales of miraculous stage-craft enacted in the *Lives* of Saint Martin and Saint Foy; some bear striking similarities to miracles attributed to Thomas Beckett or Frideswide. These repetitive patterns, the topoi or tropes that hagiographic authors sought to emulate, served in part to garner greater authority and distinction for their saint.[62] But tropes of the miraculous are also what Rachel Koopmans has called plotlines of the "Christian saint metanarrative."[63] These plotlines, in which a divine intervention furnishes a solution to a health-related problem, would have been repeated among all members of medieval society from a young age. They shaped how individuals interpreted their own experiences, and they informed hagiographers' translation of those experiences into nar-ratives. In this way, miracle stories are less about the saint than about pos-sibilities of the self, about how one could learn to gain the personal effects of a saint's favor.[64]

The repetition of healing miracles generated potential realities, prompt-ing people to imagine options for healing.[65] The constant revival and adapta-tion of tropes highlight their effectiveness; if authors were recycling tropes, and healing communities repeating them (and vice versa, as it was a mutually informing process), then it was because they were effective, not just entertain-ing.[66] They promoted knowledge about the acquisition of health resources in intellectually and emotionally satisfying ways. In the thirteenth-century low-lands, miracle stories that drew on hagiographic topoi centered on the power of certain *women* to wield cure. In other words, in this region and this time, individuals shared stories about finding therapeutic resources at the hands of local religious women, living and dead. They sometimes related their experi-ences with those women—and apparently *not* their experiences with men—in hagiographic impressions, adapting common plotlines from hagiographic

---

62. Koopmans, *Wonderful to Relate*, 28.

63. Koopmans, 31.

64. Koopmans adapts a model from the social sciences, calling this form the "personal miracle story." *Wonderful to Relate*, 23–25.

65. Marcus Bull, *The Miracles of Our Lady Rocamadour: Analysis and Translation* (Suffolk: Boydell & Brewer, 1999), 35.

66. Simone Roisin also argued that the tropes familiar in Cistercian hagiography were adapted and fitted into local circumstances. Trope is never mere trope. Simone Roisin, *L'hagiographie cisterci-enne dans le diocèse de Liège au XIIIe siècle* (Louvain: Bibliothèque de l'Université, 1947), 210–12.

topoi.[67] But the fact that authors adapted biblical and hagiographic topoi to represent lived experiences of a saint does not render them into fictions of hagiographic craft. In the case of the thirteenth-century *liégeois* corpus, those tropes reveal how hagiographic craft intersected with new modes of acquisition of health resources. They suggest that communities began to commemorate and express gratitude for the religious women in their midst who, as we will see in the next chapter, followed an apostolic model of active charity that encouraged them to provide care to the infirm by working in hospitals, leprosaria, monastic infirmaries, and in informal settings such as homes and even on city streets.[68] Hagiographers in the thirteenth-century lowlands devised their stories to encourage trust in religious women's efforts and abilities, to advertise their therapeutic treatments, and perhaps also to defend them from potential detractors. But we are not quite there yet. For now, let us turn to those first testimonies, to the tales of therapeutic power uttered after the death of saintly mulieres.

The Tomb as Site of Healing

The posthumous miracle stories position the saint's tomb as a site of expectation for her supplicants. This shared understanding of the tomb as a site of therapeutic assistance is reflected in deliberations after the death of Lutgard of Aywières in 1246. When the saint's dead body was laid on the bier for her funeral service, some question arose about the location of her planned burial.[69] The appointed visitor of Aywières, the abbot of Aulne, was present during these discussions and ordered that Lutgard should be

---

67. Thirteenth-century Italy venerated its living saints who worked in hospitals and other care-giving institutions differently. Margaret of Cortona (d. 1297), Angela of Foligno (d. 1309), Aldobran-desca (d. 1309), and Ubaldesca (d. 1206) all worked in hospitals and received textual hagiographies. But so did Franciscan men who dedicated their lives to hospital work. These men include Raimondo Palmerio of Piacenza (d. 1200), Omobono of Cremona (d. 1197), Gerard Tintori of Monzo (d. 1207), and Walter of Lodi (d. 1224). A thorough study of gender and bodywork in this corpus is needed to offer any solid conclusions. See André Vauchez, *Sainthood in the Later Middle Ages* (Cambridge: Cambridge University Press, 1997), 200–201.

68. Ronald Finucane also sought to explain why pilgrims would seek saints as what he called an "alternate" form of cure, assuming a hierarchy of resort in which shrines and relics were secondary to "doctors or medicines." He called attention to "the expectation of miracles" or the "psychogenic" mode of healing. In this mode, according to Finucane, "the force which caused healing at shrines or through vows to saints was expectant faith." See Ronald Finucane, *Miracles and Pilgrims: Popular Beliefs in Medieval England* (New York: St. Martin's, 1977), 79–81.

69. The *Lives* of Lutgard and Ida of Nivelles provide exacting detail about the nuns' mortuary practices. They washed the body, recited the *Commendatio animae*, ushered her body to the church, then laid the body on the bier where they recited psalms in wake all night. In the morning, they celebrated Mass and conducted the body to burial.

interred in the church so that "she can be worthily visited by everyone."[70] During her life, Thomas recalled, Lutgard had predicted that her tomb would be accessible, that a community would grow around it. Harkening back to a conversation between Lutgard and her sisters when she was alive, Thomas remembered that the sisters queried her on how to prepare for her death, fearing that they would not survive in the absence of her prayers. Lutgard responded by instructing them to go to her tomb where she would be "present to [them] in death as I was in life."[71] This story primes readers and listeners that, indeed, the living Lutgard had promised a continued access to her presence after death; it assured them that they would discover aid at her tomb. Thomas further instructed his audience on how to find her at the tomb; he asserted that "anyone who invoked her *with faith in their heart*" could access her grace of healing.[72] While this insistence on the saint's accessibility after death is a familiar trope, it is one worth investigating further when it is deployed by a hagiographer with the theological savvy of Thomas. In fact, as we will see, the interplay of skepticism and confidence in the therapeutic power of the saintly mulieres is a critical feature of the stories of posthumous cure.

For instance, the cultivation of faith at the tomb appears repeatedly in plotlines that unfold around the burial site of Ida of Nivelles. Before Ida's body was entombed, a young girl who attended the funeral reported experiencing a painful toothache. Her participation in Ida's burial ceremony aroused in the girl a sense of "firm hope" (*spem habens firmam*) for recovering her wholeness.[73] Beaming with confidence and a steady grip, she snatched a tooth from Ida and applied it to her aching cheek. Thereupon, the girl instantly experienced relief. In this brief account of remedy, the hagiographer, Goswin of Bossut, introduced an important component of Ida's healing miracles, one that he repeated throughout the miracle stories. He emphasized the role of hope in the saint's salutary presence beyond the grave. His stories featured the presence of the saint, in relics or at her tomb, as the mechanism through

70. *VLA* III.20, 261; trans., 292: "ubi digne possit ab omnibus frequentari."

71. On this accessibility of the saint in life and death, see also Natalie Zemon Davis, "Hosts, Kin, and Progeny: Some Features of Family Life in Early Modern France," in *The Family*, ed. Alice Rossi, Jerome Kagan, and Tamara Hareven (New York: Norton, 1978), 87–114; and Peter Brown, *The Cult of Saints: Its Rise and Function in Latin Christianity* (Chicago: University of Chicago Press, 1981), esp. 1–20. *VLA* III.20, 262; trans., 293: "ad tumulum, inquit, meum confugite; ibi vobis adero mortua sicut vivens."

72. *VLA* III.20, 262; trans., 293: "fido corde eius adjutorium" (emphasis added).

73. Brussels, KBR, MS 8895–96, fol. 33r: "intolerabili dolore dentium." It should be noted that Henriquez's edited version of the *Life* of Ida of Nivelles omits certain passages, particularly in the posthumous miracles. This phrase, for example, is not included.

which the sick petitioner triggered a transition in her passions, generating affects that were conducive to the therapeutic process.

Another nun of La Ramée underwent this very process at Ida's tomb. This unnamed sister had suddenly become deaf. Seeking assistance, she made a petition to Ida, vowing to deliver a wax votive ear on the condition that Ida intercede on her behalf. The nun's vow to the saint was an uttered performance, an externalization of her hope.[74] By voicing the vow, the nun entered an imagined space, a space of possibility wherein she welcomed remedy from an outside authority, God via the saint. Goswin notes that the nun's request, *with its promise*, proved effective.[75] The nun's faculty of hearing was restored, at which point the nun was compelled to uphold her end of the promise—to present Ida with a votive ear at her tomb. The nun's sisters at La Ramée, however, found this offering laughable, perhaps because they could not themselves imagine that Ida was the agent of the nun's cure. They mocked the nun's intent to offer wax at Ida's tomb (*plurimum exhilarata iocosa*). Their laughter signifies that Ida's tomb was not yet considered a site of therapeutic significance by everyone at La Ramée. But the nun persevered in her own conviction, visiting the priest to gain approval for making pilgrimage to the tomb.[76] That Goswin included these mocking sisters in this story indicates the influence of the social setting in these hagiographic depictions of healing. Her sisters' doubtful scorn was *part* of the miracle story. Not only did the nun triumph in her hope and intention despite their disdain, but the mocking nuns became witnesses to the miracle and could then convey the story. They became a mechanism for augmenting knowledge of Ida's healing powers.

Once she arrived at the tomb, the nun rendered thanks and delivered the votive. The votive produced a physical sign of Ida's power, authenticating her capacity to intercede on the condition that she proffer her own physical proof by restoring the nun's faculty of hearing.[77] The votive was a material sign of Ida's success in attaining cures, a physical presence that remained at Ida's tomb even when no healing community was present to share knowledge of her therapeutic power. It performed the work of testimony, drawing

---

74. Gabor Klaniczy, "The Power of Words in Miracles, Visions, Incantations, and Bewitchments," in *The Power of Words: Studies of Charms and Charming*, ed. James Kapaló, Éva Pócs, and William Ryan (Budapest: Central European Press, 2013), 281–304.

75. *VIN* XXXV: "Quam petitionem atque promissionem."

76. The wax votive operated within a micropolitical relationship of gift exchange. Marcell Maus, *The Gift: The Form and Reason for Exchange in Archaic Societies*, trans. W. D. Halls (New York: Norton, 1990); Simon Yarrow, "Twelfth-Century Miracle Narratives," in Mesley and Wilson, *Contextualizing Medieval Miracles*, 60.

77. Bull, *The Miracles of Our Lady of Rocamadour*, 37–38.

others into conviction in Ida's authority.[78] At the tombs of saints, the votive was mobilized as a material sign of an oath, a manifestation of the trust contracted between patient and practitioner bound together in a therapeutic relationship.

Such an external sign features prominently in another miracle that Goswin relayed, one that also centered the petitioner's doubt and derision. In this story, a different nun from La Ramée was ailing with catarrh and headache during Rogation Days, a time that was important to the nun because she wished to sing for the feast of the Ascension. Despite her desire to have a clear throat for rogations, the nun issued her petition to Ida in a flippant and disbelieving manner. "Joking and laughing," she promised Ida that if she would convince God to cure her by the next day, she would deliver a votive nose of wax to her tomb.[79] Goswin may have included a description of the nun's demeanor as chuckling because it was precisely her mockery that was altered in this encounter. The nun harbored doubt about Ida's therapeutic power. When Ida delivered health (*sanitatem*) to the nun at the exact moment she specified, the nun was affectively transformed. She converted to belief, and she made no delay in visiting the tomb to deliver the promised votive.[80] Once again, the votive remained at the tomb as proof of Ida's power, an externalization of her ability to heal.[81] It was a physical verification upon which others could muster greater hope.

Goswin's miracle stories demonstrate a gradually swelling network of believers in Ida's capacity to heal, a community developing as stories of her tomb-side interventions were transmitted orally. Goswin conveyed the predilection for doubt that many people likely entertained before they assented to a saint's healing powers, particularly those of a local and unofficial saint

---

78. In this sense, the votive is similar to what Stacey Langwick has called "alternative materialities." This phrase builds on Bruno Latour's observation that aspects of the world that are not visible become material and visible through the process of scientific experimentation. Langwick extends this observation beyond the realm of Western science to show that therapeutic relationships lead to the materialization of maladies and bodily threats, to new articulations of affliction. In the example of votives, the alternative reality that is made visible is the ingredient of trust necessary to the therapeutic relationship. See Stacey Langwick, *Bodies, Politics, and African Healing: A Matter of Maladies in Tanzania* (Bloomington: Indiana University Press, 2011), 151–65; and Bruno Latour, *Science in Action: How to Follow Scientists and Engineers through Society* (Cambridge, MA: Harvard University Press, 1988).

79. Brussels, KBR, MS 8895–96, fol. 34v: "Jocando atque ridendo." This phrase is omitted from Henriquez's edition.

80. For more on the cultural function of the votive, particularly outside of the Christian context, see the essays in Ittai Weinryb, ed., *Ex Voto: Votive Giving across Cultures* (New York: Bard Graduate Center, 2015).

81. Yarrow, "Miracle Narratives," 43.

like Ida. All of these stories occurred at La Ramée; they involved nuns from her abbey, and took place shortly after her death. The miracles thus showcase people who would have known Ida during her life, those most inclined to trust her. And yet Goswin presents their doubt as a central feature of her healing miracles. Even among her most intimate associates, her spiritual sisters, doubt of Ida's therapeutic power appeared to be a roadblock. His miracle stories portray an arc, a gradual coming into confidence in Ida's tomb as a source of recovery. For example, a third nun with fever approached Ida's tomb with complete incredulousness and an utter lack of hope for regaining health.[82] She nevertheless made petition at Ida's tomb, perhaps going through motions recommended by those who had already found success. Alternatively, she may have noted the votives at Ida's tomb and decided to take a chance for herself on the therapeutic exchange they signified. Goswin stated that this nun made a request for recuperation of her health (*sanitate recuperanda*), but "doubt was in her as she said it: distrust about Ida's intercession, distrust about her own cure."[83] Again, Goswin here emphasizes the nun's doubtful interior constitution. He staged her disbelief as an opportunity to instruct his readers and hearers on how properly to approach the saint. Chastising the nun for her "ambivalence" and "distrust," Goswin offered a lesson to petitioners on how to approach the saint for remedy.[84] Rather than doubting, and thus filling the self with despair or scorn, he asserted, petitioners should greet Ida with confidence, stating instead, "I hope by your mediating suffrage to be restored to health."[85] This authorial interjection allows Goswin to train readers and auditors. For him, Ida's miracle stories should dispel their doubt and encourage confidence in her therapeutic power.

Thomas of Cantimpré also played on the need for confidence in his subject as a source of therapeutic power and instructed readers to cultivate it when advancing to her tomb. He recounted in the *Life of Margaret of Ypres* that her confessor, Friar Zeger, often spent time sitting near Margaret's grave. While there, a woman once queried him about how she might cure her arm. Thomas indicates that this exchange "was the custom in such matters"—a comment that foregrounds the role of the saint's confessor as a critical catalyst of the healing community and suggests that visits to grave sites were

---

82. *VIN* XXXV: "nullam omnino spem habens de sanitate recuperanda propter incredulitatem suam."

83. *VIN* XXXV: "Haec autem dubitans dicebat, dissidens de intercessione virginis et curatione sua."

84. These words are omitted from Henriquez. In MS 8895–96, fol. 34v they are "incredulitatem" and "verbii ambiguita"

85. In MS 8895–96, fol 35r: "spero vestro suffragio mediante in sanitatem restitui."

an ordinary means of seeking healing intervention.[86] Zeger informed the woman, whose arm was swollen from the shoulder to the hand, that she should visit Margaret's grave, ordering her to deliver a cure. Zeger assured the woman that Margaret would obey this command, as it originated with him, who held authority over her when she lived; Margaret would obey him in death as she had in life. The woman followed Zeger's instructions and received a successful outcome, a restored arm, in the presence of many witnesses.[87] This occasion served as an opportunity for Thomas to praise the power of clerics over their saintly protégés, even extending their authority beyond the term limits of life just as Zeger had done in the graveyard and Thomas had done with his textual authority. But the story also reveals a typical pattern of health-related behavior in which the sick and afflicted searched for therapeutic options among gravesites.[88] An individual with knowledge of a certain resource then convinced her that, with confidence, the tomb of Margaret would yield results.

The miracles included in the *Life* of Lutgard mirror these tomb scenes in which petitioners undergo internal affective transformation as they negotiate a remedy. For example, a nun named Oda appeared at Lutgard's tomb complaining of a dire headache that she had endured for some time. Thomas included the important detail that Oda had famously avoided Lutgard's tomb because she loathed the scent of lilies, which emanated from the site.[89] That the tomb was covered with fresh, fragrant lilies over the long course of Oda's illness indicates that it had become a gathering site for sick petitioners and that Oda was aware of the community that assembled there in search of cure. She knew, after all, to avoid the lilies. Moreover, Thomas remarked that Oda was his own blood relative. Given Thomas's special affection for Lutgard—as the proud possessor of a bone from her little finger—he must have encouraged Oda to visit the tomb for relief.

Oda's awareness of Lutgard's therapeutic power, communicated to her by Thomas and others in her community, eventually convinced her to visit the tomb. At first, Oda only very timidly peeked her head in the direction of the

86. *Vita Margarite de Ypris* (*BHL* 5319), in Gilles G. Meersseman, "Frères prêcheurs et movement dévot en Flandre au XIIIe siècle," *Archivum Fratrum Praedicatorum* 18 (1948): 106–30; hereafter *VMY*; *Life of Margaret of Ypres*, trans. Margot King and Barbara Newman, in Newman, *Thomas of Cantimpré*, 163–208. *VMY* 128–29; trans., 204: "Ut fieri solet in talibus consilium expostulans."

87. *VMY* 129.

88. On their relationship, see John Coakley, *Women, Men, and Spiritual Power: Female Saints and Their Male Collaborators* (New York: Columbia University Press, 2006), 222; and Dyan Elliott, *Proving Woman: Female Spirituality and Inquisitional Culture in the Later Middle Ages* (Princeton: Princeton University Press, 2004), 54–55.

89. *VLA* III.26.

tomb, testing the site. In the presence of Lutgard's lilies, Oda experienced none of the ordinary resulting repugnance. She therefore stepped in further, closer to the saint's corpse; still no maladroit reaction. Having now gained confidence in Lutgard's salutary presence, in which Oda was relieved of her typical aversion, Oda then approached the tomb, and "feeling absolutely no pain in her head," she became increasingly convinced of Lutgard's powers.[90] Oda then returned to the tomb to seek assistance, at which point, while prostrate, she fell upon a candelabrum and stabbed herself in the eye, experiencing a sensation as if the eyeball had ripped directly out of its socket![91] Thereupon, she cursed Lutgard, flummoxed by the fact that she had "left with affliction where [she] looked for remedy."[92] Her injury diminished her willingness to believe. In this way, Thomas reported the tale as one in which Oda experienced her pain as linked to her own disbelief and wavering certainty. Her suffering was only relieved after the frustration subsided, when she was "fully restored to health and retained absolutely no weakness or pain."[93]

Oda's cure represents a story of doubt removed. At the site of Lutgard's tomb, Oda and other petitioners entered a relationship with the saint and with her community of believers. Oda was a reluctant part of that community, refusing to approach the lily-laden tomb and thus hesitant to assent to Lutgard's power over her own body. Her experiences of pain and relief were directly linked to her participation in a community of belief, the healing community surrounding Lutgard. Oda's story suggests something of the emotional and psychological dimensions of healing that played out among saints and their petitioners. Lutgard's tomb was rendered as a site for potential transformation. It possessed an abundance of significance for her healing community. Flowers, votives, and the sharing of healing miracles coded it as a site that could be accessed for remedy. These material remnants worked in tandem with healing stories. Both worked to encourage trust. The healing community coached sick petitioners in the appropriate confidence with which they should arrive at the saint's tomb. In this sense, hearing stories of miracle cures was part of the therapeutic process. These stories educated petitioners in the saint's therapeutic power, directed them to the site of her tomb, and encouraged them to place confidence in her.

---

90. *VLA* II.26, 262; trans., 295: "nullum penitus capitis dolorem sensit."

91. *VLA* II.26, 262.

92. *VLA* II.26, 262; trans., 295: "inde molestiam retuli, unde remedium praestolabar."

93. *VLA* II.26, 262; trans., 295: "plenissime restituta sanitati, nihil languoris pertulit vel doloris."

Tales of incubation reported at the tombs of the *liégeois* saints participated in this dynamic of encouraging salubrious passions.[94] The *Life* of Ida of Nivelles includes the healing story of a young man affiliated with La Ramée who had been sick with a fever.[95] The liturgical time is noted as vespers, when the young man was pained with fever and had not eaten. In this condition, he turned his thoughts to Ida and "the many sick people who came to Ida's tomb and were healed of their infirmities."[96] This statement suggests that several stories of her healing powers were circulating in the area. As a familiar of the community, the man was aware of numerous sick people (*multi infirmi*) visiting Ida's tomb. Such evidence worked on his imagination, endowing him with hope in this time of need. He decided to visit Ida's tomb, barefoot, to pray for relief. Sleeping next to the tomb, he awoke fully restored to health (*sanatum se omnino reperiens*). Goswin reports this healing event in terms of the man's altered passions. He returned fully cured to the guesthouse where he served, experiencing delight (*gaudio*) where there had been dolor.[97]

Stories of incubation express the continuous temporality maintained between the living and the dead, in which actions in life trigger effects after death.[98] For example, when a plague afflicted the monastery of Aywières, one of the nuns experienced a dream vision in which a crowd attacked the monastery church. Thomas's sentence construction places the violent crowd in direct parallel to a "fatal plague" (*pestis morientium*). Long suffering, one of the nuns "saw in a vision that a crowd was insolently attacking the monastery

---

94. Domenico Mallardo, "L'incubazione nella cristianità medieval napoletana," *Analecta Bollandiana* 67 (1949): 465–98; Natalio Fernández Marcos, *Los Thaumata de Sofronio: Contribución al estudio de la incubatio Cristiana* (Madrid: Instituto Antonio de Nebrija, 1975); Gabor Klaniczay, "Dreams and Visions in Medieval Miracle Accounts," in *Ritual Healing: Magic, Ritual, and Medical Therapy from Antiquity to the Early Modern Period*, ed. Ildikó Csperegi and Charles Burnett (Florence: SISMEL, 2012), 147–70.

95. This person's status is ambiguous. Goswin clearly marks lay brothers, so he is probably not a lay brother. But Goswin does attach him to the abbey: "Iuvenis quidam in eodem monasterio."

96. *VIN* XXXV; trans., 97: "coepit cogitare quod multi infirmi ad sepulchrum beatae Idae venientes ab infirmitatibus suis sanabantur."

97. *VIN* XXXV; trans., 97: "sanatum se omnino reperiens, ad domum hospitum ubi minister fuerat deputatus, doloris expers, cum gaudio recurrit."

98. On alternative temporalities, see Shahzad Bashir, "On Islamic Time: Rethinking Chronology in the Historiography of Muslim Societies," *History & Theory* 53.4 (2014): 519–44. On this particular cure, note that, rather than a tale of incubation, it might also be understood as a dream cure. The *Life* of Juliana reports a similar "dream cure" in which a woman who was a true devotee of Juliana while she lived had become very ill. She dreamed of Juliana standing beside her and instructing her to prepare to receive grace. Just as Juliana had predicted, the woman fell into an ecstasy of grace at Mass the next morning, and when she returned to her senses she was overflowing with grace, and her weakness had been banished. *VJM* II.ix.54.

church."[99] The plague was therefore experienced as a physical assault on the solemnity of their space. To meet this assault, the nun, while still in visionary mode, perceived Lutgard "[rising] from her tomb and [driving] them all from the church with the greatest violence."[100] Thomas then explained that the vision "took effect." Her vision was realized in that the contagious plague subsided.[101]

In this communal healing story, the nun's imagination conjured Lutgard's presence. Lutgard's power was understood to cure even epidemics, not just singular afflictions.[102] The narrative provides insight into patient experience during times of widespread illness. Whatever was infecting the monastery, it was experienced as a violent plague. Moreover, Thomas indicates that the presence of the plague was not random and that the nuns knew its exact cause. Lutgard herself had foretold its occurrence when she chastised her sisters for their lack of attention in performing the canonical hours. Note that it was the sisters in the *infirmary* that Lutgard singled out for their lack of liturgical fastidiousness, a reflection of Lutgard's presence in the communal infirmary and her management of communal prayer for the health of its inhabitants.[103] When nuns began dying suddenly, they knew the cause and reacted swiftly. The locutions that Thomas used to describe the plague connote vengeance, punishment, and disorder. He refers to it as "a grievous plague that raged in the convent," "aveng[ing]" this defect in the sisters."[104] Spreading among the nuns in the infirmary, it affected an already weakened population. Fourteen nuns died "in a short time," and two of them "at the *same* instant."[105] This rapid mortality posed the problem of an efficient means to bury the dead. Thomas reports that he had to travel to Aywières to assist with Masses for the dead and the digging

---

99. *VLA* III.iii.22, 262; trans., 294: "in visione vidit quod multi ecclesiam monasterii insolenter irruerent."

100. *VLA* III.iii.22, 262; trans., 294: "vidit quod pia Lutgardis surrexit de tumulo, et omnes cum maxima violentia ab ecclesia propulsaret."

101. *VLA* III.iii.22; trans., 294: "Nec mora effectum suum visio."

102. On saints as practitioners in the fight against epidemics, see Peregrine Horden, "Disease, Dragons, and Saints: The Management of Epidemics in the Dark Ages," in *Epidemics and Ideas: Essays on the Historical Perception of Pestilence*, ed. T. Ranger and P. Slack (Cambridge: Cambridge University Press, 1992), 45–76.

103. More on her infirmary wanderings in the following chapter. *VLA* III.14, 259: "Frequenter sorores in infirmaria Moniales redarguerat eo quod minus bene et minus attente Canonicas Horas Deo solverent divinitus constitutas."

104. *VLA* III.14, 259; trans., 286: "defectum istum in sororibus manus Domini vindicabit . . . pestilentia gravis in conventu Monialium mox grassatur."

105. *VLA* III.14, 259; trans., 286: "infra brevissimi temporis spatium;" "duas spiritu carneque sorores uno spatii momento migrantes" (emphasis added).

of graves, and he insisted on the burial of a few bodies together in a single grave. Throughout the plague's brief course at Aywières, its cause was certain, rooted in Lutgard's demand for an alteration of behavior. Therefore, the appropriate remedy was applied: "When the sick nuns in the infirmary had thoroughly corrected themselves by saying the Hours punctiliously, the Lord mercifully withdrew his hand, just as Lutgard had predicted, and the plague soon ceased."[106] This curt episode provides insight into the blended mode of conceptualizing premodern epidemics, one that identified and responded to contagious disease through liturgical celebration, traditional infirmary care, burial practices, altered devotional behaviors, and participation in the cult of saints. This multiplicity suggests that thirteenth-century conceptions of health were also, at their center, fundamentally multiple, including material and immaterial sources of therapeutic power, as well as individual behavior and communal responsibility.

Miracle tales in the corpus also provide a sense of the extent of the healing community, the distance to which people would travel to visit the tomb of a saint, and the depths of their stories of miraculous healing. Returning to the lay brother from Herkenrode who was cured of a hernia, note that he journeyed to Villers to pray at Juliana's tomb. Once he arrived there, he felt "completely free of his former pain, so that he could walk and ride ably and go about the business of his house."[107] The distance the lay brother traveled indicates that Juliana's tomb was well known as a source of remedy, that knowledge about her therapeutic power had spread throughout Liège.[108] A single posthumous miracle recorded in the *Life* of Christina Mirabilis also raises questions about the span of geographic mobility in accessing a saint's tomb as a healthcare resource. This cure was not recorded by Thomas himself, but rather comprises an anonymous addition to the *Life*, appended after the second exhumation and translation of Christina's corpse. The miracle reports that, in 1249, after a divine revelation urged a monastic priest and his affiliated community to exhume Christina's bones and place them next to the altar, "immediately" a very sick woman living near the monastery (*in vicino monasterii*) undertook to visit her there. She had heard

---

106. *VLA* III.14, 259; trans., 286: "Nec mora post haec, cum se debiles in infirmaria, in dicendis solicite Horis, plenissime correxissent; manum suam, secundum quod pia Lutgardis praedixerat, Domino misericorditer revocante, pestilentia mox cessavit."

107. *VJM* II.9, 477; trans., 297: "se sensit ab angustia pristina quasi totaliter liberatum; ita ut pedes ire posset, et equitare competenter, et domus suae negotia procurare."

108. As it was a Cistercian women's community, it makes sense that stories of Juliana's healing, particularly those that took place at her Villers tomb, would be shared there. As I show below, however, her healing community certainly extended beyond Cistercians.

stories of Christina's powers and, "excited by the fame of these occurrences and trusting more firmly in them," she asked her husband to transport her to the monastery where she was buried.[109] At Christina's grave, the woman stood up with her limbs unharmed (*membris omnibus sospitata surrexit*). Because this is the only specific healing miracle recorded in Christina's *Life*, the woman's immediate impulse to seek cure from her suggests the possibility that other stories were circulating orally. Although Thomas asserted that Christina possessed the grace of healing and bestowed it upon those who visited her tomb, he made the choice not to record any of these reports as healing miracles, stating that he could not "pursue these matters." At the time Thomas wrote her *Life* (mostly in 1232, completed after 1239), he appears to have sought to stifle the development of a healing community. Thomas thus made a choice not to transmit stories of her posthumous therapeutic power in text.

Whether or not the healing miracles were recorded, it appears that, as members of the saintly mulieres' immediate surroundings began to accept them as legitimate sources of therapeutic power and promulgated their *fama* as such, gradually individuals living at a distance from their tombs began to learn of their powers. Goswin provides another example of this long-distance sharing of healing stories when he reports on a woman and her fevered young daughter. The mother had traveled to several churches to beg for suffrages from the saints, but she had found no cure and concluded that there simply was no hope for her daughter.[110] During her fruitless wonderings, however, she was told by some folks (*quibusdam*) that Ida's tomb was a worthy resource. When the child was cured by Ida's intercession, the mother expressed her gratitude and returned to "her own home."[111] Goswin noted how the woman shared the story of her child's illness at various shrines and tombs, searching for a cure. She happened, felicitously, upon some folks who had knowledge of Ida's therapeutic power, who encouraged her to travel to her tomb and invest faith in the saint. This story of the mother learning about Ida through other reports of her power accentuates the role of community in the procurement of saints' cures. The healing story itself was part of the healing process, a preparation for the petitioner to begin to trust, a resource for determining the best local options for care.

---

109. *VCM* 59, 660; trans., 156: "Fama ergo tantae rei confidentius excitata, orat virum suum, ut ad monasterium deferatur."

110. Henriquez neglects to include much of the mother's search. See MS 8895–96, fol. 35 for the complete tale.

111. *VIN* XXXV: "ad propria remeavit."

This story also casts additional light on the familiar hagiographic trope that opposed physicians' cures to those of saints. In stories featuring this trope, the sick person has already exhausted the remedies offered by physicians, only to find cure at the hands of a saint. In Ida's cure of the young child, Goswin stressed that other *saints* were ineffectual. While stories of the failures of other saints also represent a trope, its appearance here serves a specific purpose for Goswin. The healing miracles that he attributes to Ida hinge on a kind of faith in cure that only she can provide; they rely on convincing the sick, through the process of story itself, to place their faith in her as a viable source of cure. We cannot know the exact identity of the unnamed group of people who informed the desperate mother of Ida's power, but we can imagine how their knowledge circulated through stories of healing success. Other saints might fail to cure just as physicians often fell short of desired outcomes; multiple resources were necessary. This comparative appears again in Ida's miracles when Goswin explains, "The work that could not be done by healers of the body was brought to completion by the supreme healer, Christ, thanks to the merits of his handmaid Ida."[112] This comment does not portray saints' cures at odds or in competition with that of physicians and other healers. Instead, it reflects what Julie Orlemanski has called "variegated and overlapping therapeutic competencies" that developed highly local hierarchies of expertise.[113] The stories of therapeutic success generated at the tombs of saints demonstrate how the healing community worked as an agent in guiding patients to specific healthcare resources, the material remains of saintly mulieres religiosae.

The Relic as a Healing Technology

As a stationary locus of healing, the saint's tomb was powerful because of the visibility of the saint in effigy or a stone marker, and in votives, the memorials of her success. But the distribution of relics mobilized the saint's therapeutic power. It is through the distribution of relics that we can see an expanding conviction in the saintly mulieres as legitimate sources of care. As a therapeutic technology, saints' relics operated in part through the healing stories that circulated with them, that attached to them and attracted new petitioners. The *Life* of Juliana, for example, tells of several cloth relics that

---

112. *VIN* XXXV; trans., 98: "Sicut factum est, ut quod per medicos corporum fieri non potuit, per summum medicum Christum meritis."

113. Julie Orlemanski, *Symptomatic Subjects: Bodies, Medicine, and Causation in the Literature of Late Medieval England* (Philadelphia: Pennsylvania University Press, 2019), 54.

were in possession of a female "religious person" (*religiosam personam*).[114] In the story, two beguines with severe toothache sought this religious woman for aid. When they arrived, the woman wielded the handkerchief and other linens belonging to Juliana, touching these items to the cheeks and faces of the beguines, actions that produced salutary results. This story positions the "religious person" as a healer, a specialist in manipulating relics for the purpose of health. That the possessor of relics was named as a female "religious person" rather than as a specific medical practitioner suggests that her placement in a religious house superseded her identification as a caregiver; or alternatively, that her identification as a female "religious person" encompassed her identification as a healer. But the story leaves no doubt that people outside of this woman's immediate religious community recognized her and pursued her for therapeutic ends. They sought her because Juliana's relics were already recognized as salutary implements. While we do not know how the two beguines learned of this healthcare option, it is clear that stories were spreading that transmitted knowledge about Juliana as an effective source of treatment.

Another miracle performed through Juliana's relics underscores this category of practitioner who was skilled in relic-induced healing. The miracle tale only indicates that a mother wrapped her sick baby in a piece of cloth that she had been given for the purpose of curing it.[115] Again, this story confirms that contact relics from Juliana were circulating for unequivocally therapeutic purposes, and that a healing community in the region had knowledge of whom to seek to access their power. A similar comment about Marie indicates that "when women in labor are wrapped in her clothing, they are freed from the danger of death."[116] Like the "religious woman" who had charge of Juliana's linens, these unnamed healthcare practitioners in possession of Marie's clothing did not earn occupational titles associated with academic medicine; nevertheless, in these narrative sources, they appear as valued caregivers and repositories of healthcare knowledge.[117]

---

114. *VJM* II.ix.53. The name of the monastery or church where she was located is not given.

115. *VJM* II.ix.53, 476.

116. This comment appears in "The History of the Foundation of the Venerable Church of Blessed Nicholas of Oignies and the Handmaid of Christ Mary of Oignies," trans. Hugh Feiss, in *Mary of Oignies: Mother of Salvation*, ed. Anneke Mulder-Bakker (Turnhout: Brepols, 2006), 172.

117. Noting that practitioners skilled in the use of relics for the purpose of healing were not captured by official medical monikers, Nicole Archambeau has proposed the term "miracle mediators" to signal people who had knowledge of how to procure, protect, and apply relics for therapeutic purposes. Nicole Archambeau, "Miracle Mediators as Healing Practitioners: The Knowledge and Practice of Healing with Relics," *Social History of Medicine* 31.2 (2017): 209–30.

Despite their lack of visibility in traditional medical sources, it is clear that healing communities placed tremendous value on the material remnants of the mulieres religiosae of this region. For example, Thomas of Cantimpré testifies that the nuns of Aywières clamored over Lutgard's belongings, including belts, robes, and veils, which they then used to achieve various cures. The case of Beatrice de Raive is illustrative here. Beatrice was a noble nun who had endowed the monastery of Aywières. She suffered from an ulcer on her neck, which physicians diagnosed as a carbuncle. That Beatrice sought assistance from Lutgard's relics after her diagnosis suggests that she sought various options for relief, from physicians and saints. When Beatrice placed Lutgard's veil on her neck, the swelling subsided immediately.[118] In this case, Thomas did not single out an individual as the guardian or practitioner of relics, but it is clear that the nuns oversaw a whole cache of them, which they used for therapeutic purposes. Thomas unabashedly rendered this cure into a marketing opportunity, advertising the therapeutic treasures to be unleashed at Aywières. Commenting on Lutgard's cure of Beatrice, he gushes, "O gracious Lutgard, you acted altogether justly and worthily, so that she whose temporal goods you received in this life might reap your spiritual ones after you died."[119] Thomas's construction indicates the framework for a therapeutic economy. Beatrice's endowment of Aywières merited her Lutgard's posthumous intercession; patrons might expect salutary cure in return for their donations.

Aywières must have been a site known for its varied supply of relics on hand for therapeutic purposes. Sick travelers and patrons appear to have sought out the community for their collection of relics. For example, a monk of Valdieu, a Cistercian abbey about fifty-five kilometers to the east of La Ramée, once swallowed a perch bone, which became lodged in his throat rather painfully. Not knowing how to treat this condition, the monk stopped at Aywières, where a sister counseled him that a white veil belonging to Ida of Nivelles might assist him.[120] The nuns of Aywières were thus in command of relics other than those belonging to Lutgard, and they associated each of these relics with specific treatments. They made a therapeutic choice in directing the monk to Ida's veil.[121] In other circumstances, Lutgard's

---

118. *VLA* III.xxiii, 262; trans., 294: "anthracem, quem carbunculum physici dicunt . . . et perniciose turgens inflatio visibiliter mox aufugit."

119. *VLA* III.xxiii, 262; trans., 294: "O pia Lutgardis, et digne per omnia hoc fecisti, ut tua post mortem spiritualia meteret, cuius in hac vita temporalia suscepisti."

120. *VIN* XXXV.

121. This story probably occurred shortly after Ida's death in 1231. Because Lutgard did not die until 1246, the nuns did not have the option to use Lutgard's relics. But the story illustrates the logic

relics were chosen. For example, Dom Alard, while serving as chaplain at Aywières, used Lutgard's relics to treat his swollen thumb, binding them to the impaired appendage.[122] And the subprioress of Aywières, Oda, bound her arm to Lutgard's relics when she suffered from a swollen arm.[123]

Just like Ida's relics, Lutgard's circulated outside the monastery of Aywières, where they attracted numerous laypeople. That the nuns of Aywières designated specific relics for the treatment of specific afflictions is evident in the example of a noble matron who, when experiencing a difficult labor, made use of a horsehair belt that Lutgard had worn to lacerate her body. When Lutgard's belt was placed on the matron's womb, she finally delivered safely and painlessly. Thomas asserts that this same treatment had been proven as efficacious in relieving a difficult labor "in diverse places and by diverse persons."[124] With this comment, Thomas implies that Lutgard's belt was by this point widely recognized beyond her immediate community as an effective resource in facilitating childbirth.

Thomas's interest in relaying the efficacy of Lutgard's belt for the parturient raises important questions about how this particular relic and its healing story functioned. It is possible that the parturient journeyed to Aywières to access the belt and the childbirth assistance of the nuns. As I will discuss in chapter 5, manuscript evidence suggests the possibility that some Cistercian women's abbeys could serve as ad hoc lying-in hospitals where poor pregnant women found rest and care. During those times, the recitation of Lutgard's healing miracles to the sick or parturient may have served as part of the therapeutic process. Alternatively, a priest associated with Aywières may have carried the belt with him to women in need, just as the priest at Fosses-la-Ville brought Saint Foillan's belt to local women "any time" they suffered in labor and feared for the child's life.[125] Other monastic institutions in the region also served as custodians of relics that worked as therapeutic technologies in childbirth. For example, Marie of Oignies's clothing was said to serve as a method of securing a "happy birth"; at Nivelles, the belt of Saint Gertrude was considered a means of easing pain from childbirth, and at Michelsberg abbey in Bamberg, women in labor sought the belt and mantle

---

of visiting a religious community in search of an effective relic and that the nuns of Aywières had relics on hand for such purposes. It also illustrates the extension of knowledge about Ida as a healer.

122. *VLA* III.xxv.

123. *VLA* III.xxvi.

124. *VLA* III.xxxviii, 262; trans., 296: "Hoc idem in diversis locis, et in diversis personis efficaciter est probatum."

125. Hillinus, *Miraculi sancti Foillani,* in *AASS* Oct. XIII (1883): 420; Robert Bartlett, *Why Can the Dead Do Such Great Things? Saints and Worshippers from the Martyrs to the Reformation* (Princeton: Princeton University Press, 2015), 246.

of Saint Cunigunde.[126] Additionally, Thomas wished to educate priests on how they might instruct midwives, relaying a series of childbirth recipes and obstetric procedures in his *Liber de natura rerum* for this purpose.[127] This evidence points to a collaborative network, a healing community, that mobilized in times of difficult labor to provide appropriate relics, prayers, and sometimes shelter for parturient women. It shows that, outside of the limited reach of professional midwifery and obstetric medicine, parturient care was a situated form of knowledge transmitted through local stories and practices. The ethnographic level of detail offered by Thomas's miracle stories captures the therapeutic uses of relics as well as the motives for relying on them.[128]

These childbirth practices suggest the cooperation of religious women and men in the exercise of relics as a therapeutic technology. Though the gender identity of the person in control of access to Lutgard's belt is unclear from Thomas's assertions about its efficacy, at other times when women's relics circulated they were clearly placed in the hands of figures identified as male. For example, in the posthumous miracles included in the *Life* of Margaret of Ypres, Friar Zeger managed to wrest control over her curative relics. Thomas of Cantimpré recalled that after Margaret died, Friar Zeger acquisitively sought from her mother all of the saint's belongings, including even her shoelaces. When the mother delivered the requested items, Zeger noted that Margaret's headdress was missing from the collection. After her mother explained that she had buried the headdress because of its putrefaction, Zeger commanded that she dig it up and deliver it to him. Behold! When unearthed, the headdress, which was once saturated by the ooze from Margaret's head wound, now gleamed white and emitted a dulcet fragrance. Thomas reported that Countess Marguerite of Flanders wished to possess the headdress, but Zeger jealously guarded it and refused her advances. He added that the headdress was the vehicle that launched numerous miracle

---

126. On these obstetric aids, see Iliana Kandzha, "Female Saints as Agents of Female Healing," in *Gender, Health, and Healing*, ed. Sara Ritchey and Sharon Strocchia (Amsterdam: Amsterdam University Press, 2020), 67–92; and Bonnie Effros, "Symbolic Expressions of Sanctity: Gertrude of Nivelles in the Context of Merovingian Mortuary Custom," *Viator* 27 (1996): 1–10.

127. Monica Green, *Making Women's Medicine Masculine: The Rise of Male Authority in Pre-modern Gynaecology* (Oxford: Oxford University Press, 2008), 139; Thomas of Cantimpré, *Liber de natura rerum* (Berlin: De Gruyter, 1973), I.76. Green notes that Thomas's recipes derive from the abbreviated version of Muscio's *Gynaecology*, the *Non omnes quidem*, which had been in circulation since the eleventh century.

128. These observations on situated medical knowledge and the motivations captured in ethnographic descriptions of health-seekers are inspired by Monica Green, "Gendering the History of Women's Healthcare," *Gender & History* 20.3 (2008): 487–518.

cures.[129] Because Margaret was not cloistered, Zeger may have regarded his clerical position as a strengthened stance from which to protect her relics, lest they be trampled by hordes of petitioners visiting her mother's home. We have already seen how he often spent time at her tomb and occasionally mediated therapeutic access to it. His desire to control Margaret's legacy points to one of the ways that stories of her therapeutic competence and healthcare outreach were inflected by, indeed saturated with, appeals to her spiritual merit. Like all of the saints discussed in this chapter, Margaret was a cleric's spiritual protégé. The significance of her labor, both in life and after death, was determined in part by her relationship to clerical authority, not only that of Zeger, but that of Thomas as well.

While clerics like Friar Zeger and Thomas of Cantimpré certainly sought to direct sick petitioners to the relics and tombs of their saintly subjects, and they therefore recognized and endorsed their therapeutic competence, these men also conveyed stories of their curative success in spiritual, rather than medical, terms. They translated therapeutic events into stories of miracle cure. They situated the locus of therapeutic power in a divine source, one earned through their protagonists' spiritual merit or virginal holiness. It was their spiritual grace that distinguished the therapeutic efficacy of the saintly mulieres, according to hagiographic tradition, from that of material medicine. For example, Goswin of Bossut tells the story of a young boy who was troubled by a fistular ulcer on his eye. His parents had consulted many healers (pluribus medicis), but none were able to alleviate his condition. When the boy and his parents encountered a lay brother from La Ramée who carried with him Ida's tooth, his ulcer began to heal upon contact. Goswin then attributed this cure to "the merits of [Christ's] handmaid, Ida."[130] Goswin ensured his readers that this relic practice was only an effect, through the material vector of the tooth, of a spiritual power. He distinguished Ida's expertise as a power of "completion" that she was able to accomplish because of her spiritual merit. Although Ida was certainly a recognized healer by the time of the promulgation of this story, Goswin did not include her in the broad category of healer signified by the term medici. He clarified that medici were healers of bodies (medicos corporum) who worked on a strictly material plane. To Goswin, Ida was categorically different: a handmaid of Christ, a holy virgin, a saint.

---

129. VMY liv: "sed per eandem mitram sanitates fieri."

130. VIN XXXV: "Meritis ancillae eius." Goswin describes the ulcer's shrinking as a gradual effect: "paulatimque gravis ille morbus coepit annihilari."

As we conclude this chapter, let us return to the question raised at its beginning, Why would well-educated clerics with access to the most recent expositions on natural theology portray religious women in this way, as sources of divine remedy? At the forefront of their stories of posthumous healing is a problem of belief. The posthumous healing miracles of the *liégeois* corpus center skepticism and situate the act of sharing the stories themselves as a therapeutic resource. They seek repetition, pronouncement, and conviction. Two final examples will demonstrate this, as well as transition us to the next chapter, in which we can continue to pursue some answers. First, an autobiographical example proffered in Thomas of Cantimpré's *Life* of Lutgard of Aywières. Thomas recounts that when Lutgard learned of his intention to cut off her hand after her death, she was bewildered. "I cannot imagine what you plan to do with my hand!" she exclaimed, whereupon Thomas quickly informed her that it would be healthful for his soul and his body for him to possess it.[131] Lutgard assured him that her little finger would be more than sufficient for fulfilling this purpose, but Thomas insisted that he required either her whole hand or else her head: "No part of your body could be enough for me, mother, unless I had your hand or head to comfort me when I am bereft of your whole self."[132] After Lutgard had died, two lay brothers plotted to remove her finger and sixteen of her teeth. When Thomas discovered that her little finger had been amputated by such means, he interpreted this news as a prophetic fulfillment. Lutgard had promised him that finger! He quickly journeyed to Aywières to beg Abbess Hadewijch for the relic, but she was not willing to part with it. It was only after Thomas promised to translate Lutgard's life into an official text, her *Life*, that he was able to take possession of his prized relic. For him, Lutgard's little finger was a site of an encounter, the locus through which her grace might affect his body and soul. Her *Life* authorized and legitimized this power and licensed the proliferation of healing miracles that issued from her tomb and relics, a pattern we will have occasion to revisit from the perspective of manuscript transmission in chapter 5.

Thomas told another story that illuminates the therapeutic codependence of hagiographic texts and the relics and tombs at which patients reported receiving salutary treatment. In his supplement to the *Life* of Marie of Oignies, Thomas introduced the cardinal bishop of Ostia, Hugolino of Segni (who would later become Pope Gregory IX), who acquired Marie's book and a relic of her finger. Hugolino had confided in

---

131. *VLA* III.xix, 261; trans., 290: "tu autem quid de manu mea facere cogites multum miror."

132. *VLA* III.xix, 261; trans., 290: "nihil inquam, mihi ex tuo, Mater, corpore sufficere porterit, nisi manum aut caput habeam, quo tunc relever toto orbatus."

Jacques de Vitry that he was extraordinarily burdened by a spirit of blasphemy. The spirit wreaked violence on his soul so that food, drink, and sleep eluded him and drove his body to near destruction. Jacques, being a "prudent and experienced man" (*vir prudens et expertus*), knew that what the cardinal bishop truly required for his remedy was a good *exemplum*, a good story. He thus recounted for Hugolino the memory of his friend Marie of Oignies, who "had obtained a special grace of expelling blasphemous spirits."[133] He insisted that the grace she exhibited in life was accessible after her death, and sent away Hugolino with a copy of her *Life* so that he could read examples of her grace for himself. Jacques's gesture reveals that he understood the very act of reading saintly exemplars as a method of therapy, a means to drive out the afflicting spirit and thus to repair his exhausted body. By reading her *Life*, Hugolino transmitted Marie's grace. Taking the book with him, Hugolino troubled Jacques for one additional favor: Would he loan him Marie's relics to include in his therapeutic routine? The generous Jacques was pleased by this request and conceded that "there is a finger of hers enclosed in a silver case which is constantly hanging from my neck. It has always kept me safe in various dangers and during crises at sea."[134] Though Jacques had apparently kept Marie's relic with him for apotropaic purposes, for Hugolino it worked, in conjunction with her *Life*, as a means of curing his passions. Thomas concludes this episode in the supplement with the extraordinary recovery of Hugolino, who "found wondrous hope and peace for himself [by reading her *Life*] and from the relic that remained with him he derived great mental confidence."[135] The *Life* of Marie operated together with her finger bone to goad affective transformation within the distraught bishop. The coupling of book and bone signaled Marie's presence, access to her salubrious grace.

These two final examples demonstrate that the material locus of the saintly mulier in relics and tomb represented an earthly instantiation of her grace. But they operated, they *worked*, in collaboration with the saint's story, her *Life*, a narrative of her grace. The therapeutic power of the saintly mulieres in the thirteenth-century southern Low Countries depended on stories told about them. Those who wished to control the distribution of their grace

133. *Thomas Cantipratensis Supplementum*, ed. R. B. C. Huygens in *Vita Marie de Oegnies*, ch. 15, 187–88; trans., 154: "a domino obtinuerat gratiam in effugandis blasphemie spiritibus specialem."

134. *Supplement*, ch. 15, 188; trans., 155: "digitus eius, argenteo locello reconditus, assidue michi suspensus ad collum, qui me utique in diversis periculis et inter marina discrimina semper tutavit illesum."

135. *Supplement*, ch. 15, 188; trans., 155: "in ea quidem miram spem et sui quietem inveniens, [et lectionem vitae eius] de reliquo quod restabat fiduciam magnam animo iam exultante concepit."

had to become authorities over their stories, recapitulating them for others, convincing patients of their merit, their virginal holiness.

We have examined in this chapter the miracle stories that form an outermost layer of hagiographic production in the *liégeois* corpus, which re-present community memories of the mulieres religiosae. They reflect, albeit distantly, the stories told by health-seekers in proximity to the saint's religious community. While they first circulated orally, often generated "immediately" after the death of the saint, they are preserved now as formal texts. These healing stories thus present translations, interpretations, re-presentations in the service of regulating cult and the diffusion of saintly graces. Just as Augustine first posited about miracles, these stories produced a "new truth" about certain religious women in the region. They transformed their vestiges—their memorializations, their legacy—into legitimate therapeutic resources within the grasp of clerical control. The "new truth" about these women, however, also affords partial insight into communal negotiations that took place on peripheries of clerical supervision. Read from the perspective of the healing community, the stories of miracle cure disclose the ways that sisters, neighbors, and other proximate individuals remembered certain mulieres religiosae and expressed gratitude for their work.

CHAPTER 2

Bedside Comforts

The Social Organization of Care

In 1218, when Count Louis II of Loon was convalescing on his deathbed, he cried out for assistance to a local holy woman, Christina of St. Trond, with whom he had developed an intimate friendship. Count Louis was said to have called Christina "Mother" because he found such comfort in her presence. He always followed her *consilia* and was deeply affected by the words of her prayer.[1] As he lay dying, the count demanded Christina's maternal presence. When she arrived in his bedchamber, he dismissed his servants and guests and implored Christina to remain with him until death. Louis then mustered what little physical strength he had remaining to prostrate himself at Christina's feet. There, he wept profusely as he divulged to her his sins in a final act of confession before dying.

Throughout the thirteenth- and early fourteenth-century lowlands, we find tales of the presence of mulieres religiosae like Christina bringing comfort and care to bedchambers and infirmaries. In the previous chapter, I explored stories of miracle cure attributed to a select few of those women and observed the formation of healing communities, which make visible otherwise unnamed healthcare practitioners and healthcare resources such as the "religious woman" in possession of Juliana's efficacious linens. I turn

---

1. *VCM* IV.xxxi: "Quam excitantia verba habuit"; *VCM* IV.xix: "oris gratia." Christina's *consilia* is mentioned in IV.xxx and IV.xxxiii; trans., 148–49: "et ejus consiliis ac colloquiis sinceriter inhaerere."

now to the caregiving behaviors attributed to mulieres religiosae during their lives. The focus of analysis transitions, then, from assertions of posthumous therapeutic success shared in stories of miracle cure to efficacious caregiving practices attributed to living religious women.

Despite the attention to hagiographic sources, my interest here is not in saintly heroines. Rather, I am drawn to the many unnamed religious women who likely organized their days according to routines similar to those represented in the *liégeois* corpus; additionally, I am interested in the broader community members, laypeople like the Count of Loon, who interacted with them in times of need and who supported the institutions in which they lived. While the process of rendering certain of the mulieres religiosae into saints translated their caregiving interactions into exemplars of Christian charity and compassion, those interactions with the poor and sick were hardly unique. Hundreds of religious women throughout the region engaged in these behaviors. The caregiving relationships portrayed throughout the *Lives* produce a composite picture of the kinds of therapeutic acts practiced by mulieres religiosae. Although those acts of care are idealized and rendered in hagiographic terms, their translation into hagiographic tropes nevertheless suggests that the caregiving of mulieres religiosae was highly valued. My goal in this chapter is to think through this translation process, to use the hagiographic impressions in order to envision the broad range of caregiving practices undertaken by the many, often anonymous, mulieres religiosae. For this reason, I supplement hagiographic portrayals of caregiving acts with sources from the many caregiving institutions in which mulieres religiosae were often embedded. These institutions include hospitals, leprosaria, and monastic infirmaries where the sick, poor, indigent, and dying found care in its various forms, from feeding and bathing to wound maintenance and healing prayers.

These caregiving interactions took place in an intellectual and social arena far removed from the analytic categories of scholastic textual production.[2] They were not recorded in texts that have been handed down to us in medical genres, nor were their caregiving practices described in the terminology of Latin physica. Read collectively, however, a vivid picture emerges of how beguine and Cistercian women in the southern Low Countries provided healthcare resources to a population undergoing transformation. In Flanders, Hainaut, Brabant, Namur, and Liège, cities comprised roughly 30 percent of the total population, and were becoming more populous throughout

---

2. Pablo Gómez, *The Experiential Caribbean: Creating Knowledge and Healing in the Early Modern Atlantic* (Chapel Hill: University of North Carolina Press, 2017), 11.

the thirteenth and fourteenth centuries as the textile industries expanded
into Brabant and copper wares from the Meuse valley found trading outlets
across western Europe.[3] This demographic transformation brought greater
visibility to the urban poor, a spectacle of vulnerability that theologians and
preachers readily addressed. Early in his pontificate, around 1202 or 1203,
Pope Innocent III issued two treatises on poverty and charity in which he
urged that almsgiving should be motivated by genuine love of Christ in
one's neighbor as a form of "prayer with works, not words."[4] Shortly after
the Fourth Lateran Council confirmed Innocent's reform agenda, Jacques
de Vitry would begin delivering sermons that ridiculed ill-gained material
goods, championed the ennobling effects of almsgiving, and encouraged the
poor to persevere with patience and dignity.[5] It was precisely at this moment
that the region underwent, in parallel with other European urban centers, a
steep rise in the establishment of hospitals, leprosaria, and almshouses dedicated to providing shelter, meals, and general comfort and care to the sick,
poor, and indigent.[6]

As part of the process of boosting charitable support for these institutions and, moreover, channeling personnel to continue the enactment of
charitable caregiving within them, the labors of ordinary religious women
who regularly worked in those institutions were often translated into hagiographic impressions of supernatural healing and spiritual virtue. I argue in

---

3. Solid numbers prior to the mid-fourteenth century are shaky. For Ghent, we can estimate
sixty-four thousand inhabitants by the third quarter of the fourteenth century; Bruges was roughly
forty-six thousand; Brussels had an average of twenty thousand, and Liège was probably fairly similar
in size. See Paul Hohenberg and Lynn Hollen Lees, *The Making of Urban Europe, 1000–1950* (Cambridge, MA: Harvard University Press, 1985); Peter Stabel, *Dwarfs among Giants: The Flemish Urban
Network in the Middle Ages* (Leuven: Garant, 1997); and Pierre de Spiegeler, *Les hôpitaux et l'assistance
à Liège: Aspects institutionnels et sociaux* (Paris: Les Belles Lettres, 1987), 55. On the expansion of trade,
see Walter Simons, *Cities of Ladies: Beguine Communities in the Medieval Low Countries, 1200–1565* (Philadelphia: University of Pennsylvania Press, 2001), 5; and Herman Van der Wee, "Industrial Dynamics
and the Process of Urbanization and De-Urbanization in the Low Countries from the Late Middle
Ages to the Eighteenth Century," in *The Rise and Decline of the Urban Industries in Italy and the Low
Countries*, ed. Herman Van der Wee (Leuven: Leuven University Press, 1988), 307–81.

4. Innocent III, *Libellus de eleemosyna*, in *PL* 217:745–62. See also the *Encomium charitatis*, in *PL*
217:761–64.

5. Jessalyn Bird, "Medicine for Body and Soul: Jacques de Vitry's Sermons to Hospitallers and
Their Charges," in *Religion and Medicine in the Middle Ages*, ed. Joseph Ziegler and Peter Biller (York:
York Medieval Press, 2001), 95.

6. In northern France, of 151 leprosaria, 22 percent were twelfth-century foundations, 54 percent were thirteenth-century foundations, and 24 percent were fourteenth. Michel Mollat, "Floraison
des fondations hospitalières," in *Histoire des hôpitaux en France*, ed. Jean Imbert and Michel Mollat
(Paris: Privat, 1982), 35. Leprosaria tended to be established earlier than the flurry of hospitals and
hospices that were founded in the thirteenth century. See James Brodman, *Charity and Religion in
Medieval Europe* (Baltimore: Johns Hopkins University Press, 2009), 56.

this chapter that charitable caregiving was central to the identity of many mulieres religiosae. Their healthcare labor, however, has been historically obscured because of the hagiographic impressions through which it has been transmitted. Reading hagiographic sources on the mulieres religiosae alongside those of the viri religiosi brings into focus caregiving acts; it highlights how the care these women provided became a source of their veneration. At the end of this chapter I will turn to the lives of the viri religiosi to contemplate the gendered division of caregiving labor. Before doing so, however, I place these narrative sources next to administrative documents, such as foundational charters, statutes, and testaments, which will enable us to envision how acts of care that were narrativized in hagiography might have been put into practice in institutional settings.

Women's Institutions of Care

We can gain a more complete picture of religious women's healthcare services by putting into conversation narrative depictions of caregiving from the *Lives* with records from the institutions in which mulieres religiosae lived and worked. What stands out in this picture is religious women's maintenance of what Peregrine Horden has called a "non-natural environment." These women oversaw diet and hygiene, offered soothing words, and provided opportunities for comfort and rest. By hearing informal confessions, uttering prayers, and caring for the body, many of the mulieres religiosae who gained extant textual *Lives* helped to garner the health of patients or, when death was certain, to create the conditions for a good death. The social value of their labor is demonstrated not only in bequests to their communities but also in the range of hagiographic material generated about their provision of care. That is, their caregiving contributed to their perceived sanctity and circulated in stories of their Christian virtue *because* certain sectors of the population valued it.

Medieval hospitals functioned largely as relief shelters for the poor, sick, and aged.[7] Virtually anyone with means could found them.[8] In the cities and

---

7. Most recently, Adam Davis, *The Medieval Economy of Salvation: Charity, Commerce, and the Rise of the Medieval Hospital* (Ithaca: Cornell University Press, 2019); and Davis, "Hospitals, Charity, and the Culture of Compassion," in *Approaches to Poverty in Medieval Europe: Complexities, Contradictions, Transformations, 1100–1500*, ed. Sharon Farmer (Turnhout: Brepols, 2016), 23–45; Peregrine Horden, *Hospitals and Healing from Antiquity to the Later Middle Ages* (Aldershot: Ashgate, 2008). For the Islamic world, see Ahmed Ragab, *Medieval Islamic Hospital: Medicine, Religion, and Charity* (Cambridge: Cambridge University Press, 2018).

8. Miri Rubin, *Charity and Community in Medieval Cambridge* (Cambridge: Cambridge University Press, 2002), 103.

towns of the Low Countries, members of the rising bourgeoisie facilitated the foundation and maintenance of hospitals and leprosaria, since existing charitable institutions, unsystematically governed by bishops, were inadequate for a growing urban population.[9] The oldest formal hospital in the southern Low Countries was probably in Huy, founded in 1066, with those in Louvain and Wanze following shortly thereafter.[10] By the twelfth century, there were hospitals with charters and endowments established in Brussels, Cambrai, Arras, Bruges, Ypres, and Ghent, and leprosaries in Cambrai, Bruges, Ghent, Tournai, Ypres, and Liège. By the thirteenth century, bishops, lay confraternities, monastic institutions, other townspeople, and members of the aristocratic classes all responded to the needs of a surging urban population, in what André Vauchez called a "revolution in charity," by founding additional institutions of care, especially small home hospices, quasi-regular hospitals, and independent hospitals.[11] Originally, the individuals who staffed hospitals were both religious and secular or semireligious personnel. But by the thirteenth century, under the direction of episcopal reformers like Robert of Courson, European hospitals in this region increasingly conformed to a monastic model, as staff were expected to live communally and to adopt a monastic rule, most often the Augustinian Rule, and to wear the religious habit.[12] The move toward regularization of thirteenth-century hospitals under episcopal jurisdiction also points to the varied services they provided. Hospitals in this era were not primarily medical institutions, but also chapels, shelters, retirement homes, and temporary rehabilitation clinics.[13]

---

9. Spiegeler, *Les hôpitaux et l'assistance*; Daniel Le Blévec, "Le rôle des femmes dans l'assistance et la charité," in *Cahiers de Fanjeaux 23: La femme dans la vie religieuse du Languedoc (XIIIe–XIVe s)* (1998): 171–90.

10. Brodman, *Charity and Religion*, 55–62; Paul Bonenfant, *Hôpitaux et bienfaisance publique dans les anciens Pays-Bas, des origines à la fin du XVIIIe siècle* (Brussels: Société belge d'histoire des hôpitaux, 1965), 13. The hospital of St. Nicholas at Fosses was founded on the collegial chapter of St. Feuillien during the reign of Bishop Henry of Verdun (1075–91). See Spiegeler, *Les hôpitaux et l'assistance*, 67n58.

11. Davis, *The Medieval Economy of Salvation*; Bonenfant, *Hôpitaux et bienfaisance publique*, 3–44; Spiegeler, *Les hôpitaux et l'assistance*, 89–99; André Vauchez, *La spiritualité du Moyen Âge occidental (VIIIe–XIIIe siècle)* (Paris: Seuil, 1994), 118. For other regions in Europe, see Martin Scheutz et al., eds., *Europäisches Spitalwesen: Institutionelle Fürsorge in Mittelalter und Früher Neuzeit / Hospitals and Institutional Care in Medieval and Early Modern Europe* (Vienna: Oldenbourg Verlag, 2008).

12. The monastic model was by no means homogenous and universal throughout the region, of course. Davis, *The Medieval Economy of Salvation*, 226; Bird, "Medicine for Body and Soul," 98–99. Bird cites Robert of Courson's statutes for the reform of religious houses, which influenced the content of statutes adopted in Flanders-Brabant and northern France. In Liège, the statutes of St. Christopher are found in A. Borgnet and S. Bormans, *Ly myreur des histors ou chronique et geste de Jean des Preis dit d'Outremeuse* (Brussels: Publications de la Commission royale d'Histoire, 1864–87), 5:249–52.

13. Davis, *The Medieval Economy of Salvation*, 4.

The caregiving practices that took place in small-scale hospices and leprosaria are best understood from the perspective offered by the non-naturals in medieval medical theory. Thirteenth-century hospitals were largely sites at which practitioners managed the non-natural environment, seeking to restore the body's humoral balance and providing general comforts.[14] Hospital staff managed a healthy regimen for those who could not provide for themselves by feeding, clothing, housing, and praying for the infirm, the poor, and the needy.

Examining the infrastructure and administration of hospitals in Liège, Pierre de Spiegeler concluded that, in these hospitals, men outnumbered women as caretakers, a pattern that was mirrored among hospital staff elsewhere in Europe.[15] But Spiegeler's evidence derived from late fourteenth- and fifteenth-century hospital records that reflected the activities of benefactors and administrators rather than caretaking staff. In addition to these official positions, ranks, and institutions, religious and semireligious women served the bodily needs of the poor, elderly, sick, and impaired in a less official capacity, which has been obscured from the historical record. As Adam Davis has discussed, hospital sisters were often needed to minister to women among the sick poor, and a *magistra* or prioress was required to oversee hospital sisters and to enforce gender segregation among patients and staff.[16] Davis's study of hospital statutes from Champagne reveals a gendered division of labor in which women were the principal caretakers of the sick, while chaplains and choirboys maintained administrative records and performed the canonical Hours and Masses.[17] Alain Saint-Denis has observed a similar pattern, demonstrating that while hospital brothers at the Hôtel-Dieu in Laon were the original caretakers of the sick, by the thirteenth century, they had outsourced caregiving labor to hospital sisters so that they could devote attention to the temporal administration of the hospital.[18] Meanwhile, Elma Brenner has found that, in the hospitals and leprosaria of Normandy, while men appear

---

14. Peregrine Horden, "A Non-natural Environment: Medicine without Doctors and the Medieval European Hospital," in *The Medieval Hospital and Medical Practice*, ed. Barbara Bowers (London: Routledge, 2007), 133–46.

15. Spiegeler, *Les hôpitaux et l'assistance*, 156–57.

16. On the invisibility in the sources even of hospitals' *magistrae*, see Davis, *The Medieval Economy of Salvation*, 206–7.

17. Davis, 210–11. At Tonnerre, for example, the charter states that the sisters should care for the sick and oversee washing and bedding, while chaplains and choirboys perform the Hours and Mass. At Gonesse, the master and brothers tended the hospital's properties and workers, while the prioress and sisters cared for the sick.

18. Alain Saint-Denis, *L'hôtel-Dieu de Laon, 1150–1300* (Nancy: Presses Universitaires de Nancy, 1983), 97.

as founders, administrators, and visiting physicians, it was women who provided the bulk of daily care, nursing, and practical duties.[19] Sharon Farmer has similarly shown that Jacques de Vitry's sermons and exempla for hospital workers indicate that women provided prolonged physical contact with the sick.[20] Indeed, when observing apostolic and penitential behaviors in Umbria, Jacques singled out women's roles as hospice workers, a behavior that, he noted, distinguished them from the friars. Describing these religious women as "abid[ing] together in various hospices near the cities," Jacques may have been writing to support the religious women in Liège who exercised their penitential calling in a similar fashion.[21] As Catherine Mooney has asserted, the traces of these women who worked in hospices have been largely erased from history because they never received the civic or ecclesiastical approval and institutional support that enabled male communities like the lesser brothers to flourish.[22]

Scholars can resist that erasure by focusing attention on traces of evidence for religious women's presence in ad hoc, ephemeral caregiving institutions, recasting our gaze from large-scale, civically and ecclesiastically sponsored hospitals like the hospital of St. John in Brussels to more modest home hospices and communal infirmaries.[23] In smaller-scale hospitals serviced by religious women, the institutional supports for women's labor were constantly shifting. For example, some assisted the sick and dying in

---

19. Brenner focuses on La Madeleine, the principal hospital in Rouen dedicated to care of the sick poor. Elsewhere she examines the gender dynamic of healing in the city's leprosaria. See Elma Brenner, *Leprosy and Charity in Medieval Rouen* (Woodbridge: Boydell, 2015), 52, 89.

20. Sharon Farmer, "The Leper in the Master Bedroom: Thinking through a Thirteenth-Century Exemplum," in *Framing the Family: Narrative and Representation in the Medieval and Early Modern Families*, ed. Diane Wolfthal and Rosalynn Voaden (Tempe: Arizona Center for Medieval and Renaissance Studies, 2005), 95–96. For Jacques's exempla, see Thomas Crane, *The Exempla or Illustrative Stories from the Sermones vulgares of Jacques de Vitry* (London: The Folklore Society, 1890). Farmer notes that, among seven charitable exempla in Jacques's hospital sermons, three were about men giving property, and four were about corporeal works of mercy in which two featured men and two featured women, but women appear as the sustained handlers of sick bodies.

21. "Mulieres vero iuxta civitates in diversis hospitiis simul commorantur." The recipient of the letter remains unknown. See Letter I in Jacques de Vitry, *Lettres de Jacques de Vitry, 1160/70–1240 évêque de Saint-Jean d'Acre*, ed. R. B. C. Huygens (Leiden: Brill, 1960), 71–78. On the interpretation of the letter as it relates to the "lesser sisters" and Clare of Assisi, see Catherine Mooney, *Clare of Assisi and the Thirteenth-Century Church: Religious Women, Rules, and Resistance* (Philadelphia: University of Pennsylvania Press, 2016), 30–48.

22. Mooney, *Clare of Assisi*, 48.

23. Although it should be noted that women caretakers *also* factor more prominently in the larger-scale civic and ecclesiastic hospitals, such as St. John in Brussels. See Davis, *The Medieval Economy of Salvation*, chs. 3 and 5. On the female practitioners of St. John, see Tiffany Ziegler, "The Hospital of St. John: Exploring Charitable Distribution in High Medieval Brussels," *Ëa: Journal of Medical Humanities and Social Studies of Science & Technology* 3 (2011): 1–32.

private homes that were transformed into caregiving shelters, such as when Marguerite, a widow of Ypres, converted her home into a hospice in 1227 or when the sisters Ida and Oda of Lauw donated their home in 1243 to beguines serving the hospital in Tongres. Other women worked in independent or quasi-regular hospitals that were only later regulated as formal civic or ecclesiastical institutions or from which the women were later separated entirely because of monastic enclosure practices. For example, Grand-Vaux, a mixed-community pilgrim hospital, was transferred around 1229 to Argenton, where the women who once served the hospital became affiliated with the Cistercian order.[24] The ad hoc and ephemeral nature of feminine circuits of care has meant that religious women's healthcare practices and caregiving identities have been easily overlooked. But careful attention to documentary sources reveals that beguines and Cistercian nuns were involved in caregiving and that the lay and clerical communities in which they were embedded valued their healthcare practices, endowing them with material support.

This process of gradual erosion of the identifying connection between religious women and caregiving can be illustrated in the example of the Refuge of the Blessed Mary in Ath. In May of 1220, Joan, the Countess of Flanders and Hainaut, informed the bailiff and aldermen of Oudenaarde that she had granted to the women living at the hospital of Notre-Dame the right to build an attic in the enclosure of its building so that they could sell cereals as a means of supporting themselves.[25] The women of the hospital appear to have continued to operate in this manner until at least 1224, when Walter of Marvis, the bishop of Tournai, imposed on the inhabitants of the hospital, women and men, the obligation to maintain vows of poverty, chastity, and obedience and required them to adopt the religious habit.[26] By the following decade, we see efforts to further regulate the women in

---

24. Jean-François Nieus, "La route, les pauvres et le prince: L'hôpital rural de Grand-Vaux à Balâtre/Boignée; Approche historique (XIIIe–XVIe siècles)," in *Voyageurs, En Route! Au detour du chemin, trouver le vivre et le couvert*, ed. Aurélie Stuckens (Bouvignes-Dinant: Maison du patrimonie médiéval mosan, 2019), 91–109.

25. Theo Luykx, *Johanna van Constantinopel, gravin van Vlaanderen en Henegouwen: Haar leven (1199/1200–1244), haar regeering (1205–1244) vooral in Vlaanderen*, Verhandelingen van de koninklijke Vlaamsche Academie voor Wetenschappen, Letteren en schoone Kunsten van België, Klasse der Letteren, 5 (Antwerp, 1946), no. 13, 543–44: "quod illi de hospitale de Aldenardo faciant solarium in domo sua, ubi segetes uendantur ad usus suos, sicut melius uiderint expedire."

26. The original can be found in Oudenaarde at the Archief van het Openbare Centrum voor Maatschappelijk Welzijn (OCMW), Fonds Onze-Lieve-Vrouwehospitaal 669; it is edited in Aubertus Miraeus and Joannes Foppens, eds., *Opera diplomatica et historica* (Louvain: Diplomatum belgicorum nova collectio, 1723–48), 3.100, 85–86.

particular.[27] In January of 1232, Joan approved an act to build a small Cistercian abbey adjacent to the hospital of Notre-Dame for the use of the hospital sisters.[28] By 1234, this situation, too, was deemed inappropriate, and Joan approved the transfer of the nuns from their little abode (*mansiunculus*) to a more suitable dwelling near the town of Ath, where they became known as the Refuge of the Blessed Mary.[29] Although they were physically removed from the hospital of Notre-Dame at Oudenaarde by some fifty kilometers, the women of the Refuge nevertheless sought to maintain connections with their former community. In 1235, for example, the countess confirmed a donation on behalf of the nuns to the hospital community where they once lived. Their former connection to the hospital is iterated when they are identified in the donation as the abbey of nuns who once lived next to the hospital at Oudenaarde.[30] That is, they continued to identify and to be identified with their roots in hospital work even after their transformation into a Cistercian abbey.

Similarly, at the Cistercian women's abbey of Marquette, a hospital sat at the door of the monastery and was supported by extensive donations. The hospital had served the sick poor among the laity (*domum hospitalis pauperum infirmorum de seculo*) since the time of its construction in 1224. In 1236, Countess Joan released the nuns from care and regimen of the hospital, as well as from the donations that had sustained it.[31] However, it was not until 1249 that the abbess of Marquette, Marie I de Raisse, acknowledged and accepted that the abbey no longer retained rights to the hospital, which had been transferred to Lille.[32] While we do not know precisely how the hospital functioned in those intervening years, it is possible to imagine that the hospital's status remained unconfirmed for over a decade due to persistent, perhaps willed, ambiguity on the part of the nuns, who may have wished to continue their service and foundational connection to the institution of care.

---

27. A similar anxiety about women in less than fully regulated conditions in hospitals is detectable in a document of 1222 when Pope Honorius III transferred a woman living in the leprosarium at Cambrai to the Cistercian abbey of La Brayelle. C. A. Horoy, *Honorii Romanorum pontificis opera omnia* (Paris, 1879–83), vol. 4, no. 143, col. 364.

28. Henry Raepsaet, *Archives de l'hôpital Notre Dame, à Audenarde*, in *Messager des Sciences historiques de Belgique* (Ghent: Hebbelynck, 1832), 358.

29. The original no longer exists. A copy is edited in Miraeus and Foppens, *Opera diplomatica et historica*, 82:201–2.

30. Luykx, *Johanna van Constantinopel*, 44, 573: "abbatie monialium, tunc tempore existencium iuxta hospitale de Aldenardo predictum."

31. *Cartulaire de l'abbaye de Marquette*, ed. Maurice Vanhaeck (Lille: Secretariat de la Société, 1937), vol. 1, no. 89: "cura et regimine hospitalis."

32. *Cartulaire de l'abbaye de Marquette*, vol. 1, no. 156.

While some communities of women, like those of Marquette and the Refuge, became physically separated from the communities of care that originally brought them together, others managed to incorporate hospital work into their monastic communities. For example, in May of 1221 Mathilda of Béthune, lady of Dendermonde, donated land to the hospital of St. Gilles. By 1223, with the support of Bishop Godfrey of Cambrai, she had transferred the hospital to the Cistercian nuns of Zwijveke.[33] In the following years, the nuns received support and issued prayers on behalf of the souls of their benefactors, especially Robert of Béthune, son of Mathilda, who continued to extend the holdings of Zwijveke after his mother's death.[34] That the nuns remained at least peripherally involved in extraclaustral business is shown in a document of 1234, when Pope Gregory IX forbid the nuns of Zwijveke the ability to be summoned to appear at a distance of more than two days' journey from their monastic property without an apostolic letter of permission.[35] This act, though not explicitly related to their healthcare practices, suggests a degree of permeability that would have facilitated their healthcare mission. A request from the abbess of the Cistercian community of Nieuwenbos supports this picture of mobility in the service of healthcare in early Cistercian women's abbeys.[36] A document of 1229 expressed her wish to release her community from service to the hospital in Ghent because of the dangerous distances the nuns were required to travel in order to fulfill their caregiving functions there.[37] But the abbess's insistence on the "love of mutual devoted affection" (caritatis mutuae devotus affectus) between the hospital of Notre-Dame and her community, which will "preserve more firmly into perpetuity," suggests that they maintained supportive connections.[38] In their absence, the nuns of another Cistercian women's community, the Bijloke, began to

---

33. *Cartulaire de l'abbaye de Zwyveke-lez-Termonde*, ed. Alphons De Vlaminck (Ghent: Annoot-Braeckman, 1869), nos. 1 and 3.

34. On the spiritual economy in which donations for care of the sick poor benefited the souls of the wealthy, see Jean-Claude Schmitt, *Ghosts in the Middle Ages: The Living and the Dead in Medieval Society* (Chicago: University of Chicago Press, 1998).

35. *Cartulaire de l'abbaye de Zwyveke-lez-Termonde*, no. 30.

36. On the permeable walls of Nieuwenbos as they related to healthcare, see Erin Jordan, "Roving Nuns and Cistercian Realities: The Cloistering of Religious Women in the Thirteenth Century," *Journal of Medieval and Early Modern Studies* 42.3 (2012): 608. Jordan points out the two other Cistercian abbeys for women in this region, Flines and Marquette, maintained hospitals.

37. Leopold Van Puyvelde, *Un hôpital du Moyen Âge et une abbaye y annexée: La Biloke de Gand; Étude archéologique* (Ghent: University of Ghent, 1925) no. 9, 108–10.

38. Van Puyvelde, *Un hôpital du Moyen Âge*, no. 9: "in posterum firmius perseuerent."

serve the hospital of Notre-Dame.[39] A 1233 charter issued by Countess Joan established that the Cistercian house of the Bijloke was inseparable from the hospital. The foundation charter stipulated that the number of nuns in the abbey hospital was not to exceed twenty-five, with only as many lay sisters as necessary to fulfill their caregiving functions. In addition to ensuring that the number of nuns did not exceed the community's resources, this measure also concentrated the community's income on the hospital's caregiving functions.[40] A separate charter of 1246 records the nuns of the Bijloke purchasing a parcel of land from the Ghent leprosarium, and the abbot of Clairvaux in that same year recalled that the Bijloke could house no more than forty choir nuns, raising questions about their expansion.[41] Both of these documents suggest that the Bijloke was expanding in order to further accommodate caregiving provided by the nuns and lay sisters.

At La Ramée, the infirmary became the center of a controversy that lasted over two years. In 1231–32, the bishop of Liège, Jean d'Eppes, had tied the income of La Ramée's infirmary to the curé of Marilles, working under the assumption that the sisters' services were too modest to be of any significant use to the sick.[42] By 1252, however, their needs were so great that this meager income was no longer sufficient, and the nuns convinced the bishop to devise a more favorable funding structure.[43] In order to create additional revenue for the infirmary, the nuns were allowed to dispose of a portion of the income derived from the properties held by Marilles.[44] This act led to a series of contentious negotiations in which a Master Barthelemy, who is identified repeatedly in the sources as the doctor of the Duke of Brabant,

---

39. The Count and Countess of Flanders and Hainaut, Ferrand and Joan, announced their intention to found an abbey adjacent to the hospital in Ghent in 1228.

40. Luykx, *Johanna van Constantinopel*, no. 42, 570–72: "et quicquid ultra necessitatem tot monialium de bonis eiusdem loci poterit esse residuum, in usus infirmorum et indigentium convertetur, ita quod percipua solicitudo habitantium in loco eodem sit semper erga pauperes et infirmos . . . nostramque precipuam intentionem ac pium desiderium super receptionem paucarum monialium et larga provisione multorum infirmorum et pauperum nullis temporibus pretermittant firmiter et fideliter observare."

41. The original is still preserved in Ghent, Stadsarchief [SA], Bijloke E 58; transcribed from Walters's edition in the Diplomatica Belgica database, DiBe ID 27151. Jozef Walters, *Geschiedenis der Zusters der Bijloke te Gent* (Ghent: Veritas, 1929–30), vol. 2, 3n137, 330.

42. Jules Tarlier, *Geographie et histoire des communes Belges: Province de Brabant* (Brussels: Decq, 1865), 2:258.

43. Georges Despy and André Uyttebrouck, *Inventaire des archives de l'abbaye de La Ramée à Jauchelette* (Brussels: Archives générales du Royaume, 1970), 180.

44. On this affair, see Marie-Élisabeth Henneau, "Entre terres et cieux . . . le temps des fondations (XIIIe–XIVe siècles)," in *La Ramée: Abbaye cistercienne en Brabant Wallon*, ed. Thomas Coomans (Brussels: Éditions Racine, 2002), 31.

laid claims on the land, income, and other goods of La Ramée.[45] The affair finally seems to have been resolved in July of 1254, but the persistence of the nuns' claims, and the will of their supporters, demonstrate that the sisters of La Ramée were deeply attached to their provision of care, and that various classes of people in the vicinity of their community found themselves involved in debating the needs of their communal infirmary, some even seeking to sustain and extend their care. Cistercian women were thus integral to healthcare concerns that included members both of their own religious communities and of the larger lay community.[46]

While Cistercian abbeys like Zwijveke, Nieuwenbos, Marquette, and the Bijloke maintained hospitals within or adjacent to their walls, others provided salutary outreach to their communities in less formal structures and relationships, sometimes collaborating with beguines in this effort. Collaboration with local beguines in the provision of *salus* is demonstrated, for example, in the charters of Salzinnes, which include several instances when the care and prayer work of the nuns was supplemented by that of local beguines. In March of 1271, a canon of Saint Lambert in Liège confirmed, along with a knight Nicholas of Refail, that François of Aische had provided material support to the nuns for the celebration of an office in his memory on the day before the feast of Saint Gregory (11 March). The document notes that, should the nuns falter in this responsibility, the obligation would be executed by the beguines of the hospital of Jambes.[47] By this point, the abbey had long established strong connections with beguines in the region who identified with charitable care. In 1248, Imène, the abbess of Salzinnes and daughter of the Count of Loon, learned that Juliana of Mont-Cornillon had been ousted from the leprosarium where she served as prioress. Juliana was then living in a small house next to the beguine hospice in Namur. Imène thus arranged for a pension to be commuted to them.[48] Guiard of Cambrai advised the women to submit to Imène's authority, thereby formally connecting the legacy of Juliana and her companions with the operations of Salzinnes. In fact, the abbey of Salzinnes enhanced their outreach not only to two hospitals in the

---

45. Despy and Uyttebrouck, *Inventaire*, 181.

46. On the role of women as active, acknowledged participants in the delivery of services that promoted health and healing, see Deborah Harkness, "A View from the Streets: Women and Medical Work in Elizabethan London," *Bulletin of the History of Medicine* 82.1 (2008): 52–85.

47. Émile Brouette, *Recueil des chartes et documents de l'abbaye du Val-Saint-Georges à Salzinnes (1196–1300)*, Cîteaux: Commentarii Cistercienses (Achel: Abbaye cistercienne, 1971), no. 148, 190–91. In 1238, Countess Joan provided for the construction of an abbey church with chapel in Salzinnes for her soul and the soul of her second husband, Thomas of Savoy. Brouette, no. 73.

48. Barbara Walters, "The Feast and Its Founder," in *The Feast of Corpus Christi* (College Park: Penn State University Press, 2006), 28.

region but also to Namur's poor table. The abbess Imène confirmed a donation from Thomas of Saint Aubin to continue provisions for the poor at
the anniversary of his death and to make a regular contribution to the poor
table in Namur.[49] In another instance, the poor table of Namur, the hospital
of Jambes, as well as the friars minors, crosiers, and canons of Saint Aubin
accused the nuns of Salzinnes of negligence in their anniversary prayers,
which had been funded by a beguine, Catherine of Lesve.[50] That so many
religious communities in the region banded together to ensure the proper
execution of the nuns' anniversary prayers testifies to the importance of
those prayers for the maintenance of postmortem health and demonstrates
the spiritual collaboration between beguines and Cistercian nuns in ensuring their delivery. The urgency to fulfill those anniversary prayers locates
them, and the women responsible for them, in a broad salutary economy
that included spiritual and physical forms of caregiving for persons both
living and dead. Recognizing thirteenth-century Cistercian women's institutional ties to these broad forms of care assists in the reconstruction of the
meaning and purpose of their labor.

Among beguines in the region, we find similar arrangements in which
their houses received donations in land and rents for the purpose of supporting care of the sick and indigent in their infirmaries.[51] These transactions show that their livelihoods were built on relationships of obligation
to provide caregiving, that these women were component to a recognized
and valued system of healthcare. Communal support of beguine caregiving institutions dates from at least the mid-thirteenth century, during Renier
of Tongres's tenure as protector of beguinages in the region.[52] Prior to his
appointment as provisor and procurator to unaffiliated (that is, uncloistered)
mulieres religiosae in the Diocese of Liège, Renier had served as the priest-
provisor of St. Jacques' hospital in Tongres from 1236 to 1241, then as supervisor of the beguines in that city.[53] His experiences in these roles fostered in
him a deep respect both for the hospital as a charitable institution and for the
extraregular women who provided occasional and ad hoc healthcare services
in the city. In a gesture of appreciation for their work, he left in his will one
mark to the poor beguines of St. Christopher at Liège and to their hospital,
as well as one bonnier for the beguines at St. Catherine in Tongres and one

49. Brouette, *Recueil des chartes et documents*, no. 129, 159–60.

50. Brouette, no. 153, 196–99.

51. Simons, *Cities of Ladies*, 77.

52. Ernest McDonnell, *The Beguines and Beghards in Medieval Culture: With a Special Emphasis on the Belgian Scene* (New Brunswick: Rutgers University Press, 1954), 165.

53. McDonnell, *The Beguines and Beghards*, 165.

for the poor in their hospital.[54] To be sure, Renier included gifts to several institutions in the diocese, but these donations nevertheless make explicit a wish to sustain beguines' caritative mission.

This support for beguine hospitals is evident elsewhere in the region. In Liège, Pierre Tirebourse founded a hospital in 1267 for old and sick beguines, which was gradually enfolded into the beguinage.[55] A leprosarium, established sometime before 1304, was also attached to the beguinage of St. Christopher, annexed to the hospital and reserved for leprous beguines.[56] At the hospital of St. Elizabeth in Valenciennes, there were so many beguines that Countess Marguerite intervened to secure the cooperation of the monks of St. Saulve in assigning three chaplains there.[57] The presence of hospital sisters working in conjunction with the canons of St. Pierre in Notre Dame at Lille is clear from a 1245 charter issued there; and in 1247, the women at the hospital are referred to clearly as "beguines" and the hospital as "Hospitali Beghinarum."[58] At Cantipret in Mons, Countess Marguerite established in 1245 a hospital for sick beguines, and then, along with her son Jean, began in 1249 to provide it with thirty *livres de blanc* annually.[59] In addition to those mentioned here, Walter Simons has enumerated the hospitals and infirmaries maintained, founded, and staffed by beguines, showing that the court beguinages of Borgloon, Ghent, Lille, Mechelen, Tongres, and perhaps also Bruges were founded by beguines working as nurses in or near a preexisting hospital.[60] Additionally, hospitals for the care of sick and elderly women were the explicit purpose of the foundation of beguinages in Antwerp, Arras, Bruges, Brussels, Ghent, Louvain, and Ypres. And at the court beguinages of Antwerp, Assenede, Cambrai, Diksmuide, s'Hertogenbosch, Maubege, and Mons, the infirmary was one of the original, foundational buildings.[61] These hospitals were established on small scales. But their proliferating presence should serve as a reminder of the everyday caregiving actions taking place among beguines who cared for one another, as well as for other poor

---

54. McDonnell, 168–69.

55. Liège, Archives de l'État, Béguinage de Saint-Christophe, no. 477. Documents on the beguinage of St. Christopher and the hospital of Tirebourse are collected together in the state archives in Liège.

56. Spiegeler, *Les hôpitaux et l'assistance*, 80.

57. The original is preserved in Lille, Archives départementales du Nord [AD], 40H 630/1839; transcribed in Diplomatica Belgica Database, DiBe ID 22561.

58. Miraeus and Foppens, *Opera diplomatica*, vol. 3, no. 39, p. 594.

59. *Cartulaire du béguinage du Cantipret à Mons*, ed. Léopold Devillers (Brussels: Archives Générale du royaume, 1865 [repr. 2001]), 139–40 and 146–48.

60. Simons, *Cities of Ladies*, 76.

61. Simons, 77. See also his Appendix 1, pp. 253–303.

and indigent townspeople. The provision of shelter, meals, and basic human comforts, including the assurance of regular prayer, was central to their identity as beguines.

The growth of the community serving the hospital of St. Catherine in Tongres exemplifies how, throughout the thirteenth century, citizens of Brabant-Liège made provisions to sustain beguine caregiving. In 1243, Renier provided the stipulations for two sisters, Ida and Oda of Lauw, who lived adjacent to the hospital of St. James in Tongres, to establish a house for beguines (figure 1).[62] The beguines of this small house maintained strong ties with the hospital. They attended chapel services there and shared with the hospital the fees they garnered from providing prayers and other assistance at local funeral services.[63] By 1245, their numbers had swelled so greatly that the hospital could no longer accommodate them. The women thus prepared to move to a spot of land close to the Jeker River. However, wishing to maintain ties to the hospital, a beguine, Mechtild or "Mella," made provisions in her will for some additional beguines to remain in the original house established near the hospital, and named in this document as the convent of St. James. Mella's testament specifically designated that the house be used for care of the poor in the infirmary.[64]

Even after moving away from the hospital of St. James, the beguines wished to preserve their commitment to hospital care. For example, because the hospital was in disrepair, the brothers and sisters requested a twenty-day indulgence for those who provided assistance in rebuilding the hospital.[65] Meanwhile, the beguines of St. Catherine's also transferred their interest in providing care to their mission in the new foundation. For example, the testament of Gerard Poytevin sought to fund the construction of an infirmary within the new beguinage.[66] Additionally, a beguine named Mettula de Niel left an acre of land to its infirmary in her testament of 1264.[67] These documents, though sparse in detail, indicate that, throughout the thirteenth century, provision of care to the sick and elderly remained central to the mission of the beguines.

---

62. Stadsarchief Tongeren, Begijnhof, 21 May 1243. I am grateful to archivist Steven Vandewal for making documents available to me. See also the document dated 21 October 1236 in the Tongeren Gasthuis collection.

63. Stadsarchief Tongeren, Begijnhof, 24 October 1245.

64. Stadsarchief Tongeren, Begijnhof, 5 March 1273.

65. Stadsarchief Tongeren, Sint-Jacobsgasthuis, 12–1246.

66. Stadsarchief Tongeren, Begijnhof, 17 February 1263.

67. Stadsarchief Tongeren, Begijnhof, 3–1264.

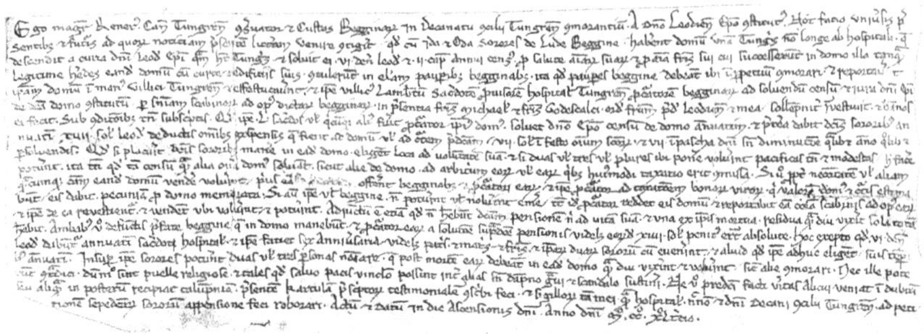

FIGURE 1.   Gift of Ida and Oda of Lauw. Stadsarchief, Tongeren, Begijnhof (1), 21 May 1243.

Wills and testaments from throughout the thirteenth and early four-teenth centuries demonstrate a high degree of community support for the caregiving services that beguines provided. These sparse economic transac-tions validate public recognition of and, moreover, desire for the medical services provided by beguines. For instance, in Douai in 1246, Gervasius of Villa, a local burgher, founded a hospital for the care of poor women "com-monly called beguine."[68] By the following year, they had use of an oratory for the celebration of Mass.[69] In Leuven, records from the small beguinage indicate that an infirmary was established by 1275.[70] Secular support for the work of the infirmary is demonstrated in a ducal deed of that year, which referred to it as "St Gertrude's."[71] At Vilvoorde, a 1288 donation from "Gertrude" to the local beguinage specified that her inheritance be used for the court beguinage to care for poor and indigent beguines; it was at this beguinage in Vilvoorde that an image of Mary was used to provide "comfort" to elderly beguines, a gift given for this very purpose by Sophie of Thuringia, wife to Duke Henry II of Brabant.[72] Beguines thus provided care to the sick and indigent in small-scale foundations. Often they operated within their own communities, sometimes expanding or acquir-ing land for the explicit purpose of building a small foundation dedicated

68. Georges Espinas, *La vie urbaine de Douai au Moyen Âge* (Paris: August Picard, 1913), vol. 3, no. 73, p. 53: "hospitale unum pauperum mulierum, que Beguine uulgariter appellantur."

69. Modeste Brassart, *Notes historiques sur les hôpitaux et établissements de charité de la ville de Douai* (Douai: Adam d'Aubers, 1842) n. 33, 304–5.

70. Rijksarchief Leuven, Klein Begijnhof, 1st series, no. 146.

71. Rijksarchief Leuven, Klein Begijnhof, 1st series, no. 108: Gertrudis in Iovanio.

72. On the image, see Philippe Numan, *Miracles Lately Wrought by the Intercession of the Glorious Virgin Marie, at Mont-aigu*, trans. Robert Chambers (Antwerp: Arnold Coinings, 1606), 11.

to sick care. In other cases, however, they served the sick by visiting them at larger nearby hospitals; in all cases, they received donations for the purpose of caring for the sick and in return for their prayers. That is, the lay communities in which they were embedded regarded beguine prayers as efficacious and connected that efficacity to the healthcare labor they performed.

In Brussels, documents from the hospital of St. John provide an example of how beguines from Wijngaard and Ter Arken were connected in a therapeutic economy that shared revenue and personnel. The hospital kept administrative records of patrons who made donations to the infirmary of the beguinage, as well as land records that indicate a relationship between the beguinage and the hospital.[73] The cartulary records that a beguine, Hedwige van der Maerct, gave a bonnier of land to the hospital of St. John with the stipulation that, after her death, they would pay a rent of five sous to the sick in the infirmary of Ter Arken.[74] It also reports that, in 1277, a woman named Elizabeth bequeathed land to the magistra of the infirmary at the beguinage at Wijngaard in order to support its healthcare work.[75] These documents support a vision in which personnel from the Brussels beguinages cooperated with the administrators of the hospital of St. John in maintaining charitable healthcare and serving the poor in Brussels. Although such land and wealth transfers between multiple institutions were common, the recognition of these economic transactions, when paired with narrative evidence, suggests the establishment of networks of cooperation to ensure the sustenance of care.[76]

---

73. *Cartulaire de l'hôpital Saint-Jean de Bruxelles*, in *Actes des XIIe et XIIIe siècles*, ed. Paul Bonenfant (Brussels: Publications de la Commission Royale d'Histoire, 1953).

74. *Cartulaire de l'hôpital Saint-Jean de Bruxelles*, no. 165, 210–11.

75. *Cartulaire de l'hôpital Saint-Jean de Bruxelles*, no. 183, 236–37: "ad opus ejusdem infirmarie tria bonaria terre." Note that Cistercian nuns of La Cambre were also integrated into the healthcare economy at St. John. A testament of 1228 made by Michael, a citizen of Brussels, gave monetary gifts to the canons of St. Gudule, the nuns of La Cambre, and the hospital of St. Jean. The dean of the chapter of St. Gudule designated a priest for St. Jean's chapel. We can envision through such transactions a kind of network of prayer enveloping caregiving work in the city.

76. City of Brussels Archives I, Ancien beguinage. On Ter Arken, see also Michelle Tasiaux, "L'hospice Terarken, à Bruxelles des origins à 1386," *Annales de la Société Royale d'Archéologie de Bruxelles* 57 (1980): 3–37; Simons, *Cities of Ladies*, 269. Wijngaard was also an important source of healthcare services in thirteenth-century Brussels. Records for Wijngaard indicate that there was a hospice for the sick and infirm attached to the beguinage and named "infirmary of Wijngaard." They also testify to the existence of a poor table serving needy beguines at Ter Arken, which was founded as a hospice for poor beguines. Carole Rawcliffe has shown that the givers and receivers of hospital care could often be blurred, as hospital attendants who became ill or feeble could receive care just as the more able-bodied patients might assist with caregiving. See Rawcliffe, "Hospital Nurses and Their Work," in *Daily Life in the Late Middle Ages*, ed. R. H. Britnell (London: Stroud, 1998), 63.

The proliferation of women's communities that served the poor, sick, indigent, and dying furnishes a more granular picture of the particular forms of care they provided, the epistemologies that informed their care, and the reason their care was valued by the broader urban communities in which they lived. The religious women of the region were involved in caritative networks, and donated and received property at a high rate in order to sustain their involvement in caregiving. These documents reveal that beguinages often included infirmaries or hospitals for the care of the poor, sick, and indigent as a central component of their founding mission. The women who lived there identified closely with this foundational purpose, and their surrounding community, both cleric and secular, recognized and supported that caregiving mission, creating legal and fiscal documentation to ensure that their care would endure. Bequests in support of religious women's communities demonstrate that the care work provided by Cistercian nuns and beguines was perceived by their neighbors as valuable. For them, it worked not only as care, but in some instances also as a means to recovery, to cure. In this way, religious women were positioned within communal structures of obligation that incorporated the health of the body and soul, individual and community, life and afterlife. Economic transactions in the form of land and rents given in exchange for women's prayer and care constituted mutually beneficial therapeutic relationships.

Care and Cure in the *Lives* of Religious Women

In the corpus of thirteenth-century *Lives* from this region, individuals identified as women are described as remaining at the bedsides of the dying, as curing passersby and petitioners, and as otherwise tending to the bodies of the sick.[77] To be clear, this examination of the hagiographic corpus does not assert that women *more frequently* cared for the sick. Rather, as I will discuss momentarily, in stories of sanctity from the region, women's caregiving actions were depicted as an integral component of their sanctity in a way they simply were not for men. Put another way, although men and women both

---

77. On the work of gender among the *Lives*, see Alison More, "Convergence, Conversion, and Transformation: Gender and Sanctity in Thirteenth-Century Liège," in *Representing Medieval Genders and Sexualities: Construction, Transformation, and Subversion, 600–1530*, ed. Elizabeth L'Estrange (Surrey: Ashgate, 2011), 33–48; and Martha Newman, "Crucified by the Virtues: Monks, Laybrothers, and Women in Thirteenth-Century Cistercian Saints' *Lives*," in *Gender and Difference in the Middle Ages*, ed. Sharon Farmer and Carol Braun Pasternack (Minneapolis: University of Minnesota Press, 2003), 182–209.

worked in healthcare institutions and provided charitable caregiving, those behaviors are attributed only to religious women (and one man, Guerric) in the narrative hagiographic sources from the region.

Recall that when Ida of Leuven treated a dying man's tumor, her actions were celebrated in her community as a function of her "virginal holiness." A pattern throughout the *Lives* of female living saints from the region reveals that caregiving actions such as Ida's were consistently translated into tropes of female sanctity. In part, it was their reputations as chaste virgins that enabled these women to provide caregiving at all, to enter homes and lay hands on ailing bodies. Allusions to their chastity, virginity, and pious widowhood affirmed a perception of them as impermeable vessels of grace and enabled them to enter homes, to sit at bedsides, to comfort by their very presence.[78] Their hagiographic construction as "handmaids of Christ" built community trust in the mulieres religiosae as providers of medical services. Although hagiographic sources are riddled with tropes praising their charity and compassion, nevertheless they also offer rich detail on women's interactions with the sick, and reveal their familiarity with prognosis, regimen, symptoms, and duration.

These tropes about religious women in the southern Low Countries also make visible their involvement in the everyday business of health and healing. The hagiographers in this corpus appear to have celebrated some of the mulieres religiosae as particularly skilled treaters of the ensouled body and of the soul at the body's most vulnerable moments of sickness, death, and emotional torment. The caregiving practices conveyed in these stories have been overlooked as acts of care largely because they are inseparable from hagiographic motifs highlighting spiritual virtues. Furthermore, the caregiving acts practiced by religious women have been difficult to differentiate as therapeutic because they are so deeply enmeshed in the expected social behaviors of religious women, their nurturing, praying, mourning, and management of serenity and spiritual delight. The caregiving services described in the hagiographic corpus become more evident as services when we pair them with the caregiving institutions in which they often unfolded. Read alongside the institutional records described above, women appear in these stories as active participants in the delivery of goods and services that promoted communal health. Those goods and services included prayers, burial,

---

78. On virginity tropes and healing, see Naoë Yoshikawa, "The Virgin in the Hortus conclusus: Healing the Body and Healing the Soul," *Medieval Feminist Forum* 50.1 (2014): 11–32.

entertainment, and comfort.[79] But because they were not often transacted as fee-for-service exchanges, they do not show up in the same way in medico-economic records. These therapeutic services are further distinguished by their attention to body and soul, that is, by hagiographic translations that tend to shift the locus of therapeutic power to a supernatural source.

Deathbeds/Deathcare

The mulieres religiosae of the thirteenth- and fourteenth-century southern Low Countries developed reputations as care providers through their prayers for the dead and their proximity to dead bodies. The form of charity in which they were skilled, and for which they were celebrated, positioned them as uniquely qualified to tend to both body and soul. This specialty over the matrix of body and soul is most evident in the care they provided during moments surrounding death, those moments when treatment of both soul and body was most urgent. For example, beguines guarded corpses and prepared them for burial, escorted bodies to burial grounds, and made a routine practice of praying for the dead. Indeed, Jean-Claude Schmitt has shown that beguines in the Upper Rhine were the expected social group to care for the dead.[80] The Rule of Wijngaard in Bruges, for example, stipulated that beguines guard and pray for corpses as well as chaperone them to burial.[81] When a member of the beguinage at Wijngaard died, half of the community kept wake for part of the night, then the other half took over until dawn.[82] Walter Simons has uncovered testaments summoning groups of beguines to homes on the night of their testator's death in order to utter prayers, recite psalms, and remain with the body until its burial. For example, at Tournai, provisions were made for beguines to guard the body of a local woman, Catherine Boineffant, and to recite psalms and prayers until her burial.[83]

---

79. On the recognition of women as acknowledged participants in the delivery healthcare services, see Harkness, "A View from the Streets," 56; and Richelle Munkoff, "Poor Women and Parish Public Health," *Renaissance Studies* 28.4 (2014): 579–96.

80. Jean-Claude Schmitt, *Mort d'une hérésie: L'Église et les clercs face aux béguines et aux béghards du Rhin supérieur du XIVe au XVe siècle* (Paris: Mouton, 1978), 46–48.

81. Joanna Ziegler, *The Sculpture of Compassion: The Pietà and the Beguines in the Southern Low Countries, 1300–1600* (Brussels: Institut Historique Belge du Rome, 1992), 143. The 1290 Bruges Rule is transcribed in Rodolphe Hoornaert, "La plus ancienne règle de béguinage de Bruges," *Annales de la Société d'Émulation de Bruges* 72 (1930): 1–79; another example is the 1328 memorandum describing the beguinage of St. Elizabeth in *Cartulaire du béguinage de Saint Elisabeth à Gand*, ed. Jean Bethune (Bruges: Zuttere, 1883), 74.

82. Hoornaert, "La plus ancienne Règle," 62, in Simons, *Cities of Ladies*, 78.

83. Simons, *Cities of Ladies*, 78–79; Schmitt, *Mort d'une hérésie*, 44–48.

Another will from Tournai requested that twenty beguines attend a woman's wake, while several other wills provided funding for burial in cemeteries maintained by beguines.[84] Because the public was aware of the beguines' daily practice of performing the Aves and the psalter of the Virgin, they associated beguines with aptitude in these prayers, and therefore considered them as efficacious caretakers of the dead.[85] Women were responsible for the prayers and rituals that gave cultural meaning to death, that managed for the community the transition of their members from life to death, which they fashioned according to Christian custom as a new life, an everlasting life, even a more real or true life.[86] In their most fragile moments of human vulnerability, the citizens of the Low Countries pursued religious women, particularly the highly mobile beguines, for the care of their body and soul. The request for beguine presence at these dying moments reflects a broader conceptualization of deathcare as part of healthcare insofar as the health of the soul required a "good death" in order to ensure well-being in the Christian afterlife. The comforting presence of a thoughtful caregiver extended beyond the dying patient to ease the suffering of family members and friends by ensuring them that, through their efficacious prayers, the souls of the dead would be well cared for.

The feminization of mortuary prayer and ritual is reflected in narrative descriptions from the *Lives* of the *liégeois* saints. In the *Life* of Marie of Oignies, for example, Jacques de Vitry characterized Marie by her proximity to the dying and the effects of her prayers on the souls of the dead. In a section of tales dedicated to her assistance to the dying, Jacques asserts that Marie "spent many sleepless nights praying for [the sick]."[87] For this reason, she was often present at the bedside of the sick at the moment of extreme unction.[88] Jacques offers the example of her constant aid to the mother of a

---

84. Christine Guidera, "The Role of Beguines in Caring for the Ill, Dying, and the Dead," in *Death and Dying in the Middle Ages*, ed. Edelgard DuBruck and Barbara Gusick (New York: Peter Lang), 57.

85. Simons, *Cities of Ladies*, 78.

86. On cultural meanings of illness and death, see Peregrine Horden and Richard Smith, eds., *Locus of Care: Families, Communities, Institutions, and the Provision of Welfare since Antiquity* (London: Routledge, 1997).

87. VMO II.3, 106; trans., 89: "super infirmos pia gestans viscera circa quos aliquando noctes insomnes ducebat."

88. VMO II.3. We can imagine the specific role Marie and others like her would have played in death and mortuary ritual. When someone died in the religious community, monks or nuns assembled at the bedside of the dead to recite the creed, litanies, and other prayers. The body was washed and clothed, then laid on a bier on sackcloth with their hands crossed over the breast. All the while, the community would continually chant the Psalms. After a Mass for the dead, the body was carried to a burial place with the community in procession, censed with holy water, then buried. See

canon from Oignies whom Marie accompanied at bedside until she finally died. In another instance, Jacques reports on her tending to the sickbed of the dying John of Dinant. In memory of him, she bowed at his gravesite in Oignies each time she passed it. When the sister of an Oignies canon was dying, Marie could penetrate into her soul to see that demons were harassing it, and she wielded prayers successfully to scatter them. On another occasion, Jacques insisted that Marie once perceived, as a woman's corpse was being taken away from her home for burial, that she was in dire need of prayer for the health and future of her soul. Marie thus hastily arranged for prayers on the woman's behalf.[89] Stories such as these suggest that Marie was known for the efficacy of her prayers for the sick and dying. They point to Marie's ongoing proximity to the dead and dying, providing them with comfort, and concerning herself specifically with the prayers performed for them after their deaths. Marie was understood to have a special aptitude for relieving the purgatorial punishment of souls for whom she prayed, and thus she was sought as a facilitator of a "good death," one in which sins were confessed and reconciliations made. In the eyes of her community, Marie's prayers rendered real effects; they were therapeutic.

The community that shared stories about Juliana of Mont-Cornillion portrayed her assistance to the dead in a similar manner. Juliana was said to be gifted with a unique power to discern when the sick were approaching death and to offer comfort as they transitioned. For example, when a sister Ozilia became extremely ill, Juliana happened to be far away in another town. Nevertheless, when the bell rang to offer Ozilia the viaticum, Juliana immediately sensed that her friend was nearing death and thus prostrated herself in prayer.[90] Once when Juliana was conversing in the dormitory with her friend Eve, the two began to pray for another friend who was dying at that very moment. When Eve asked Juliana how she knew of this imminent death, she learned that Juliana routinely experienced pain when someone she loved was dying.[91] This way she knew when to commence her prayers.[92] Stories about the ability to perceive and prophecy impending death are not unique to the

---

Christopher Daniell, *Death and Burial in Medieval England, 1066–1550* (New York: Routledge, 1998); Geoffrey Rowell, *The Liturgy of Christian Burial: An Introductory Survey of the Historical Development of Christian Burial Rites* (London: Alcuin Club, 1977); Fredrick Paxton, *Christianizing Death: The Creation of Ritual Process in Early Medieval Europe* (Ithaca: Cornell University Press, 1990).

89. Jacques discusses these events under the heading "On [her] spirit of piety," in *VMO* II.3, 101–16.

90. *VJC* I.v (25).

91. *VJC* I.v (26).

92. She would likely have recited the *Commendatio animae*.

women in this corpus; as we will see, there are similar predictions in the *Lives* of the viri religiosi, particularly among the lay brothers Arnulf of Villers and Simon of Aulne, and they are replicated in *Lives* from outside this region as well.[93] But the stories about Marie and Juliana, stories that their communities told about their skills in communicating between the living and the dead, center the therapeutic efficacy of their prayers. These stories reflect that it may not have been the power of prophecy that their communities valued, although hagiographers certainly appeared to have reveled in elaborating their prophetic power; rather, their friends, neighbors, and family members entrusted these women with efficacious prayer-making as they transitioned from life to death.

Juliana's mortuary knowledge extended from knowing when a loved one stood on the brink of expiration; she also knew exactly how to pray for the dead. Once when Juliana understood that a woman dear to her was dying, she immediately began to recite the vigil of the dead. Shortly thereafter, the woman appeared to her posthumously in a vision to confirm that her vigil had indeed aided the health of her soul.[94] A tale like this one certainly served the hagiographer's purpose—to convince others of Juliana's sanctity and to enforce liturgical conformity. But it also conveys the cultural perception of the labor performed by religious women who provided prayers for the dead. It suggests that religious women's prayers eased communal anxieties about sickness, death, and the soul's afterlife. Some of the most potent forms of medicine took effect on another ontological plane.[95] These stories point to the ways that thirteenth-century *liégeois* society organized around shared commitments to remembering the dead, including caring for their souls. Those social organizations centered around the prayers of religious women as therapeutically efficacious treatments for the living and the dead.

The hagiographic depiction of women as seeing or communicating with the souls of the dead often stemmed from their proximity to the dead and dying in their caregiving activities during life. But it also stemmed from a related practice: their expression of penitential piety. In other words, the penitential practices of the mulieres religiosae were a component of their

---

93. Vincent Ferrer and Bernardino of Siena were also said to have intuited the deaths of friends and neighbors.

94. *VJC* I.v (27), 453: "vigilias virginis sibi plurimum profuisse."

95. On the effects of medicine beyond life in this world, see Pamela Klassen, "The Politics of Protestant Healing: Theoretical Tools for the Study of Spiritual Bodies and the Body Politic," *Spiritus: A Journal of Christian Spirituality* 14 (2014): 68–75.

healthcare services, aimed at aiding the health of the soul after bodily death. Because religious women were culturally associated with penitential prayer—either as a result of lived practice or, as Dyan Elliot has suggested, because they were useful clerical tools for showcasing this sacramental necessity—they frequently appear in stories about the status of the souls of the dead.[96] The example of Christina Mirabilis is instructive here. Thomas of Cantimpré depicts her as engaging in elaborate, even "horrifying" performances of penance staged in grief for damned souls.[97] At the same time, when she walked through town, she could perceive the souls of those who would receive salvation, and for these folks she leapt with glee. Thomas asserts that townspeople "could easily mark by her joy or sorrow what would happen to the dying in town."[98] Communal appreciation for religious women's maintenance of penitential obligations was shared in stories of their dutiful prayer and their affirmations of the status of the souls of the dead. As religious women were considered custodians of the soul, their prayers and penance could ease the afterlife of the beloved dead. In times of the most profound discomfort and fear, residents of the lowlands thus called on religious women, most often beguines, for assistance and assurance in matters of body and soul. Their presence at the bedsides of the dying, and in stories of the dead, reveals their status as valued caregivers.

Hagiographic narratives about the interactions of the mulieres religiosae with the dead and dying underscore the significance of their presence for thirteenth-century mortuary practice. Individuals preparing for death clearly harbored concerns about unconfessed sins and the performance of prayer at death and burial. The charitable practices and prayer life of the mulieres religiosae must have assured many that, in religious women's care, their bodily remains would be handled appropriately and their souls would receive the most efficacious forms of prayer, that their earthly lives would be remembered, valued, and safeguarded. The mobility of beguines, in particular, allowed them to offer deathbed services throughout towns and cities so that beloved laypeople, such as the mother of a canon of Oignies or Count Louis of Loon, could benefit from mortuary practices generally reserved for

---

96. Dyan Elliott argues that hagiographic portraits of living female saints undergoing highly somatic penitential acts were useful to post–Lateran IV clerics, who were increasingly concerned with policing Christian orthodoxy. See her *Proving Woman: Female Spirituality and Inquisitional Culture in the Later Middle Ages* (Princeton: Princeton University Press, 2004), 9–13.

97. On Christina's power to evoke horror in her audience, see Smith, *Excessive Saints*, 48–82.

98. VCM III.26, 655; trans., 142: "facile animadvertere poterant in gaudio vel moerore, quid in urbe esset morientibus affuturum."

those living within the cloister.[99] Women remained by the bed of the dying uttering prayers until their final breaths; they elicited confession from the dying; they chanted the Psalms and the Office of the Dead after their passing; they prepared their bodies for burial, and accompanied them in procession to the cemetery to oversee their final repose. In providing an opportunity for confession and care, religious women helped to dispel the anxiety of the dying and of their family members by creating a serene non-natural environment for death.

Sickbeds/Sickcare

At bedsides in abbeys, beguinages, and private homes religious women nursed and prayed for the sick and dying, and occasionally traveled some distance to lend their assistance when beckoned. Take, for example, the case of Ida of Nivelles, who visited a sick woman in her home in the village of Kerkom. While engaged in harvest in the grange at Kerkom, Ida began to languish, purportedly from withdrawal from the Eucharist. Because she required medicine (*medicinam eius dolori*), Goswin notes, God furnished her with an opportunity for personal healing. It so happened that an old woman in a nearby village had just become ill, and when the nuns passed her house, they determined that they should visit her.[100] Tending to the woman, the nuns were certain that she would die, a detail that suggests some familiarity with prognosis. Therefore, they called for a priest to administer the viaticum, but he arrived too late. Lo! Ida's "medicine" was delivered when she received the consecrated host intended for the dead woman. Although this story emphasizes cultural understandings of the Eucharist as remedy, it also reveals the nuns' comfort with visiting the sick in their homes.

When Ida and her sisters called upon the sick woman, they most likely did so out of attention to the care of the non-natural aspects of her health. They would have provided the woman with pleasant conversation that might lift her spirits, perhaps assisting her with minor household tasks. Religious women were particularly valued for their skill in modulating the passions of the soul, that is, the emotional or affective life of patients. Stories of therapeutic practice attributed to mulieres religiosae often involve their use of meditation, song, and prayer as central to their caregiving. These techniques drew on the passions of the soul. They aroused salubrious affects

---

99. In this way, they provided an experience for laypeople of monastic mortuary ritual. Daniell, *Death and Burial in Medieval England*, 28.

100. *VIN* XX, 248–49.

such as joy, hope, or delight, and dispelled noxious ones such as fear. That religious women might be regarded as experts in affective forms of caregiving should come as no surprise. As Sarah McNamer has shown, religious women were instrumental in designing affective forms of meditation that trained audiences in feeling certain desirable emotions, such as joy, grief, or pity.[101] Descriptions of women visiting the sick in infirmaries and private homes characterize their affective forms of prayer as bearing specific therapeutic effects. This hagiographic evidence suggests that their communities ascribed to them a kind of performative therapeutic efficacy. Their prayers and meditations, as I will discuss in greater detail in the following chapters, could be used to directly alter or dispel negative emotions, or to intensify healthful ones.

An example of religious women's affective caregiving techniques can be found in the *Life* of Ida of Leuven (d. c. 1290).[102] Ida, extremely ill and bedridden, received nursing services from a beguine who visited her every day for the duration of a two-week illness. The beguine brought Ida bread, made her bed, and performed other chores for her.[103] These healthcare services fall under the umbrella of the maintenance of the non-naturals—ensuring that the patient was eating properly, was housed in a clean environment, and that her other bodily comforts were met. When Ida again became ill "for some days" she relied on the nursing care of a sister. During her time of convalescence, Ida was subjected to regulatory customs catered to her illness.[104] The *Life* does not provide specifics on who prescribed this health routine for Ida, though psalters from the region supply evidence that women's communities maintained medical regimens, so it is possible that the infirmarian or magistra adapted a regimen for Ida's illness.[105] The *Life* does indicate that the sister helped Ida by performing such services (*obsequii*) as the illness seemed to require.[106] Among these services was the effort of Ida's nurse to exhort the patient (*infirmantem*) and "revive her with comforting conversation."[107]

---

101. Sarah McNamer, *Affective Meditation and the Invention of Medieval Compassion* (Philadelphia: University of Pennsylvania Press, 2009).

102. Her *Life* was written by an anonymous author who claimed to have assembled it from notes left by her Cistercian confessor at Roosendaal abbey.

103. *AASS* April II, 157–89 (*BHL* 4145); hereafter *VILeuv*; *VILeuv* III.34, 167. The beguine also guided Ida on refreshing walks.

104. *VILeuv* III.40, 169: "Morem gerens infirmitati."

105. I explore this evidence in chapter 4.

106. *VILeuv* III.40, 168–69: "pro ut sua requirere videbatur infirmitas."

107. *VILeuv* III.40, 169: "exhortationis allocutionisque solatio recreavit." Ida's nurse in this assistance was also a patient in the infirmary, a detail that affirms Carole Rawcliffe's observation that some patients acted as caregivers.

This aspect of Ida's care points to nuns' and beguines' efforts to create a non-natural environment conducive to recovery, in which the passions were suitably consoled so that patients' fear or sorrow was transformed into a more salutary affect.[108]

Lutgard, too, was rather expert in regulating the passions of patients' souls in the abbey infirmary. A young woman of Aywières, Elizabeth, who was convalescing in her sickbed, once begged Lutgard for her healing prayers. Elizabeth had been in the infirmary for many years, burdened by a need to eat every hour and so weak that she was unable to stand. She longed to join the community, to perform the monastic discipline with her sisters, but she was simply too weak. Lutgard agreed to pray for Elizabeth, with the result that the patient soon healed, "raised from her sickbed and resurrected to full health."[109] After offering this anecdote, Thomas launched into its moralization. He instructed readers on the most useful kinds of caretaker, asserting that "by this it was meant that the sick in the infirmary are subject, willingly or not, to those who minister to them, not only to the good and gentle but also to those who are irritable."[110] Thomas interpreted the interaction between Lutgard and Elizabeth as a lesson on the proclivity of the sick to heal more readily when they are nursed by cheerful practitioners. He portrayed Lutgard as a dutiful and effective assistant to the sick because her presence provided patients with hope for recovery.

In another sickbed story, Thomas relayed that when John of Cantimpré believed he was dying of dropsy, the brothers of his community placed him in a sickbed, and Iueta, the prioress of Prémy, took over his care to relieve the monks who had been reciting vigils for him. As she was praying for him, John reportedly received a vision of the Virgin Mary, which he communicated to Iueta using medical terminology: he had "scarcely enough vital heat to survive."[111] This seemingly obscure detail suggests something of how Thomas grappled with health and healing in gendered bodies. In medical theory, the soul provided vitality through heat and spirits; vital heat was life heat, the heat that circulated through the body and

---

108. On entertaining conversation and other delights as a means of bodily therapy, see Glending Olson, *Literature as Recreation in the Later Middle Ages* (Ithaca: Cornell University Press, 1988); and Naama Cohen-Hanegbi, *Caring for the Living Soul: Emotions, Medicine, and Penance in the Late Medieval Mediterranean* (Leuven: Brill, 2017).

109. *VLA* II.20, 248; trans., 255: "Elisabeth elevandam, et consurrecturam in sanum statum."

110. *VLA* II.20, 248; trans., 255: "quibus in infirmaria debiles, non tantum modestis, verum etiam discolis subjici ministris oportet, voluntarios pariter et invitos."

111. *Vita Ioannis Cantipratensis*, in Robert Godding, "Une oeuvre inédite de Thomas de Cantimpré, la 'Vita Ioannis Cantipratensis,'" *Revue d'Histoire Ecclésiastique* 76 (1981): 257–316; hereafter *VIC*. *VIC* III.ii, 309; trans. 114: "nec erat vitalis calor quo diutius possem advivere."

distinguished all living, active bodies from cold, dead ones.[112] The enlivening power of heat was gendered as masculine according to Aristotelian concepts of physiology and embryology, which positioned "vital heat" as originating ultimately in the generative capacity of male semen, the animating factor that mixed with the passive material seed of a woman to create an ensouled human. That his contact with a woman reignited John's heat, then, suggests a gender reversal in this deathbed interaction. As the vision unfolds, the female practitioner before him, the Virgin Mary, questioned "how or where [he] felt the pain," and after he described his symptoms, she provided a vial of "holy medicine" and applied it to his abdomen. "At her touch came healing," Thomas declared.[113] In this Marian vision, John was healed by a woman who inquired into his symptoms and prescribed a potion accordingly. While it cannot be assumed that Iueta performed the medical tasks that John attributed to the Virgin Mary, we can understand his interaction with Iueta as premised on the gendered expectation of sickbed care, a kind of care that restored his vital heat. As I will explore in the next chapter, this production of vital heat may have stemmed from Iueta's ability to stimulate salubrious passions of the soul. It is impossible to know. What is clear is that, although only Iueta attended him, John perceived Mary as preparing powerful medicine. Moreover, when John really did die, he chose to spend his final days in the care of the nuns at Prémy.[114] It seems that in these most vulnerable moments in his sickbed, only one gender would do.[115]

Hospices and Leprosaria

The *Lives* of the thirteenth-century Cistercian nuns and beguines of the southern Low Countries often locate their saintly subjects and admirable deeds in proximity to and within the walls of hospitals and leprosaria. This proximity reflects the presence of those institutions in the lives and everyday behaviors of religious women. For instance, the *Life* of Ida of Nivelles

---

112. The classic essay on this subject is James Bono, "Medical Spirits and the Medieval Language of Life," *Traditio* 40 (1984): 91–130.

113. *VIC* III.ii, 309; trans., 115: "ubio vel quid dolorem corpore requisivit . . ."; "sacro medicamine . . ."; "cuius tactum salus."

114. *VIC* III.vii.

115. On questioning such moments when "only one gender will do," see Mary Fissell, "Introduction: Women, Health, and Healing in Early Modern Europe," *Bulletin of the History of Medicine* 82.1 (2008): 15.

proclaims that she was active in serving the sick in the hospitals of her hometown, St. Sépulchre and St. Nicholas. Prior to joining the Cistercian order at La Ramée, Ida lived for nine years in a beguine community that served the hospital of St. Sépulchre.[116] The author of her *Life*, Goswin of Bossut, asserts that, prior to taking orders as a Cistercian nun, Ida spent time with the sick at the hospital of St. Nicholas. She frequently remained in the vicinity of the hospital to beg on behalf of others for clothing, footwear, bread, meat, and cheese, and she distributed these items to the needy. When Ida learned of a sick woman lacking any necessity, such as bread, clothing, or medicines, Goswin reported, she would beg so that she might remedy the patient's privation. Ida must have appeared to her peers as constantly doting on the patients at St. Nicholas because, according to her *Life*, one of them sought to trick her.[117] Testing the source of Ida's caregiving—to determine whether it stemmed from genuine charity or performed sanctimoniousness—a young convalescent named Oda called attention to her own bodily needs. When Ida immediately fled the hospital to beg on the girl's behalf, Oda was convinced of Ida's true charity. This brief "trick" conveys the expectation of Ida's reliable presence at the hospital during the years of her life as a beguine. It also suggests how the performance of charitable caregiving was seen as a marker of feminine sanctity. Oda wondered if Ida's charity was real or just a simulation for the sake of earning a reputation, a mere performance of living sanctity, the enactment of a hagiographic trope.

An interest in the motivations of charity and the public performance of works of mercy grew considerably in the late twelfth and thirteenth centuries in Europe.[118] In response to several social, economic, and religious transformations, theologians and canon lawyers began to define the involuntary and the "true" or "deserving" poor according to levels of ability and infirmity.[119] The urban population throughout western Europe rose steadily; for example, in Liège, the population may have doubled from roughly ten

116. See Jean-Luc Delattre, "La foundation des hôpitaux de Saint-Nicolas et du Saint-Sépulchre à Nivelles au XIIe siècle," in *Hommage au Professeur Paul Bonenfant (1899–1965)* (Brussels: Université Libre de Bruxelles, 1965), 595–99.

117. *VIN* I, 203: "Quedam puella que tunc temporis infirmabatur in hospitali ad sanctum Nicolaum Oda nomine, tentabat eam verbis iocosis, utrum vellet aliqua sibi mendicare, quare ad manducandum vel ad bibendum ei erant necessaria."

118. Davis, *The Medieval Economy of Salvation*.

119. Brian Tierney, "The Decretists and the 'Deserving Poor,'" *Comparative Studies in Society and History* 1.4 (1959): 360–73. Rufinus and Hugguccio are especially noted as distinguishing the deserving from the undeserving poor. The deserving poor were sick, orphaned, widowed, or impaired, while the undeserving were merely actors who refused to work.

thousand to twenty or twenty-five thousand.[120] As a result, the wandering poor were becoming increasingly visible at precisely the same time that mercantile activities and the growth of the textile industries led to new concentrations of wealth and their public display. While charity had been an imperative of the Christian community since the conversion of Constantine, Christians found ever more creative and urgent means of practicing charity, spurred in part by the formalization of the doctrine of purgatory at the Second Council of Lyon in 1274 and the concurrent proliferation of the mendicant orders.[121] Hospitals, leprosaria, chantry chapels, poor tables, and confraternity services burgeoned as outlets for distributing alms and for enacting the seven corporal works of mercy, which by the thirteenth century appeared as seven clearly outlined gestures: feeding the hungry, providing drink to the thirsty, giving hospitality to strangers, clothing the naked, visiting the sick, visiting prisoners, and burying the dead.[122] But while canonists delineated gradations in the "worthy poor," devotional writers showed concern for the motivations of charitable behavior.[123] Oda's "trick" appears as a reversal of attempts to decipher the merits of the poor. She sought to expose Ida's false piety; but instead, according to Goswin, she learned that the saint's caregiving was inspired by true love of Christ and compassion for the poor, sick, and needy.

Throughout the remainder of her *Life*, Goswin continued to connect Ida's *caritas* to her genuine compassion. Stating that her "works of charity" had begun at a young age, prior to her conversion to the Cistercian order, Goswin

---

120. Jean-Louis Kupper, "La cité de Liège," in *Fête-Dieu (1246–1996): Actes du Colloque de Liège, 12–14 septembre 1996*, ed. André Haquin (Louvain-la-Neuve: Institut d'Études Médiévales de l'Université Catholique de Louvain, 1999), 19–26.

121. On the shift in patterns of charity in late antiquity, see Peter Brown, *Through the Eye of the Needle: Wealth, the Fall of Rome, and the Making of Christianity in the West, 350–550* (Princeton: Princeton University Press, 2012); on the rise of profit and charity, see Lester Little, *Religious Poverty and the Profit Economy in Medieval Europe* (Ithaca: Cornell University Press, 1978).

122. Twelfth-century theologians outlined six "good deeds" from Matthew 25:35–36 as corporeal works of mercy that were required for admission to heaven (feeding the hungry, providing drink to the thirsty, giving hospitality to strangers, clothing the naked, visiting the sick, and visiting prisoners). In the later twelfth century, a seventh work was added: burying the dead, which originated in Tobit 12. The first reference to the seven works appears in Peter Comestor, *Historia scholastica*, PL 198, cols. 1613A-B. In the thirteenth century, Alexander of Hales enumerated the seven "spiritual works" to match the corporal works in *Glossa in quatuor libros sententiarum* IV 233–34 (IV.dist. 15, 14). On the works, see Federico Botana, *The Works of Mercy in Italian Medieval Art* (Turnhout: Brepols, 2011), 2.

123. On suspicion and mistrust of beggars and the poor, see Michel Mollat, *The Poor in the Middle Ages: An Essay in Social History*, trans. Arthur Goldhammer (New Haven: Yale University Press, 1986), 102.

illustrated their flowering within the cloister in acts of care such as Ida's regular ministration to the sick in their beds at the infirmary, praying for them through the night, and attending the wakes of her dead sisters.[124] He also asserted that she would break her moments of contemplation when necessary to provide charitable services for her neighbors.[125] Goswin's language is suggestive. Addressing Ida's ministrations, he clearly marked her "sisters" (*sororibus*) as the recipients of her care; but in the following sentence, when he described Ida's charitable service, he noted that she would "dismiss" in order to assist those he specified as her "neighbors" (*suis proximis*), suggesting the possibility that she managed to serve those in the vicinity of La Ramée who were not a regular part of the cloistered community.[126] These activities were "signs of her perfect charity," which Goswin related to her compassion.[127] When she was made aware of another person's affliction, he explained, the "fire of charity" would ignite her soul, which melted into compassion, "and this [compassion] was for her a salubrious remedy."[128] Throughout the *Life*, Goswin portrayed Ida's caregiving as an expression of her *caritas*, and through the lens of her love of Christ, as his virgin *ancilla* (handmaiden). Therefore, Ida's acts of care are inseparable from the Christian virtue with which Goswin imbued them; they were completely intertwined both in terms of his construction of her as a saint and in her forms of caregiving. The point, for Goswin, was to convey the stories of charity that her community generated about her. That these stories stemmed from her location in the infirmary is indicative both of her presence there and of her community's memory of, and gratitude for, her care. As a beguine, Ida treated patients at the hospital of St. Nicholas, and as a Cistercian nun, she spent much of her time in the infirmary. Her reputation for sanctity was inseparable from her care for the sick and dying.

A similar picture of Christian virtue mediating religious women's acts of care emerges from the *Life* of the widow Yvette of Huy (d. 1228), who "gave

---

124. *VIN* XXX, 277: "sciendum est igitur quod ab ipsis pueritiae annis charitatis operibus fuit dedita"; XXX, 279–80: "circa aegrotantes in infirmitorio . . . vigiliis monialium defunctarum instanter adesse."

125. *VIN* XXX, 280: "sic interdum Deum propter Deum dimittere ut proximis suis per charitatem deserviret."

126. The term *proximo* here may intentionally evoke the Gospel of Mark 12:31: *diliges proximum tuum tamquam te ipsum*. In this reading, Ida would be turning her attention to those around her, presumably the nuns, rather than outsiders. In either case, Ida is described as engaged in caregiving; the change in noun, however, suggests the possibility that the recipients of her care were not her sisters.

127. *VIN* XXX, 278: "perfectae autem charitatis signa."

128. *VIN* XXX, 279: "hoc erat ei salubre remedium."

herself wholly over to the sick."[129] In 1181, Yvette left her family and her home to reside at a leprosarium just outside of Huy on the river Meuse. She remained there for eleven years.[130] Her friend, the Premonstratensian canon Hugh of Floreffe, recorded her *Life* at the request of his abbot, John, who had served as Yvette's confessor.[131] The *Life* provides details of the care Yvette practiced in the leprosarium, known as Grandes Malades.[132] She ministered to the sick, providing services that even the "vilest persons" disdained to engage.[133] She prepared their food, laundered their soiled linens, and washed broken and repugnant bodies. Hugh also described Yvette as assisting the leprous in finding a comfortable position in bed at night, and in helping them to rise safely in the morning. Her identification with the sick bodies that she served was so acute that at one point Hugh fashioned Yvette as wishing to contract leprosy, bathing in the waters of the leprous, dining with them, and even infecting herself by mixing her blood with theirs.[134] This characterization was intended to promote Yvette's fervid desire to enact Christian virtue; Yvette wished to inhabit the social category of *pauperes Christi*, which gave spiritual status to the poor, indigent, and leprous.[135] But in doing so, the *Life* translates into the language of Christian virtue the care she provided for

---

129. *Vita Beatae Juettae reclusae* (*BHL* 4620), in *AASS* January II, 145–69; hereafter *VBJ*; translated by Jo Ann McNamara as "The Life of Yvette, Anchoress of Huy," in *Living Saints of the Thirteenth Century*, ed. Anneke Mulder-Bakker (Turnhout: Brepols, 2011), 49–141. *VBJ* 152; trans, 93: "coepit velle ex toto se ad eosdem transferre infirmos."

130. Despite the prevalence of the term *lepra* in these sources, I avoid as much as possible the term "leper." As Carole Rawcliffe has demonstrated, the term "leper" acquired a social stigma in imperialist nineteenth-century England, which persists in English uses of the term. On the terminology and identification of leprosy in medieval sources, see Carole Rawcliffe, *Leprosy in Medieval England* (Woodbridge: Boydell, 2006); Luke Demaitre, *Leprosy in Premodern Medicine: A Malady of the Whole Body* (Baltimore: Johns Hopkins University Press, 2007); and François-Olivier Touati, *Maladie et société au Moyen Âge: La lèpre, les lèpreux, et les lèprosaries dans la province ecclésiastique Sens jusqu'au milieu du XIV siècle* (Paris: De Boeck, 1998).

131. On these relationships see Anneke Mulder-Bakker, *Lives of the Anchoresses: The Rise of the Urban Recluse* (Philadelphia: University of Pennsylvania Press, 2005), 55–59. There are no extant medieval manuscripts of Yvette's *Life*. It does not appear to have circulated widely, outside of Liège, or in the vernacular. Her name is not included in the thirteenth-century saints' calendar from Huy identified by Maurice Coens, "Les saints vénérés à Huy d'apres un psautier récemment rapatrié et le martyrologe de la collégiale," *Analecta Bollandiana* 76 (1958): 316–35.

132. See Joseph Daris, "Notes historiques sue Huy," *Analects pour Server à l'Histoire Ecclésiastique de la Belgique* 14 (1877): 36–77. Yvette would have followed the *Praeceptum* of Augustine and his *Ordo monasterii* as the foundational regulations of the Premonstratensian canons. Anneke Mulder-Bakker considers her leprosarium at Huy as one of the oldest forms of beguinage. See Mulder-Bakker, *Lives of the Anchoresses*, 67.

133. *VBJ* 11.36, 152: "viles personae."

134. *VBJ* 11.36, 152: "Siquidem huius rei desiderio et gratia manducabat et bibebat cum leprosis, lavabatque se de aqua balnei ipsorum: minuebat quoque eis ipsamet sanguinem ut sanguine eorum inficeretur."

135. Mollat, *The Poor in the Middle Ages*, 102.

patients in the leprosarium—feeding, bathing, and one might assume from the remark about blood, facilitating with bloodletting.[136] Hugh's attention to Yvette's virtue is attached to and inseparable from her daily ministrations as an attendant at the leprosarium. Even when she left the sick in her care, she remained at Grandes Malades, attached to an anchor-hold on the west side of the chapel.[137]

Service in a leprosarium is a feature shared in many of the Lives of mulieres religiosae from the region and one that is not mirrored in the Lives of viri religiosi. For example, Marie of Oignies began her ministry at the leprosarium at Willambroux in 1191, ten years after Yvette was working in Liège. Margaret of Ypres was also said to have felt enormous compassion for those suffering from leprosy. She joined them in begging and gave to them all that was offered to her.[138] And Juliana of Mont-Cornillon joined the leprosarium there around 1207, after she was orphaned at the age of five. She lived at the Boverie, a farmhouse attached to a hospice that was run by a community of religious women and men at Mont-Cornillon.[139] While Juliana was young, she assisted the sisters who acted as nurses at the hospital, cooking for them and performing menial tasks. Juliana must have had considerable exposure to the services these women provided for leprous patients.[140] She became prioress of the community around 1222, and assumed a role as "maid, mother, and nurse" to the patients there.[141] As prioress, she would have overseen the house of healthy sisters who served the leprous women, in particular.

---

136. Phlebotomy was considered one of the most effective treatments for leprosy, working to purge corrupt humors. Luke Demaitre, *Medieval Medicine: The Art of Healing from Head to Toe* (Santa Barbara: ABC Clio, 2013), 106. According to Elma Brenner, in women's leper houses in northern France, it was required that a competent female bloodletter be on hand. Brenner, *Leprosy and Charity*, 93.

137. It should also be noted that Yvette was a formidable founder of the leprosarium. When she moved there in 1181 it was little more than an old chapel with shelter for those identified as "lepers." Under her fundraising and donations, however, Grand Malades was transformed into a functioning hospital with a new convent and a church served by three priests. Mulder-Bakker, *Lives of the Anchoresses*, 66.

138. VMY, para. 22.

139. On the management of the hospice, see Robert Hankart, "L'Hospice de Cornillon à Liège," *Vie Wallonne* 40 (1966): 5–49; Pierre de Spiegeler, "La léproserie de Cornillon et la cité de Liège (xiie–xve)," *Annales de la Société Belge d'Histoire des Hôpitaux* 18 (1980): 5–16.

140. Simons, *Cities of Ladies*, 76.

141. VJM, ch. 1, para. 2, 457: "Non dominam se exhibebat, sed ancillam, sed matrem, sed nutricem." Under Juliana's tenure as prioress, the community at Mont-Cornillon followed the Augustinian Rule. But Juliana would soon come into conflict with the burghers of Liège, who claimed the foundation of the property and for whom Henry of Guelders acted to support.

We know that Yvette, Marie, Margaret, and Juliana interacted intimately with the leprous as caregivers, and yet the hagiographic narratives reported about them do not provide recognizable details of their medical authority. Rather, in each case, we find tales of feminine virtue, of their outsized *caritas*, their penitential sacrifice, and guarded chastity. That their healthcare provision was recorded not as "medical" but as "saintly" suggests the kinds of historical trajectories through which communities remembered and recorded religious women's caritative and therapeutic acts. The caregiving services provided by these women were transmitted in stories of compassion, humility, and charity located at bedsides of the sick. Taking place in these sites far removed from the construction of medical commentaries or *consilia*, stories of their therapeutic caregiving were not rendered in medical terminology but in terms of compassion and piety, in terms of the phenomenological and emotional experience of the patients they assisted.

One such bedside is visible in the *Life* of Alice of Schaarbeek (d. 1250), which relates the story of a Cistercian nun of La Cambre who herself contracted leprosy. The author of her *Life* introduces Alice's leprosy with a flair for drama, as a gift sent from God. He explains her affliction with the disease as part of a divine plan hatched not as "the fault for some crime, nor in any vindictiveness," but as a way of secluding her for himself, "as a sign of his perfect love."[142] Building on the drama of the tortured beloved, he describes God as snatching Alice away from her family: "He beat her heavily with an incurable disease, one few could wish for: namely leprosy itself!"[143] The remainder of Alice's *Life* relates the distortion and damage wrought on her body as she was removed from the community, thus allowing her to become more intimate with her jealous and violent lover.[144] While the association of a living saint with leprosy might evoke hagiographic tropes,

---

142. *Vita beatae Aleyde Scharembekana* (*BHL* 0264), in *AASS* June II, 471–77; hereafter *VAS*; *The Life of Alice of Schaerbeek*, trans. Martinus Cawley (Lafayette, OR: Guadalupe Translations, 2000). *VAS*, ch. 2, para. 9, 479: "non tamen ob alicuius criminis culpam vel vindictam, sed causa visitationis et more sponsi, sponsae suae arrham tribuentis in signum perfectae dilectionis."

143. *VAS*, ch. 2, para. 9, 479: "morbo incurabili, paucis desiderabili, lepra videlicet, ipsam graviter percussit."

144. Significations of rape are clear in this scene, particularly when read within the context of romance narratives that would have been familiar to readers and auditors of Alice's *Life*. On French rape narratives, see Kathryn Gravdal, *Ravishing Maidens: Writing Rape in Medieval French Literature and Law* (Philadelphia: University of Pennsylvania Press, 1991). The scholarship on rape in English literature has been particularly powerful of late, especially as it develops genealogies of survivor silence and the *longue durée* of rape culture. I call attention in particular to Carissa Harris, *Obscene Pedagogies: Transgressive Talk and Sexual Education in Late Medieval Britain* (Ithaca: Cornell University Press, 2018); and Suzanne Edwards, *The Afterlives of Rape in Medieval English Literature* (New York: Palgrave, 2016).

such as Francis of Assisi's kissing of a leper, other moments in the text point to lived practice.[145] For example, the *Life* indicates that after Alice became infected with leprosy, a maid from within her community served and nursed her in a little house built especially for her.[146] This detail suggests that at least one of the Cistercian nuns of La Cambre would have been comfortable, and even competent, in nursing the diseased in this manner. It also suggests a recognition that some diseases simply cannot be cured, some disabilities not overcome, even in the presence of saints and miracle cures. In these cases, it seems, responsible care came in the form of the maintenance of caregiving duties as well as in crafting a narrative of belonging and desirability.

This *Life* would have made for excellent narrative content among communities of women dedicated to providing care to the leprous; it may have been read to the leprous, who were counted as sisters and brothers among servants in leprosaria.[147] Documents of practice reflect religious women, especially Cistercian nuns like Alice, in close proximity to the leprous, and thus suggest why this *Life* may have served as edifying reading material. Foundation charters and wills from northern France and the southern Low Countries show that Cistercian convents were often founded adjacent to small leprosaria and hospices or involved themselves in mutual support networks.[148] The nuns of Marquette, for example, supported the leprosarium at Lille as well as the hospital of St. Nicholas at Lille, with a muid of wheat annually.[149] The nuns of Joie-Notre-Dame in Soissons originated from a community of women living among the leprous at Berneuil.[150] Even in Constance Berman's

---

145. On this trope, see Carole Rawcliffe, "Learning to Love the Leper: Aspects of Institutional Charity in Anglo Norman England," *Anglo-Norman Studies* 23 (2001): 231–50. The Gospel account of Christ's contact with lepers (Matthew 5:8) provided earlier biblical precedent. Rawcliffe also discusses the famous example of another male saint who was said to visit leprosaria, Hugh of Lincoln (d. 1200), who "would kiss the men one by one, bending over each of them and giving a longer and more tender embrace to those whom he saw worse marked by the disease" (239). His service to lepers, in turn, cured his spiritual illnesses. The tale of Saint Martin, who healed lepers by kissing them, also resonates here. See Catherine Peyroux, "The Leper's Kiss," in *Monks, Nuns, Saints, and Outcasts: Religion in Medieval Society; Essays in Honor of Lester K. Little*, ed. Sharon Farmer and Barbara Rosenwein (Ithaca: Cornell University Press, 2000), 172–88.

146. *VAS*, ch. 2, para. 12, 479: "Cumque domus, quae propter singularem ipsius infirmitatem illi specialiter fuerat deputata."

147. Touati, *Maladie et société au Moyen Âge*, 298, 360. Touati also discusses the small size of many leprosaries.

148. Anne Lester, *Creating Cistercian Nuns: The Women's Religious Movement and Its Reform in Thirteenth-Century Champagne* (Ithaca: Cornell University Press, 2011), 211–14.

149. *Cartulaire de l'abbaye de Marquette*, vol. 1, no. 85, 76–77.

150. Louis Carolus-Barré, "L'abbaye de la Joie-Notre-Dame á Berneuil-sur-Aisne (1234–1430)," in *Mélanges à la mémoire du père Anselme Dimier*, ed. Benoît Chauvin (Arbois: Chauvin, 1984), 487–504.

highly skeptical interpretation, which insists that houses of Cistercian nuns were not deeply tied to leprosaria in the Diocese of Sens, examples of their confirmed association are notable, such as Cour-Notre-Dame and Piété-Notre-Dame-lez-Ramerumpt, both of which oversaw leprosaria.[151] The close proximity of Cistercian women's abbeys to leprosaria in this region and their repeated pairing in thirteenth-century charters, as Anne Lester has shown in the case of Notre-Dame-des Prés and Val-des-Vignes, opens up the possibility that they sustained caritative relationships that escaped, perhaps intentionally, textual confirmation by male authorities.[152] Hagiographic portrayals of *liégeois* women as caretakers of sick bodies translated caregiving practices into pastorally and devotionally significant tropes, saturating their bodywork in a context of Christian piety. But that Christian context was indeed central to their intertwined healthcare mission, intersecting their lives as hospice workers or dedicated exemplars and protectors of the *pauperes Christi*. Scholars have often taken as "merely" trope these hagiographic characterizations of charity, thus masking the caregiving roles provided by religious women in the thirteenth-century Low Countries.[153]

The Saintly Body as Healing Site

The hagiographic topography of illness and healing also encompassed the saint's body as a tangible therapeutic presence. Stories of living saints at sickbeds feature patients who sought contact with the body of the mulier herself as a source of restoration. These stories serve as a marker of the manual work for which religious women were noted—they touched, palpated, massaged, or otherwise came into physical contact with sick, and often sickening, bodies.[154] Yes, this kind of contact is a hagiographic trope, but it is

---

151. Cour-Notre-Dame oversaw Viluis, confirmed by the archbishop of Sens; Piété controlled the leprosarium at Ramerumpt, confirmed in 1235. Constance Berman, *The White Nuns: Cistercian Abbeys for Women in Medieval France* (Philadelphia: University of Pennsylvania Press, 2018), 196.

152. Lester, *Creating Cistercian Nuns*, 211–14.

153. Adam Davis makes this point as well in his "Hospitals, Charity, and the Culture of Compassion," 31. He notes that while charitable caregiving may be a trope, in the twelfth and thirteenth centuries it was one that reflected lives that unfolded in hospitals.

154. On laywomen and religious women's "healing with the body," see Gianna Pomata, "Practicing between Earth and Heaven: Women Healers in Seventeenth-Century Bologna," *Dynamis* 19 (1999): 119–43. Pomata argues that, in seventeenth-century Bologna, healing with the body was marginalized and ranked as an inferior form of healthcare in a medical hierarchy that privileged healing knowledge gained through academic education. In religious settings, however, healing with the body was central. The body could occupy a central place in religious healing because the rationale for its

also a fundamental distinction in the portrayal of feminine caregiving in the hagiographic corpus, one that inversely mirrors scholastic physicians' distance from menial bodywork. In these instances, compassion for the sick is so fiercely associated with religious women that therapeutic characteristics are rhetorically and conceptually absorbed into their very feminine form.[155] For example, the anonymous author of the "History of the Foundation of the Venerable Church of Blessed Nicholas of Oignies and the Handmaid of Christ Marie of Oignies" claimed that Marie's reputation for healing was earned throughout the region because she repeatedly "cured the sick, cleansed lepers, and drove out demons from possessed bodies and, what is more, raised the dead."[156] Jacques de Vitry issued the same claim. In a section dedicated to the cures she wielded while living, Jacques described the very presence of Marie as capable of generating health. Two categories of healing stand out among the many therapeutic actions Jacques detailed. First, Jacques asserts that a number of boys with broken bones were carried to Marie, who laid hands on them in order to effect repair.[157] Marie's laying on of hands also cured a significant number of throat-related illnesses. Jacques specifically names *squinancia* as an affliction that she cured by hand on multiple occasions, as well as a more generalized swelling of the throat.[158] In each of these tactile remedies, Jacques depicted patients as seeking Marie from afar. Presumably they learned about Marie's therapeutic touch in response to circulating stories about her sanctity. Repeated stories of her "tactile balm"

---

efficacy lay outside the realm of the natural. Because they were *super*-natural in their healing capacities, religious women's bodies, the bodies of saints, could still be regarded as legitimate therapeutic sources, even by physicians.

155. On humanistic elaborations of this trait, see Eva-Maria Cersovsky, *"Ubi non est mulier, ingemiscit egens?* Gendered Perceptions of Care from the Thirteenth to Sixteenth Centuries," in *Gender, Health, and Healing*, ed. Sara Ritchey and Sharon Strocchia (Amsterdam: Amsterdam University Press, 2020), 191–214.

156. "History of the Foundation of the Venerable Church of Blessed Nicholas of Oignies and the Handmaid of Christ Mary of Oignies," trans. Hugh Feiss, in *Mary of Oignies: Mother of Salvation*, ed. Anneke Mulder-Bakker (Turnhout: Brepols, 2006), 172.

157. *VMO* II.3.

158. Medieval medical manuals treated *squinancia* as a type of angina. That Marie is said to have cured it with her finger is particularly curious because medical manuals, such as Roger Frugardi's *Chirurgia*, described three different forms of angina, one of which (*squinancia*) was incurable and could only be left to God, another of which (*scinancia*) required touch, or the puncturing of a puss-filled lesion in the throat with a finger or another device for which he included an *experimentum* involving a chestnut and a filbert. The third form (*quinancia*) was extremely mild and was treated with gargling. If Marie was known locally as a specialist in these throat afflictions, she could have used a combination of prayer and touch, in addition, perhaps, to recommending a good gargle rinse.

suggest that Marie was able to achieve a kind of physical intimacy of bodily contact with her patients, a result of her chastity.[159]

In this section on Marie's healing touch, Jacques twice compared Marie's specific therapeutic techniques with those of medical doctors. After discussing the case of a boy who was constantly bleeding from the ear, he asserted that "no medical art could cure [him]."[160] His mother brought the bleeding boy to Marie, who succeeded through "the medicine of her prayers and by the laying on of hands."[161] Marie offered patients something that physicians could not, something conveyed in the intimacy of her embodied presence. A few paragraphs later, when he cited the case of Guerric, a priest of Nivelles, Jacques remarked that many doctors (medici) had attended him, but none could promise health. Everyone's "despair," however, was dispelled when Marie tried an altogether different approach. By touching her hair, Guerric "was restored to health."[162] Jacques labeled the fruits of her remedy "consolation" and "patience" (consolationem et patientiam). That is, he used affective terminology to qualify her brand of therapeutic practice and its effect. From the healing stories that Jacques reported in this section, it is clear that he wished to depict the widespread community surrounding Marie as perceiving her bodily presence—in addition to her prayers—as a source of remedy.

The Life of Lutgard offers another portrayal of a mulier as the very embodiment of therapeutic vigor. In his descriptions of Lutgard's healing touch, Thomas hints at a rationale explaining her abilities. He reasons that "God gave her the grace of healing so universal that if there were a spot in anyone's eye or any ailment in the hand, the foot, or other parts of the body, they would at once be cured by contact with her spit or her hand."[163] According to Thomas, Lutgard's ability to cause physiological transformation in others stemmed from her own capacity for grace. Unlike other healers who, according to scholastic physicians, cured by contact because their material bodies bore unique virtue in their complexion, the bodies of Lutgard and

---

159. On women and healing touch in premodern China, see Charlotte Furth, *A Flourishing Yin: Gender in China's Medical History, 960–1665* (Los Angeles: University of California Press, 1999), 266–300.

160. VMO II.3, 106; trans., 89: "nulla arte medicinali curari posset."

161. VMO II.3, 106; trans., 89: "medicina orationum eius et appositione manus sanitati perfectae restitutus est."

162. VMO II.3, 107; trans., 90: "restitutus est sanitate."

163. VLA I.12, 239; trans., 226: "Dedit ergo ei Deus ita universaliter gratiam curationum, ut si esset macula in oculo, aut malum aliud in manu, pede, vel membris aliis, ad contractum salivae vel manus illius protinus curabantur."

Marie healed through grace.[164] Lutgard's reputation for therapeutic efficacy was so esteemed, according to Thomas, that she was constantly swarmed by visitors demanding cure. The frequency with which she received requests for cure became something of a nuisance, however, because it disturbed her meditations. Lutgard thus prayed for the removal of her grace of healing and, although Thomas avers that God obliged her, Lutgard nevertheless continued to aid the sick. For example, a noble nun named Mechtild, who had lost her hearing, was cured when Lutgard inserted two fingers, wet with her own saliva, into the deaf woman's ears.[165] Thomas's estimation of Lutgard's facility with spit remedies may have derived from his understanding of the curative effects of saliva outlined by his teacher, Albertus Magnus. Albertus had theorized that "the spittle of a fasting human heals abscesses when smeared on them and removes spots and scars."[166] While his teacher posited a material explanation for this phenomenon, however, Thomas remained convinced that Lutgard's potent saliva stemmed from grace. In a peculiar reversal of her spittle remedy, Thomas also reported that Lutgard once cured a boy of his epilepsy by "put[ting] a finger in his mouth and trac[ing] a cross in his breast with her thumb."[167] Without access to the precise mechanics of her digital ministrations, it is still possible to gather from these stories that Thomas consistently depicted the neighbors of Aywières, as well as its inhabitants, as pursuing Lutgard for health-related purposes. And indeed, he insisted that stories of her ability to cure stretched far outside of her own community. At one point, Thomas related that the abbot John of Affligem brought a troubled man to Lutgard, who implored her therapeutic aid.[168] It is clear, then, that Lutgard maintained a reputation as an apt caregiver and that patients visited her from near and far for the singular purpose of healing.

Like Lutgard, Juliana of Mont-Cornillon also entertained visits from far-flung patients requesting her therapeutic touch. The range of cures attributed to Juliana suggest that she had developed something of a healing cult even prior to her death. For example, a beguine once visited Juliana because

---

164. On the bodies of *physici* as sources of healing, see chapter 3. As I will discuss there, women's bodies were constructed by scholastic physicians as naturally harmful through corrupt humors; but they were never constructed as *naturally* healthful, as men's bodies could be on occasion. Women's bodies required grace to heal.

165. *VLA* I.22.

166. Albertus Magnus, *On Animals: A Medieval Summa Zoologica*, trans. Kenneth Kitchell and Irven Resnick (Columbus: Ohio State University Press, 2018), 1447.

167. *VLA* II.28, 250; trans., 260: "Quae statim oratione praemissa, digitum illi in os posuit, et crucem in pectore pollice fixit."

168. *VLA* II.27.

she suffered from a piece of flesh that had grown from her eye, and was "doubly afflicted" by the wound on account not only of the pain but also of the humiliation from the horror it generated in onlookers.[169] Multiple sources recommended that the beguine visit Juliana, an indication of the extent of her reputation for therapeutic competence. When the beguine finally arrived at Mont-Cornillon, she reported the exact location and duration of her symptoms, "how much pain she had suffered in her eye and for how long."[170] Juliana's prescription for the ailment was to place on the beguine's eye a linen cloth soaked in her own tears. The next day, while praying at Mass, the beguine was healed.

This kind of contact relic, sourced from the living Juliana, reappears in the story of a different beguine who sought from Juliana a cure for her *horribilis acedia*, a kind of terrible languish. Juliana offered the beguine instruction in "true religious life," and she was relieved of her emotional and psychological burden. When the beguine returned to Juliana requesting a remedy for a painful sinus headache caused by a persistent cold (*rheuma*), she was then cured by wearing Juliana's cap.[171] These tales of healing performed by the living saint indicate that Juliana's neighbors understood proximity to her bodily presence as a kind of salve. In the case of Juliana, it is impossible to know from hagiographic impression the details of the treatment she provided. What is clear is that her therapies appear to have been remembered, or reported, as highly affective—she "had amazing compassion for her neighbors who were burdened in heart or body"; she "grieved with the grieving one"; she "sympathized with the patient."[172] "People came to her" seeking her therapeutic treatments, and they preserved those interactions in stories not of medical acumen, but of spiritual and affective competence.[173]

Care and Cure in the *Lives* of the Viri Religiosi

The kinds of caregiving acts attributed to those saints labeled "religious men" in the corpus of thirteenth-century *Lives* differ markedly in quantum and character from caregiving descriptions of the religious women in the

---

169. *VJM* I.6 (41), 456; trans., 223: "affligebatur igitur illa duplici."

170. *VJM* I.6 (42), 456; trans., 224: "quantam et quanto tempore toleraverat oculi passionem."

171. *VJM* I.6 (36).

172. *VJM* I.6 (37), 455: "compatiebatur mirabiliter Juliana proximis suis . . . qui cordis vel corporis gravaminibus premebantur"; I.6 (36): "dolente condoluit"; I.6 (41): "condoluit patienti."

173. *VJM* I.6 (37), 455; trans., 220: "Quis infirmatur, et ego non infirmor? . . . Unde cum aliquae personae, familiaritatis commercio seu liberationis desiderio ad eam venientes."

corpus. While the mulieres religiosae appear in these sources as tending to the bodily suffering of the poor, sick, indigent, and dying, the charitable caregiving of viri religiosi is generally demonstrated through almsgiving and indirect forms of assistance. Just like women, men staffed hospitals, leprosaria, and communal infirmaries; they also prayed for the dead, attended funerals, and practiced penance. But while male saints from the corpus were described as providing charity, rarely were their hagiographic virtues constructed around the practice of charitable bodywork.[174] What is telling, then, is that the stories of caregiving preserved in these hagiographic texts are attributed primarily to women and are often gendered as feminine acts, as evidence of their "virginal holiness." This pattern in representations of thirteenth-century caregiving does not mean that individuals identified as saintly men did not engage in acts of bodily care. It does mean, however, that the stories that codified their holiness were not those that centered on caregiving behaviors.

A brief comparison of these sources offers a more complete picture, gendering charitable caregiving practices and the distribution of everyday healthcare in the thirteenth-century Low Countries.[175] Take the example of the noble Cistercian and former knight Walter of Bierbeek (d. 1222). Walter was in charge of his monastery's infirmary. And yet none of the stories in his brief *Life* depict him tending to the sick at bedside, although he is portrayed as healing through confession, doling out coins to the poor in the street,

---

174. Anneke Mulder-Bakker, "Holy Laywomen and Their Biographers" in Mulder-Bakker, *Living Saints of the Thirteenth Century*, 7. Of the twelve *Lives* of male "living saints" in the thirteenth-century canon that Mulder-Bakker enumerates, nine were Cistercian, one was an Augustinian canon, and two were laymen. For this chapter, I examined nine of the *Lives*, which I selected because they lived during and their *Lives* circulated in the thirteenth century. This criterion eliminated three of the *Lives* enumerated in Newman's and Mulder-Bakker's canon/corpus: Peter of Villers is of uncertain date, and Gerlach of Houthem and Bernard the Knight both died in the mid- to late twelfth century. It should be noted that the hollowed-out tree in which Gerlach lived later became a pilgrimage site where dirt from his grave served as a medicine for animals and humans. Mulder-Bakker perceptively notes, however, that Gerlach was not a "living saint" like the mulieres religiosae. Interest in his sanctity developed only after his death. See Anneke Mulder-Bakker, "Saints without a Past: Sacred Places and Intercessory Power in Saints' Lives from the Low Countries," in *The Invention of Saintliness*, ed. Mulder-Bakker (New York: Routledge, 2002), 45–47. Little work has been published on the viri religiosi as a group. See Alison More, "Convergence, Conversion, and Transformation: Gender and Sanctity in Thirteenth-Century Liège," in *Representing Medieval Genders and Sexualities in Europe: Construction, Transformation, and Subversion, 600–1530*, ed. Elizabeth L'Estrange and Alison More (Surrey: Ashgate, 2011), 33–48; and Stefan Meysman, "Virilitas in tijden van verandering: Religieuze en profane mannelijkheden in de Nederlanden, ca. 1050–1300" (PhD diss., University of Ghent, 2016).

175. At the same time, we must keep in mind that while hospital brothers also provided similar forms of bodily care, analogous narrative sources detailing and sanctifying their forms of care and interactions with patients have not survived from these sites.

and exorcising demons through prayer and song.[176] In other words, although Walter clearly would have tended to the bodily needs of patients on a daily basis, the hagiographic stories about him—the illustrations of his holiness shared within his community—were not generated from those healthcare interactions. A similar pattern is evident in the *Life* of the choir monk Godfrey Pachomius (d. 1262), which praises the saint's habit of visiting the sick in the hospital every day, even in conditions of inclement weather and when his own bodily health was weak. At the hospital, Godfrey celebrated the Mass in the presence of the patients.[177] But the *Life* does not elucidate his behavior in the hospital as therapeutic.[178] Patients did not flock to him in order to touch him, converse with him, or request prayers or penitential acts. Rather, the author of his *Life*, Thomas of Villers, characterized his actions on behalf of patients in the hospital as demonstrations of his kindheartedness; his hospital visits "showed him[self] to be amiable and affable."[179]

The few instances of bodywork or caregiving attributed to the viri religiosi reveal important gender differences in the ways that communities remembered and recorded their therapeutic interactions with the women and men they regarded as holy.[180] The Cistercian lay brothers Simon of Aulne (d. 1229) and Arnulf of Villers (d. 1228), for example, attracted petitioners from faraway places to consult with them and to gain access to their prayers. Although the local public sought these men for consultation, they did not approach them for the purpose of cure, or at least they were not recorded as doing so in narrative accounts of their lives. Arnulf's hagiographer,

---

176. *De B. Waltero de Birbeke* (*BHL* 8794), in *AASS* January II, 447–50; ch. III.8, 448; ch. IV.12, 449.

177. He also frequently distributed apples and obols to the poor. See *De venerabili viro Godefrido Pachomio*, in *Analecta Bollandiana* 14 (1895): 263–68 (*BHL* 3579), chs. II, X, XI, XIII.

178. *De venerabili viro Godefrido Pachomio*. The *Life* is incomplete in this edition and is only available in a sixteenth-century manuscript in Vienna, Österreichische Nationalbibliothek MS Series nova 12854. It is worth exploring in further detail for Godfrey's contributions to healthcare. For example, the titles provided by the *Analecta Bollandiana* edition of chapters 13, 14, 16, and 24 indicate that he gathered apples for the poor, washed their feet and cleaned their clothes, pacified sinners with his prayers, and "was a servant of the sick everyday" (Godefridus servus Dei erat quodam tempore servitor infirmorum cottidie). Note that Godfrey Pachomius is the brother of Thomas of Villers, who wrote to his sister Alice in the Cistercian abbey of Vrouwenpark. I explore this correspondence in chapter 5.

179. *De venerabili viro Godefrido Pachomio*, ch. XII, 266: "Congregationi pauperum in infirmitorio hospitum languentium singulos visitando amabilem et affabilem se semper exhibebat."

180. Martha Newman and Alison More have provided nuanced readings of the *Lives* of lay brothers in the context of Cistercian hagiographic writing, readings that helpfully disrupt gender dichotomies. See Martha Newman, "Crucified by the Virtues: Monks, Laybrothers, and Women in Thirteenth-Century Cistercian Saints' *Lives*," in *Gender and Difference in the Middle Ages*, ed. Sharon Farmer and Carol Braun Pasternack (Minneapolis: University of Minnesota Press, 2003), 182–209; and More, "Convergence, Conversion, Transformation."

Goswin of Bossut, asserted that the saint's renown for holiness brought "quite a number from various places just to see him and commend themselves to his prayers. This number included persons of knightly rank from the vicinity of the grange. To some such visitors he foretold events that were to happen to them and which subsequently they did experience."[181] Like many of his contemporary mulieres religiosae, Arnulf attracted crowds of devotees during his lifetime. But those individuals who sought the saintly man came in search of his prophetic skills, not his bodily caregiving.

An anecdote in Goswin's *Life* of Arnulf provides further indication of gendered differences in modes of caregiving. He reports that a novice of Villers was afflicted with "two unbearable illnesses, the first being an almost continuous headache, such that he could scarcely keep the silence or maintain decorum until mealtime, and the second an illness that we judge too unseemly and unrespectable to publish and which we here cloak over out of decency."[182] Goswin characterized this troubled man as despairing for his health because he could find no remedy to cure it, which suggests that he had consulted with physicians or other healers prior to seeking Arnulf's aid.[183] When the novice finally reached Arnulf, it was not for the purpose of seeking cure. Instead, he "privately confided his impasse to Arnulf."[184] Arnulf then took pity on the man and prayed for him, assuring him that both illnesses would subside. Goswin did not offer this anecdote as evidence of Arnulf's therapeutic prowess or caregiving skills; instead, he delivered it among a series of tales illustrating Arnulf's visionary and prophetic abilities. Although the boy's afflictions were indeed remedied, Gowin did not portray Arnulf as the source of healing. Rather, Arnulf predicted the man's healing. The healing itself would come from another unnamed source. On display here are Arnulf's prophetic skills rather than his caregiving abilities; his prophetic expertise marked his sanctity.

---

181. *Vita Arnulfi conversi Villariensis (BHL 713)*, in *AASS* June VII, 566; hereafter *VAV*; translated by Martinus Cawley as "The Life of Arnulf, Laybrother of Villers," in *Send Me God: The Lives of Ida the Compassionate of Nivelles, Nun of la Ramée, Arnulf, Lay Brother of Villers, and Abundus, Monk of Villers, by Goswin of Bossut* (University Park: Pennsylvania State University Press, 2005), 125–98. *VAV* II.1 (2), 617; trans., 154: "plerique de diversis locis etiam quidam Milites, qui in vicinia grangiae habitabant, ad ipsum causa videndi eum venirent, et orationibus eius se commendarent. Quibus ille quaedum quae eis eventura erant praedixit."

182. *VAV* II.14 (40), 625; trans., 180: "Tribulationem et dolorem inveni: duabus siquidem [et importabilibus] infirmitatibus plurimum affligebatur, quarum altera erat dolor capitis, fere continuus, et tam validus ut silentii vix posset tenere censuram [et usque ad horam vescendi decorum sustinere] altera vero infirmitas turpis et inhonesta, cuius qualitatem [honestatis causa] non publicandam [sed palliandam] judicavimus."

183. *VAV* II.14 (40), 625: "quia nullum inveniebat remedium quod infirmitatibus suis adhiberet."

184. *VAV* II.14 (40), 625; trans., 180: "suam secretius incommoditatem intimavit."

The anonymously authored *Life* of Simon of Aulne also depicts the saint as facilitating a cure during his life, though it was certainly an unusual one.[185] Simon was a conversus at Aulne who became grange master and garnered a considerable reputation for his prophetic abilities. He was called upon by many, including Innocent III, for predictions about the future. At one point, he was reported to have resuscitated a boy who had been kidnapped by a demon and handed over to Ethiopians, who whipped him and fed him raw meat.[186] The boy's rite of confirmation finally vanquished the demon responsible for his condition. Thus his cure was attributed to sacramental intervention and exorcism. Simon's powers as an exorcist are featured again in the *Life* of Lutgard, in which he is reported to have traveled to Aywières at Lutgard's behest for assistance in a demonic expulsion.[187] In this instance, his power to treat through exorcism was represented as a supplement to Lutgard's diagnostics.

These episodes of intellection and expulsion can be considered from the social perspective of Arnulf and Simon as lay brothers rather than choir monks. Other Cistercian lay brothers were associated with similar stories of the ability to predict disease and its remedy.[188] Take the example of Herman, who lived on the Villers grange of Velp and was said to have possessed the gift of prophecy, from which he had foreknowledge of diseases and the ability to predict deaths.[189] Another lay brother of Villers, Arnold, was able to comfort a Cistercian novice by predicting that her mother would recover from illness in thirty days. His prediction is accompanied by a direct address: "Know, however, reader, that the man of God had not predicted these things through experience of the medicinal art, about which he had learned nothing, but through the revelation of the Holy Spirit who made many things

---

185. The *Life* of Simon of Aulne (*BHL* 7755) appears in Brussels, KBR, MS 8965–66; and *Vita beati Simonis: La vie du bienheureux frère Simon, convers à l'abbaye d'Aulne*, ed. Franciscus Moschus (Tournai: Desclée, 1968). Moschus's edition was first published in Arras in 1600 along with an edition of the *Life* of Arnulf and a poem about him. See Brian Noell, "Expectation and Unrest among Cistercian Laybrothers in the Twelfth and Thirteenth Centuries," *Journal of Medieval History* 32 (2006): 253–74; and Marie-Anselme Dimier, "Un découverte concernante le bienheureux Simon d'Aulne," *Cîteaux* 21 (1970): 302–5.

186. Jeroen Deploige unpacks this unusual event in "How Gendered Was Clairvoyance in the Thirteenth Century? The Case of Simon of Aulne," in *Speaking to the Eye: Sight and Insight in Text and Image 1150–1650*, ed. Thérèse de Hemptinne, Veerle Fraeters, and Mariá Eugenia Góngora (Turnhout: Brepols, 2013), 111.

187. *VLA* II.10.

188. As discussed below, see Juliana of Mont-Cornillon, Christina Mirabilis, and Lutgard of Aywières.

189. *De B. Nicolao et Sociis Narratio*, in *AASS* Nov. IV, 277–79; ch. 3, 278.

manifest to him for the profit of his neighbors."[190] This address locates the source of Arnold's skills in his clairvoyance rather than his knowledge of physica. Arnold's hagiographer presents his ability to offer prognosis as decidedly unlearned. He wanted readers to understand that this knowledge was revealed to Arnold, not learned from a book, and that it was this revelation that allowed him to provide comfort.

Similar in this prophetic manner of responding to health outcomes is the bizarre story of the priest John of Liège and his ward, Helias. John of Liège was the son of a widow-recluse named Odilia (d. 1220), about whom we have a thirteenth-century *Life* penned by an anonymous canon of Saint Lambert.[191] The *Life* of Odilia reports that John took it upon himself to adopt a boy named Helias who contracted leprosy while under his tutelage. John prayed for a cure, and the boy seemed to improve. But when Helias expressed his desire to move to Paris to continue his studies, John became irate and reversed his prayers so that he would inflict respiratory illness upon the boy. Although John once again prayed for his improvement, Helias never fully recovered and came to fear his supervisor so much that he sought to return home. John only became more aggrieved by Helias's eventual return to his family, though when John visited him on his deathbed the boy bequeathed his inheritance to the "servant of God" (*Dei famulo*).[192] While John continually prayed for the successful cure of the boy, he also ultimately exacerbated his pain. The story thus emphasizes John's strong-willed love of his adoptive son, and his prophetic abilities in matters of health; but not his acts of bodily care or therapeutic prowess.[193]

Given Thomas of Cantimpré's thorough attention to caregiving acts in his *Lives* of women, their near absence in his only *Life* of a male-identified saint, John of Cantimpré, calls for explanation. John was a priest in the chapel at Cantimpré, which had once served as a hospital; he became abbot in 1183 when the chapel was expanded into a house of Augustinian canons affiliated

---

190. *De B. Nicolao et Sociis Narratio*, in *AASS* Nov. IV, 277–79; ch. 6, 279E: "Scito tamen, lector, virum Dei hec non predixisse per experientiam artis medicinalis de qua nil noverat sed per revelationem Spiritus sancti qui sibi multa manifestavit ad profectum proximorum suorum."

191. Odilia's *Life* has been considered as a joint life with that of her son. See, for example, Anneke Mulder-Bakker's enumeration of the canon, in which she includes John as a subject of Odilia's *Life*. *Vita B. Odiliae Viduae Leodiensis*, ed. C. De Smedt, *Analecta Bollandiana* 13 (1894): 190–287 (*BHL* 6276); hereafter *VOL*. Mulder-Bakker, *Living Saints of the Thirteenth Century*.

192. *VOL* 236.

193. Jennifer Stemmle interprets the story in the context of leprosy, as one of resistance and rebellion in the face of tribulation and lack of care. Jennifer Stemmle, "From Cure to Care: Indignation, Assistance, and Leprosy in the High Middle Ages," in *Experiences of Charity, 1250–1650*, ed. Anne Scott (Farnham: Ashgate, 2015), 51–52.

with the Victorines in Paris. Acts of care appear twice in John's *Life*. Most notable is his prayerful intervention c. 1200 in the successful birth of Jeanne (Joan), the future Countess of Flanders and Hainaut. When Jeanne's mother, Countess Marie, had been laboring for nine days in grave pain, she summoned John for the assistance of his prayers. When he arrived, he "entered his oratory" and supplicated God to "bring forth a healthy heir to rule your people."[194] The countess thereupon found immediate relief, as Thomas recounted: "The girls who were assisting the countess came running to the door with immense joy and exultation announcing that their lady had given birth to a girl."[195] Note that his reference to "girls" affords these attendants no formal title; their work in assisting the countess's labor was undifferentiated from the expected behaviors attached to their identity as "girls."

What is most curious about Thomas's rendering of this event, then, is the meager interest he expresses in John's intervention as a therapeutic act, which he does not even describe as miraculous. Rather, Thomas lavishes his attention on the royal identities that John's prayer served. The tale itself is situated among a series of stories about John's illustrious connections with Countess Marie of Flanders and her husband, Baldwin. Thomas mentions that Marie baptized the child with the name of Jeanne, which he implies was in honor of the abbot. Thomas also provides a lengthy digression explaining that Jeanne would later marry Ferrand of Portugal, raise a faithful household, and found monastic institutions. The narration of the entire event reflects John's proximity to nobility rather than his caritative constancy or therapeutic acumen. His intervention might be read as royal rather than medical—his injunction was for an heir, not a cure. It is clear that John in this instance acted to restore salubrious conditions—he immediately heeded the needs of the parturient countess, came to her side, and prayed fervently on her behalf. But as hagiography, Thomas neglected to characterize these acts as virtuous in their health-giving aspects; instead, their saintly virtue derived from John's ability to ensure the reproduction of a noble lineage that preserved institutions of the faith.

Thomas's lack of attention to John's caregiving acts is brought into relief again in his description of another holy man that appears in John's *Life*, one of the six original converts who joined John's monastic house at Cambrai. Thomas identifies the man as Geoffrey from Flanders, singling out his

---

194. *VJC* III.iv, 313; trans., 118: "in regnum populi tui fructum patrie pariat salutarem."

195. *VJC* III.iv, 313; trans., 118: "ecce puelle secretarie comitisse ad ostium cum ingenti leticia et exultatione currentes, nunciant Christi famulo dominam suam feminei sexus sobolem peperisse."

devotion to the sick. In particular, Thomas notes Geoffrey's engineering of a special toilet seat to assist people suffering with a painful infirmity in their legs.[196] The absence of such hagiographic characterizations from John's own stories of sanctity suggest that his spiritual acumen was based on clerical authority rather than dedication to the sick.

Turning to the anonymously authored *Life* of Gobert of Aspremont (d. 1263), we find the blessed monk's caregiving featured as an aspect of his humility. His failure to adequately provision others serves as a lesson, perhaps suited to recent noble converts. Gobert was a noble knight who went on crusade to Jerusalem and made pilgrimage to Santiago de Compostella, during which time he underwent a deep spiritual conversion and eventually joined Villers monastery.[197] There, Gobert showed himself to be dedicated to almsgiving. He gave chickens to sick brothers and so generously distributed alms that his superiors began limiting his handouts.[198] Gobert's almsgiving is thus characterized by its limitations. For example, when he encountered a poor beguine near Villers, he attempted to provide shoes for her, but the ones he procured were so old and stiff that they were of no use to her. When he acquired oil that he planned to apply to soften them, he only succeeded in breaking the vial and embarrassing himself.[199] On another occasion, Gobert happened upon a pauper in a blizzard only to discover that he was unable to provide clothing to the threadbare and freezing man. He thus stripped off his own clothes so that he, too, could experience the frigid conditions.[200] These descriptions of failed almsgiving highlight Gobert's divestment and his personal tribulation for the sake of others' needs. They do not lead to restoration of health for others; it is Goswin who is transformed by his own actions, experiencing humility and depredation.

Gobert's caregiving acts can be usefully compared with those of Guerric, the master of conversi at Aulne. The *Life* of Guerric truly stands out among the viri religiosi for its portrayal of caregiving practices. The *Life* was written by an anonymous author around 1229, just over a decade after Guerric's death. Guerric was one of the founding members of the Cistercian abbey of

196. *VJC* I.xv, 273: "ita ut egre infirmantibus crura sua vice digestialis selle in naturalium purgationem aptaret."

197. As a reflection of the network of religious figures in this region, I note that a beguine named Emmeloth and Abundus of Villers both counseled Gobert in his decision to join the Cistercian order.

198. *Vita B. Goberti* (BHL 3570–1), in *AASS* August IV, 370–95. On his alms, see II.iv.63–65, 389.

199. *Vita B. Goberti*, II.iv.68–70, 390. He was disgraced because the oil dripping on his clothing appeared to be urine (Factus sum opprobrium hominum).

200. *Vita B. Goberti*, II.iv.71, 390.

Aulne. His *Life* extols Guerric's multifaceted contributions to bodily and spiritual care, celebrating in particular his humble almsgiving. It presents Guerric's acts of caregiving as subversive, a behavior he strove to conceal from his brothers because they often occasioned him to break with Cistercian communal regulations. For example, Guerric habitually pilfered from the monastery, snatching bits of bread, meat, butter, salt, and peas to distribute to local beggars.[201] In addition to coins and food, Guerric frequently resorted to dubious methods in order to distribute tunics and footwear, which he did in honor of Saint Martin.[202] The *Life* justifies his trickery on behalf of the poor and sick. For example, in one instance, Guerric refused to hear confession from the conversi until they produced alms; the saint demanded, "Therefore give me money that I may give to the poor / So that I may cure your wounds with the medicine of money."[203] What is significant here is that Guerric's "medicine" was not applied to the poor through alms, but to the conversi by divesting them of material attachment and thereby curing the spiritual wounds caused by wealth and greed.

Guerric's ability to aid ailing bodies is particularly pronounced in several specific episodes that his hagiographer treats with detailed attention, rather than alluding to his generic charity. In one instance, a man from Landenias, near Aulne, sought Guerric's assistance in helping his wife manage a difficult labor, which had already lasted six days. Guerric agreed to pray on behalf of the parturient woman, but urged him to have strong faith that she would deliver their child safely.[204] Here, the hagiographer issues a petition for faith similar to those found in the posthumous healing miracles of female saints. In another case, Guerric flouted a specific prohibition placed on him by the abbot of Aulne and allowed petitioners to gather water from the purification vessel he used to celebrate the Mass.[205] Guerric's ablution water, the *Life* attested, was efficacious in healing fevers. On another occasion, one of the lay brothers asked permission to leave Aulne because his mother was too poor to afford a cloak (*nuda*). Although forbidding the lay brother to break his vows, Guerric clandestinely arranged to send the mother his own

201. *Vita domni werrici* (BHL 8865), in *Catalogus codicum hagiographicorum bibliothecae Regiae Bruxellensis* (Brussels: Typis Polleunis, Ceuterick et Lefebure, 1886), 1:447.

202. *Vita domni werrici*, 447, 452; Guerric is said to have given away a pair of shoes every year on the feast of St. Martin.

203. *Vita domni werrici*, 449: "Ergo mihi detis nummos, quos pauperibus dem / Ut plagas vestras nummi medicamine curem."

204. *Vita domni werrici*, 456: "esto fide fortis."

205. *Vita domni werrici*, 456.

new tunic (*tunica recens*).[206] Each of these stories indicates that Guerric maintained a reputation as a source of healing in the community surrounding Aulne. Folks traveled to Aulne from nearby villages for the explicit purpose of requesting his therapeutic aid. His hagiographer indicated that this regular service to the poor was recognized by the local public, and it was a source of his perceived sanctity.

It is possible that the difference presented by Guerric's *Life* can be explained in part through its form and its manuscript transmission. Unlike the other *Lives* of viri religiosi discussed here, Guerric's was composed in verse.[207] The two extant manuscript witnesses of the *Vita domni werrici* from the late thirteenth and early fourteenth centuries show that it circulated with other versified and affective texts. One of these manuscripts is KBR 4459–70, which I will discuss in detail in chapter 5, is a miscellany that contains, in addition to liturgical and sacramental material, the *Lives* of five local mulieres religiosae, thus grouping Guerric with them and associating him with their memory. A second manuscript copy appears in KBR II–1047, compiled at Aulne in the late thirteenth and early fourteenth centuries and containing an array of songs, liturgical feasts, and rhythmic texts on such subjects as contempt for the world and the significance of the Mass. The performance aspect of the texts with which it circulated, in addition to its poetic form, suggest that Guerric's *Life* was read aloud and may have participated in paraliturgical therapeutic events.[208] Guerric's *Life*, then, was not only distinct from those of the other viri religiosi in its portrayal of caregiving; the form and audience of his *Life* appear to have served a different purpose than those that were read at Villers. A purely speculative suggestion: the poetic form of Guerric's *Life* may have generated affinities with the *Lives* of female saints in the corpus, oriented as they were toward affective caregiving.

That only one person among the viri religiosi appears to have garnered any kind of significant local reputation for healing suggests some conclusions about the ways that thirteenth-century communities shared stories of the holy people in their midst, how they were remembered and recorded in

---

206. *Vita domni werrici*, 451. Guerric was noted for giving away a number of cloaks and tunics. See also 451–52.

207. Deploige, "How Gendered Was Clairvoyance?," 104. His *Life* represents the oldest hagiographic text from Aulne. Walter of Bierbeek received a verse translation in the fifteenth century. It is preserved in Brussels, KBR, MS 1780–1781, along with the prose *Life*. The *Life* of Franco of Archennes is also in verse, but the dating is inconclusive. It is recorded in the *Historia monasterii villariensis in Brabantia* II.1333–39.

208. On the oral delivery of verse texts, see Andreas Haug, "Performing Latin Verse: Text and Music in Early Medieval Versified Offices," in *The Divine Office in the Latin Middle Ages*, ed. Margot Fassler and Rebecca Baltzer (Oxford: Oxford University Press, 2000), 278–99.

their interactions with neighbors. While men involved in charitable health-care could rely on the protection of guilds, confraternities, and other pro-fessional and ecclesiastical structures, religious women wishing to fulfill a caritative mission navigated ephemeral and informal sites of care. Wills, statutes, and charters substantiate the portraits of healthcare contained in the *Lives* of mulieres religiosae and enable the construction of a picture of healthcare distribution in the thirteenth-century Low Countries, one in which women's caregiving and prayers occupied a recognized and valued position in the spectrum of healthcare options. These were hardly marginal roles within the thirteenth-century medical marketplace. Religious women's bodily care in hospitals, leprosaria, infirmaries, at sickbeds and gravesites, and through bodily contact shaped how communities perceived their care and constructed what they looked for when approaching them for salutary purposes.

Stories about the therapeutic efficacy of mulieres religiosae reflect rela-tionships of gratitude for the care and cure that religious women provided. They did not depict women as asserting universalizing claims to body knowledge. Instead, stories of feminine caregiving celebrated local, inti-mate relationships and affective efficacies. These stories portray the work-ings of medicine as a social practice, as it took place in communities removed from the elite world of scholastic physicians. In these scenarios, the man-agement of illness appears as practical and emotional rather than theoreti-cal or universal. As Goswin of Bossut explained, "Whoever comes to [Ida] weighed down and confined by any kind of sorrow and trouble can draw from her and obtain for themselves whatever consoling relief they need."[209] *Omnimode consolationis*: the maladies that religious women treated do not map clearly onto biomedical categories, and their charitable care fell in between the authoritative loci of physicians and clerics. They treated both the body and the soul, living and dead, individual and community. But they lacked the external authority to create a knowledge tradition or profession around any specific aspect of their practice.

In the absence of their own authority to explain practice and control narrative, we have hagiography. The hagiographic corpus points to diverse acts of care shared among the mulieres religiosae, modes of care that took place within their infirmaries, hospices, leprosaria, at sickbeds and burial sites, and in private homes. "While she lives, she now performs spiritual

---

209. *VIN* XXVI, 264; trans., 72: "ad quam quicumque venerint cuiuscumque gravati angustia doloris et tribulationis, haurient ab ipsa et impetrabunt levamen omnimode consolationis."

miracles; after death she will work bodily ones."[210] Thomas's adage forecasts; it translates labor into sacred terms, and in so doing, it provides cover. The miracles bodily and spiritual, the virginal holiness of feminine bodies, the insistence on the divine source of their therapies: the hagiographic corpus legitimized and enabled religious women, for some time at least, to practice acts of care.

---

210. *VLA* III.18 (9), 245; trans., 289: "spiritualia miracula in vita nunc facit; corporalia post mortem efficiet."

PART II

Therapeutic Knowledge

CHAPTER 3

Empirical Bodies

Competing Theories of Therapeutic Authority

"On bended knee," Teodorico Borgognoni
instructed, "you should say three times the paternoster, and when these
have been said, let the arrow be grasped with both hands joined as they are
and let be said, 'Nicodemus drew out the nails from our Lord's hands and
feet, and let this arrow be drawn out.' And it will come out forthwith."[1] The
instructions for this arrow-removing procedure can be found in the surgical
treatise of Teodorico Borgognoni (d. 1296), who, in addition to serving as
bishop of Bitonto and Cervia, occasionally taught medicine and surgery at
the University of Bologna. While Teodorico transmitted a small sample of
verbal remedies like this one, he confessed that they sounded to him more
like the false remedies of a *vetula* than the reasoned pharmacy of a learned

---

1. Teodorico Borgognoni, *Chirurgia*, in *Ars chirurgia Guidonis Cauliaci* (Venice, 1546), bk. I, ch. 22,
143v; *The Surgery of Theodoric*, trans. Eldridge Campbell and James Colton (New York: Appleton,
1955), 88: "Flexis genibus dicatur ter oratio dominica, scilicet pater noster: quibus dictis, accipiatur
sagitta cum ambabus manibus simul iunctis, et dicantur, 'Nicodemus extraxit clavos de manibus et
pedibus domini, et extrahatur sagitta' et exibit statim." Note that this source is available as a digital
record through the National Library of Medicine, NLM Unique ID 2249046R. It was widely translated into vernaculars, including Catalan, Castilian, French, Italian, English, and German. See Lluís
Cifuentes, "Teodorico Borgognoni," in *Medieval Science, Technology, and Medicine: An Encyclopedia*, ed.
Thomas Glick, Steven Livesey, and Faith Wallis (New York: Routledge, 2005), 95–96.

physician.[2] And yet, Teodorico was unable to jettison the remedy. After all, he understood it to work. In order to rationalize the remedy's transmission, however, he issued an apologia that shed any suggestion of its feminine origin. "It does not trouble me to write down certain empirical experiments," he confessed, explaining that "certain experienced men swear by [them]."[3] This remedy was taught to him by a learned man, not a spurious woman. Thomas's insistence on the verbal remedy's masculine origin was necessary because certain empirical remedies were already feminized, remedies that incorporated the performance of affective prayer, soothing words, and the command to have faith. As we have seen, the religious women who provided healthcare services to urban populations in the lowlands were well regarded as specialists in treating the infirm with consolatory and efficacious words and practices. When other medical practitioners relied on these methods, as they often did, they sought to distinguish their basis of authority, to ground them in a textual tradition. I turn in this chapter to masculine constructions and conceptualizations of therapeutic efficacy in a variety of discourses: medical, hagiographic, theological. Rather than resistance and contradiction, we find shared conceptual premises in discussions of the soul's effect on the health and comportment of the body, in the salutary role of hope and belief, and in the special therapeutic powers of certain esteemed individuals. A variety of thirteenth- and early fourteenth-century authoritative discourses, I show, maintained an interest in accommodating the effects of the soul on the body and in explaining unexpected bodily transformations. Their differences stem not from their authors' opposing knowledge systems, but rather from opposing constructions of diagnostic and therapeutic power.

By 1300, scholastic physicians had devised a distinct category of knowledge about the body, by which their diagnostic practices and remedies might be distinguished from those of other healers.[4] That category of knowledge was based on physical, material principles, as made clear in their chosen moniker, *physici*, or those who specialized in the physical properties that

---

2. Teodorico Borgognoni, *Chirurgia*, bk. III, ch. 1, 158v: "quia magis videntur nobis vetularum esse quam prudentis viri."

3. Teodorico Borgognoni, *Chirurgia*, bk. II, ch. 23, 143v; trans., 87: "Non piget . . . quaedam experimenta empirica scribere que quosdam peritos cum assertione plurima novimus affirmare."

4. On the triumph of scholastic medicine, see Nancy Siraisi, *Medieval and Early Renaissance Medicine: An Introduction to Knowledge and Practice* (Chicago: University of Chicago Press, 1990). Jerome Bylebyl notes that already by the ninth century, *physica* had lost its classical meaning of "natural philosophy" and was beginning to displace *medicina*. It was only during the twelfth century that *physicus* came to replace *medicus* as a medical expert. Bylebyl, "The Medical Meaning of *Physica*," *Osiris* 6 (1990): 16. See also Faye Getz, "Charity, Translation, and the Language of Medical Learning in Medieval England," *Bulletin of the History of Medicine* 64 (1990): 1–17; and Katherine Park, *Doctors and Medicine in Early Renaissance Florence* (Princeton: Princeton University Press, 1985), 58–59.

determine human health. Throughout the later Middle Ages, as *physici* circulated academic treatises on their specialized medical art, producing hundreds of commentaries on the recently translated Greco-Arabic corpus, they made marginal space for properties that could not be determined based on physical composition of substances. They sought to accommodate the unexpected, the unpredictable, the supernatural, and the divine. Take, for example, the English physician, Thomas of Fayreford, who recommended that, while preparing *materia medica*, physicians might imagine their practices in terms of biblical precedents.[5] In his recipe for gathering herbs, Thomas employed the vernacular to instruct medical practitioners to pluck herbs from the earth in the name of the Father, the Son, and the Holy Ghost. He directed them also to recite three Paternosters and Ave Marias, then, in Latin, to utter the prescribed blessing:

> Almighty, who has conceded virtue into various herbs, deign to bless and sanctify these herbs. And just as you gave your apostles the power of spurning serpents and scorpions so wherever medicine from these herbs will be presented, let every infirmity and weakness be expelled and your benign grace be bestowed on sickness.[6]

Thomas fashioned his script for a medical prayer much like the form of a sacramental. The practitioner who uttered this prayer hoped through it to channel grace into herbs. The charm induced patients and practitioners to imagine Fayreford's herbal remedy as a conveyance for divine grace. In this way, the empirical remedy relied on medical theatrics that amplified performance to the status of remedy, a mechanism for altering affective and perceptive states. Both the herbs and the words were necessary for efficacy; the words were part of the treatment.[7] The physician's prayer enhanced the herbs' efficacy, converting them into a medical ingredient, an essential component of cure.

---

5. Thomas of Fayreford was writing between 1420 and 1460. He was more of a provincial doctor, who never received a medical degree. He did, however, attend the University of Oxford. On Fayreford, see Peter Jones, "Thomas Fayreford: An English Fifteenth-Century Medical Practitioner," in *Medicine from the Black Death to the French Disease*, ed. Roger French, John Arrizabalaga, Andrew Cunnigham, and Luis García-Ballester (Aldershot: Ashgate, 1998), 156–83.

6. British Library, MS Harley 2558, fol. 63v: "Omnes qui variis herbis virtutem concessisti has herbas benedicere et sanctificare dignare. et sicut apostolis tuis dedisti potestatem calcandi super serpentes et scorpiones, sic ubicumque medicina ex hiis fuerit exibita. omnis infirmatis et langor expellatur et gratia tua benyngna infirmitatibus tribuatur." My transcription and translation are guided by Lea Olsan, "Charms and Prayers in Medieval Medical Theory and Practice," *Social History of Medicine* 16.3 (2003): 359.

7. On the use of combined words and herbs in Ghaambo, Tanzania, see Steve Feierman, "Explanation and Uncertainty in the Medical World of Ghaambo," *Bulletin of the History of Medicine* 74.2 (2000): 317–44.

A similar logic is evident in Gilbertus Anglicus's *Compendium medicinae* (written between 1200 and 1250), in which he relays a "divine charm" (*divino carmine*) that he only included, he insisted, because it had been passed down from "the ancients."[8] Known as the "Three Good Brothers" charm, it involved three brothers who were traveling to the Mount of Olives to gather herbs for a remedy that would heal wounds.[9] Along the way, according to the charm, Christ intercepted the brothers and offered them an alternative cure. But before providing them with the remedy, Christ insisted that the brothers swear on the crucifix not to receive payment for its use, which indicates a distaste for charging payment in exchange for healthcare services. Christ then proceeded to explain to the brothers that they should apply wool and olive oil to the wound while pronouncing these words:

> Just as Longinus the Hebrew pierced the side of our Lord Jesus Christ, who did not bleed nor was corrupted nor suffered pain nor decay, so do not bring that about in this wound which now I charm, in the name of the Father and the Son and the Holy Spirit. Amen. And say the paternoster three times.[10]

Here, the remedy required the practitioner to provide a material cure, oiled wool, and to inhabit a narrative by performing a biblical role. Situating themself in the *historiale* (the historical setting of the charm), the practitioner encompassed the patient in the narrative as they administered the remedy, calling the wounded one's attention to the analogous wound that Christ bore, a wound that ultimately secured human life.[11]

While the 1510 printing of the *Compendium* directs the practitioner to "believe and say" (*credite et dicite*), earlier manuscript copies omit the direction to believe.[12] Was this later insertion, which commanded the user's faith, premised on the sense that faith in such remedies had been eroded? Was

---

8. Gilbertus Anglicus, *Compendium medicinae* (Lyon: Iacobum Saccon, 1510), fol. 327r: "Quae dixerunt antiqui."

9. On the development of this charm, see Lea Olsan, "The Three Good Brothers Charm: Some Historical Points," *Incantatio* 1 (2011): 48–78. Olsan points out that the Longinus charm also circulated independent of the Three Good Brothers charm.

10. "Sicut longius ebreus cum lancea in latere domini nostri ihu. x. percussit nec sanguinavit nec ranclavit nec doluit nec putredinem fecit: nec faciat plaga ista quam carmo? In nomine patris et f. et s.s. amen. ter dicite pater noster." From Olsan's transcription of New Haven, Yale University Library, Cushing/Whitney, MS 19, fols. 44v-45r, in her "Three Good Brothers Charm," Appendix I: Charm Texts, 64–65.

11. On the *historiale* and other components of charms, see Edina Bozóky, *Charmes et prières apotropaïque*, Typologie des Sources du Moyen Âge Occidental, fasc. 86 (Turnhout: Brepols, 2003).

12. Yale University Library, Cushing/Whitney, MS 19, fol. 44vb states only, "dicite"; the 1510 print edition includes the words "credite et dicite." See Gilbertus Anglicus, *Compendium medicinae*.

it necessary to prompt practitioners and patients to inwardly assent to the externally executed words of the cure? Perhaps the instruction "to believe" was not required in earlier iterations of the cure because thirteenth-century European Christians were awash in therapeutic practices predicated upon the requirement of faith for somatic transformation. The alteration might also point to later concerns about superstitious practice, an apprehension that if performed through the words alone, without faith in Christ's wounds as the ultimate source of therapeutic power, then the charm amounted to perfidious magic.[13] Physicians understood that patients had to *believe* in the efficacy of their remedies, had to experience real hope for physical transformation. Belief in the efficacy of a remedy, confidence in the power of the practitioner, and true hope of bodily recovery were essential components of the therapeutic process. This internal conviction, a conversion of the self, was present in several localizations of cultural discourse in the later Middle Ages. It was premised on the soul's causality, the idea that the soul could effect material transformation. In this chapter, I develop an interpretive lens for capturing among these diverse discourses a shared model of the body that encompassed psychological and emotional aspects of the self. By attending to the gendered nature of these discourses, we can glimpse how the body of the practitioner emerged as the site through which therapeutic authority was negotiated.

A matrix of late medieval discourses—medical, theological, hagiographic—explored internal affective states and their potential for bodily expression, questioning the role of the soul and its accidents in generating somatic transformation. These discourses express overlapping approaches to health and care, approaches that were not necessarily incompatible, though they may have operated independently. They all affirmed that affective states had potentially profound effects on the body. These converging discourses generated ambiguities about the boundaries between the material

---

13. Only sacraments could work *ex opere operato* because God ordained that they should work, as it were, "from the work" itself. See Thomas Aquinas, *Summa Theologica*, iii.64. On growing concerns about superstitious practice in this period, see Michael Bailey, *Fearful Spirits, Reasoned Follies: The Boundaries of Superstition in Late Medieval Europe* (Ithaca: Cornell University Press, 2013). Generally speaking, the authors discussed in this chapter, all of whom were active in the thirteenth and early fourteenth centuries, did not see themselves as practicing or theorizing magic, even when they discussed verbal remedies. As Bailey, Richard Kieckhefer, and others have shown, magic was a contextual category, the meaning and contents of which changed depending on how it was used and in which historical period it was used. Kieckhefer has recently suggested that we consider magic as "an aggregating term"; he points to the encompassing elements of this conceptual category, as its various contents and associations are not linked by any single essence. See Richard Kieckhefer, "Rethinking How to Define Magic," in *The Routledge History of Medieval Magic*, ed. Catherine Rider and Sophie Page (New York: Routledge, 2019), 15–25.

and immaterial, and about which practitioners possessed the authority to administer treatments to ensouled bodies. Joseph Ziegler and Naama Cohen-Hanegbi have produced lucid monographs that detail the many mutually informing links between medical and religious discourses in the later European Middle Ages, as well as the institutions and personnel that structured them. Here I build on their insights, focusing on the place of the gendered body in those discourses. Embodied performance, I show, played a role in establishing medical authority. The body of the saintly mulier or holy virgin and the body of the learned male physician appear in these discourses as sites of concentrated therapeutic power; the therapeutic power of one was supernatural and derived from grace, while that of the other was material and naturally occurring.

Scholastic physicians' explanations of the efficacy of verbal remedies display an interest in controlling their proliferation or their use by empirical healers, the unschooled, and women. Meanwhile, hagiographers and theologians were keen to delimit the conditions of the material manifestation of grace and of the physical effects of prayer and contemplation. While physicians agreed that nonmaterial forces associated with the soul might have tremendous effects on the body, they speculated on how to predict their influence and, moreover, how to control them. At the same time, hagiographic and theological discussions of somatic transformation suggest anxiety about what their authors perceived was a diminished role of care of the soul in thirteenth-century medical practice. Taken together, these scattered discourses affirm an overarching model of the body as permeable to nonmaterial forces. Different disciplines often employed distinct terminology to give language to the unseen causes of material transformation in the world, but among all genres of discussion, the assertion of control over the mechanics of that transformation was paramount.

The Matter of Emotions in Medical Theory

Physicians categorized the charms and verbal remedies of Thomas Fayreford, Teodorico Borgognoni, and Gilbertus Anglicus as *empirica*, remedies that could be known only through experience, not by rational deduction from their material properties. Although no medical authorities condemned charms outright, as Lea Olsan has shown, their theories of causation "br[oke] down when it comes to certain areas of practice."[14] Scholastic physicians' discussions sought to explain the properties of medicine in rational, material,

---

14. Olsan, "Charms and Prayers," 343.

and universal terms. Empirica thus fit uneasily in academic medical treatises because they could not be explained by the principles of humoral medicine and thus could be known only through experience on an individual basis.[15] In twelfth-century Salerno, learned practitioners had already begun to create a new category of healer.[16] *Physici* sought to distinguish their remedies and approach to the body from the irrational prayers and remedies of unlettered folks and *vetulae*, a "demarcation of boundaries."[17] This new medical knowledge was premised on mastering a canon of freshly translated medical texts such as the *Isagoge*, the *Pantegni*, and the *Premnon physicon*.[18] Supplied with a new form of knowledge, physicians ascertained the constitution of matter and the cosmos to explain the relationship between their individual components, such as elements, qualities, and humors, and the processes of illness and health in living bodies. Scholastic physicians sought to describe bodily change according to the theory of complexion. Complexion referred to the constitution of a sublunary body's (animal, vegetal, or mineral) elements and primary qualities. Physical transformation was understood to be caused by qualitative forces of elements, their degrees of hot, cold, wet, and dry.[19]

The soul played an important role in these theorizations of bodily transformation. Greek medical tradition held that the soul's affects exerted an influence on bodily health. For instance, Aristotle's *De anima* recognized that, owing to their ensouled bodies, humans experienced physical ramifications

---

15. Magic, however, did have a rationale. See Richard Kieckhefer, "The Specific Rationality of Medieval Magic," *American Historical Review* 99.3 (1994): 813–36. Kieckhefer sorts charms into three categories: prayers, blessings, and adjurations. Of the type of charms discussed in these texts, the most useful categorization is also the most nebulous. As Kieckhefer states, "For *some* medieval people charms would count as magic. Other people would have been hard pressed to distinguish between them and purely religious prayers. And perhaps the majority of users would simply not have reflected on the question: if the charms worked, that was more important than how they worked." Richard Kieckhefer, *Magic in the Middle Ages*, (Cambridge: Cambridge University Press, 1989), 75.

16. Luis García-Ballester, "The Construction of a New Form of Learning and Practicing Medicine in Medieval Latin Europe," *Science in Context* 8 (1995): 79–85.

17. Naama Cohen-Hanegbi, *Caring for the Living Soul: Emotions, Medicine, and Penance in the Late Medieval Mediterranean* (Leuven: Brill, 2017), 71.

18. The Latin contextualization and development of medical knowledge was made possible by the translation activity of such figures as Constantine the African, Gerard of Cremona, and Burgundio of Pisa.

19. As Michael McVaugh has discussed, although the primary quality of medicines was ordinarily uncontroversial, their physiological actions within the body tended to introduce debate among physicians. Galen had recognized that clinical results vary. The Arabic corpus, particularly Al-kindī and Ibn Rušd (Averroes), theorized that the amount of hotness in a medicine depended on its degree and on the dose used. Physicians worked out their prescriptions according to the medicinal degree required of each patient, thereby altering a patient's complexion. See Michael McVaugh, "The Experience-Based Medicine of the Thirteenth Century," *Early Science and Medicine* 14 (2009): 105–30.

of their emotional lives. He linked the matter of human emotions in the body to its form in the soul.[20] To Galen, the passions of the soul were one of the six external causes that were constantly acting on the body in ways that altered the balance of the internal qualities and, ultimately, the state of humoral balance.[21] In proper proportion and magnitude, the passions promoted wellness, but out of order, they encouraged disease.[22] According to ancient tradition, then, the "passions of the soul," or what roughly corresponds to our current understanding of emotions, were a gateway, a hinge between body and soul. Beginning with the translation into Latin of the *Liber ysagogorum* of Hunayn ibn Ishaq (d. 873; Johannitius), a Nestorian Christian scholar at the Bayt al-Hikma in Baghdad, practitioners carved out a privileged place for the passions of the soul in determining the health of the body.[23] The *Isagoge*, as it was known in Latin Christendom, placed an emphasis on regimen or regulation of the six factors (*occasiones*): food and drink; sleep and waking; air; evacuation and repletion; motion and rest; and the passions of the soul. These factors determined health and, if left unregulated, caused humoral imbalance and thus illness, the contra-natural state.

In Hunayn's scheme, the passions (or "accidents") of the soul (*accidentia animae*) could produce important effects on the body by raising or lowering its natural heat and thereby causing the spirits to move away from or toward the center of the body. Scholastic physicians readily absorbed this teaching on the passions of the soul and their effects on the body. Arnald of Villanova, for example, taught that sadness and fear produced a cooling effect on the body, whereas joy and wrath caused a centrifugal movement that diffused the vital spirit and natural heat away from the heart and toward the

---

20. On the diffusion of Aristotle's *De anima* among physicians and theologians, see Cohen-Hanegbi, *Caring for the Living Soul*, 68–99.

21. See Galen's *Ars medica*, in *Opera omnia*, ed. C. G. Kühn (Hildesheim: Reprographischer Nachdruck der Ausgabe Leipzig, 1964–65), vol. 1.

22. L. J. Rather, "The Six Things Non Natural: A Note on the Origin and Fate of a Doctrine and a Phrase," *Clio Medica* 3 (1968): 339.

23. On this transmission of ancient medical tradition on the passions of the soul, see Pedro Gil Sotres, "The Regimens of Health," in *Western Medical Thought from Antiquity to the Middle Ages*, ed. Mirko Grmek (Cambridge, MA: Harvard University Press, 2002); Luis García-Ballester, "Artifex factivus sanitatis: Health and Medical Care in Medieval Latin Galenism," in *Knowledge and the Scholarly Medical Traditions* (Cambridge: Cambridge University Press, 1995), 127–50; Marie G. Balty-Guedson, "Bayt al-Hikmah et politique culturelle du calife al-Mamun," *Medicina nei Secoli* 6 (1994): 275–91. Haly Abbas connected Galen's six causes to Hunayn's six factors, labeling them as six "non-naturals" because they were external to the body and caused health or sickness. Glending Olson, *Literature as Recreation in the Middle Ages* (Ithaca: Cornell University Press, 1982), 41; P. H. Niebyl, "The Non-Naturals," *Bulletin of the History of Medicine* 45.5 (1971): 486–92.

periphery of the body.[24] It is for such reasons, he explained, that embarrassment caused the cheeks to blush. Through the estimative power, the mind judged an external object or inner thought in a positive or negative manner. The species of the image created in the mind acted on the radical spirit responsible for radical heat, generating a local movement in the heart of contraction or dilation. For this reason, the *Salernitan Regimen* commenced with instructions for patients to consider their emotional state. The first precept of the regimen advised that patients should "avoid great charges, thoughts, and cares because thought dries a man's body . . . and leaves a man's spirits in desolation."[25]

While physicians sought to establish their approach to bodily health as one dependent on rational and universal patterns in the physical world, intellectual tensions emerged over the degree of consistency with which one could trust medical remedies. Galen had recognized that the physiological effects of various therapies were open to interpretation.[26] Within the body, the physiological actions of a medicine's primary qualities were uncertain, as Roger Bacon explained in *On the Errors of the Physicians*. Bacon noted conflicts among ancient authorities on the proper dosages and known effects of certain drugs.[27] Arnald of Villanova listed for medical students an exhausting number of contingencies that affected disease states including not only the specificities of a patient's diet and complexion, but also the direction their window faced and their proximity to barking dogs.[28] In other words, the sheer number of contingent forces operating within and outside of the body meant that some laws of medicine were open to interpretation. This uncertainty compelled physicians to ponder the unpredictable effects of certain

---

24. Fernando Salmón, "The Physician as Cure," in *Ritual Healing: Magic, Ritual, and Medical Therapy from Antiquity until the Early Modern Period*, ed. Ildikó Csepregi and Charles Burnett (Florence: SISMEL, 2012), 207–8. See Arnald of Villanova's *Regimen sanitatis ad regem Aragonum*, in *Opera medica omnia*, ed. Michael McVaugh, Luis García-Ballester, and Juan Paniagua (Barcelona: Editions Universitat Barcelona, 1996), 436: "ira est motus sanguinis circa cor propter appetitum vindicte."

25. *Regimen sanitatis salerni* (London: Alsop, 1649), 2.

26. McVaugh, "The Experience-Based Medicine," 113. McVaugh cites Galen's *Commentary on Hippocrates' Aphorisms* I.1: "If someone is treated with different medicines, and improves or worsens as a result, it is not easy to decide which of these helped or harmed him; for example, if the patient sleeps smoothly and after his sleep is anointed with an epithimium, then given a cataplasm or a clyster, and finally given some dish to eat, after which he has a sudden bowel movement, it isn't easy to decide which of these things helped or harmed him."

27. McVaugh, "The Experience-Based Medicine," 114; Roger Bacon, *De erroribus medicorum*, in *Fratris Rogeri Bacon De retardatione accidentium senectutis*, ed. Andrew G. Little and Edward Withington (Oxford: Clarendon Press, 1928), 164.

28. Michael McVaugh and Luis García-Ballester, "Therapeutic Method in the Later Middle Ages: Arnau de Vilanova on Medical Contingency," *Caduceus* 11 (1995): 73–86. The list can be found in Arnald's third lectio in *Repetitio super aphorismo Hippocraticus "Vita Brevis."*

remedies. It produced a place for the medical imagination to roam. If not by supernatural forces, then how did such popular remedies as charms, amulets, and ligatures take effect on the body?[29]

Medical explanations of *empirici* hinged on the soul's influence over the body, and on the practitioner's power over the souls of patients.[30] While scholastic physicians explained the potential efficacy of verbal remedies in a variety of ways, all agreed on the necessity of internal conviction, the patient's hope for cure, and the physician's ability to inspire confidence. As Teodorico's remedy for fistula concluded, "I have set down the aforesaid because there are some who have great faith in procedures of this sort, and perchance their faith helps them."[31] Dulcet words and a convincing performance complemented the physician's material remedies, taking effect on the patient's soul. As we will see in this chapter, certain emotion states would become valuable pharmacy. But competing theories of therapeutic power would determine who was licensed to prescribe them.

The Body of the Physician

Like physicians writing in Hebrew and Arabic, those writing in Latin in thirteenth-century western Europe showed great interest in the occult or hidden properties of objects, those that could not be known or predicted by rational principles.[32] In general, thirteenth-century theologians and physicians were interested in causality, in what properties caused changes in the natural world.[33] When those causes were not explicable according to observable elemental properties, learned authors sometimes looked for explanation in occult properties or powers (*virtutes occultae*). Islamicate medical commentaries provided the intellectual foundation for Latin Christian physicians who sought to explain the effects of occult powers and unpredictable remedies that relied on them.

---

29. On these wide-ranging discussions of verbal efficacy, see the comprehensive analysis of Béatrice Delaurenti, *La puissance des mots: Virtus verborum; Débats doctrinaux sur le pouvoir des incantations au Moyen Âge* (Paris: Éditions du Cerf, 2007).

30. While verbal remedies were empirica, they were distinct from complexionate remedies, such as theriac or magnetic lodestone.

31. *The Surgery of Theodoric*, bk. III, ch. 2, 18.

32. On the process of translating and transmitting Greek, Hebrew, and Arabic magical knowledge in the Latin West, see David Pingree, *From Astral Omens to Astrology: From Babylon to Bīkāner* (Rome: Italian Institute for Africa and the Orient, 1997); and Marie-Thérèse d'Alverny, *Transmission des textes philosophiques et scientifiques au Moyen Âge*, ed. Charles Burnett (Aldershot: Variorum, 1994).

33. The manuscript transmission of Bartholomeus Anglicus's *De proprietates rerum* (c. 1230–40) is a good example of this interest. See Elizabeth Keen, *The Journey of a Book: Bartholomew the Englishman and the Properties of Things* (Canberra: Australian National University Press, 2007).

Qūsta ibn Lūqā (d. c. 910), for example, posited a continuum between body, spirit, and soul, a nexus that might respond to occult properties.[34] "The powers of the soul follow the mixture of the body," he contended. "In the case of having a well-balanced body mixture, one will have a well-balanced spirit in one's body and well-balanced activities of one's soul. In the case of having a body mixture which fails to achieve its correct equilibrium, one will have spirit and psychic activities which also fail to achieve balance."[35] His treatise *The Difference between the Spirit and the Soul* outlined the relationship between body and soul, which he understood as mediated by the spirit.[36] Seeking to reconcile Plato, Aristotle, and Galen on souls, spirits, and faculties, Qūsta proposed the existence of two spirits, which permeated the body from the heart and brain.[37] The "vital spirit" maintained life, respiration, and pulse, while the "psychic spirit" governed sensation and movement.[38] The psychic spirit was formed from the vital spirit, and the vital spirit was formed from the matter of the air. The body would remain healthy as long as the spirit was equally distributed throughout its members and organs. According to Qūsta's theory, the human being thus had one soul that imparted movement and sensation to the body by animating the vital spirit. The incorporeal soul acted on the body through the agency of the material spirit.[39] In this way, according to Qūsta, the spirit could act as a causal entity.[40] Twelfth- and

---

34. Judith Wilcox and John Riddle, "Qūsta ibn Lūqā's *Physical Ligatures* and the Recognition of the Placebo Effect: With an Edition and Translation," *Medieval Encounters* 1.1 (1995): 22. Qūsta's *Physical Ligatures* or *On Incantations, Adjurations, and Suspensions about the Neck* was translated into Latin by Constantine the African and was widely distributed in Europe (there are now fifteen extant manuscripts in European libraries). The earliest extant manuscript is from the twelfth century and includes other works translated by Constantine. Wilcox and Riddle postulate that Constantine could have translated it indirectly from Ibn al-Jazzar (27).

35. *A Philosophy Reader from the Circle of Miskawayh* (Cambridge: Cambridge University Press, 2014), 198. The philosophy reader is a translation of Oxford, MS Marsh 539, an anthology of philosophical texts that circulated in the eleventh century in the Islamicate world. It includes Arabic translations of Greek philosophical texts and Arabic works from Qūsta ibn Lūca, Farabi, and Miskawayh.

36. Qūsta ibn Lūqā, *De animae et spiritus discrimine*, 308–17, in Constantine the African, *Constantini Africani opera*, trans. Joannes Hispalensis (Basel: Henricum Petrum, 1536).

37. James Bono, "Medical Spirits and the Medieval Language of Life," *Traditio* 40 (1984): 91–30; M. D. Chenu, "Spiritus: Vocabulaire de l'ame au XIIe siècle," *Revue de Sciences Philosophiques et Théologiques* 41 (1957): 209–32; Boyd Hill, "The Brain and the Spirit in Medieval Anatomy," *Speculum* 40 (1965): 63–73.

38. Nahyan Fancy, *Science and Religion in Mamluk Egypt: Ibn al-Nafis, Pulmonary Transit, and Bodily Resurrection* (New York: Routledge, 2013), 81–84.

39. Fancy, *Science and Religion*, 83. As Fancy shows, Qūsta essentially reconciles Aristotle's and Galen's theories of the soul's relation to the body. Naama Cohen-Hanegbi explores this reconciliation among Latinate authors, such as Taddeo Alderotti. See Cohen-Hanegbi, *Caring for the Living Soul*, 78–85.

40. Bono, "Medical Spirits," 95.

thirteenth-century theologians, physicians, and hagiographers would later engage in theoretical musings about the ontology of the spirit and its role as an intermediary between soul and body, one that was capable of effecting physiological change.[41]

Qūsta's formulation of the strong bond between soul and body through the medium of the spirit also served to explain the hidden causes of bodily transformation in the presence of incantations, charms, and amulets. His *On Incantations, Adjurations, and Suspensions around the Neck* maintained that the patient's feeling of confidence in recovery was tantamount to cure. "When the human understanding is sure," Qūsta asserted, citing Plato, "even though it is not helpful to him naturally, a thing will be useful from the mere intention of mind."[42] Here, Qūsta posited that non-natural and nonmaterial agents might affect the body's health. He then proceeded to recommend that physicians enhance their material remedies with incantations, adjurations, or amulets, which secure a patient's confidence:

> It is established, therefore, that if a physician somehow helps the complexion of the soul by an incantation, adjurations or amulet, the complexion of the body will be helped too. If, moreover, to these things appropriate medicine is added, health will follow more quickly, since the body is aided by medicine [and] the soul by an incantation, in which joining of the two health for both will follow more rapidly.[43]

By the term "complexion" here, Qūsta referred to the particular constitution of elements and primary qualities in a sublunary body. Qūsta found that the most rapid recovery was achieved when the physician attended to the complexion of both soul *and* body. He recommended that physicians add incantations, adjurations, and amulets to material remedies. Qūsta then concluded his treatise by offering a number of empirica. These were seemingly irrational remedies, such as the suspension of sorrel for scrofula. He reminded readers that although they often worked, there was no rational explanation for

---

41. Bono asserts that the concept of *spiritus* "was capable of being transmitted along a range of frequencies." It appeared as a material and medical entity, as a life-giving force; and it was also theorized as a "quasi-divine substance" in theological writings. See Bono, "Medical Spirits," 99.

42. Wilcox and Riddle, "Qūsta ibn Lūqā's *Physical Ligatures*," 31; trans., 40: "Cum inquit mens humana rem aliquam licet naturaliter non iuvantem sibi prodesse certificat ex sola mentis intentionem corpus res illa iuvat."

43. Wilcox and Riddle, "Qūsta ibn Lūqā's *Physical Ligatures*," 33; trans., 41 (I adjusted the translation slightly): "Constat ergo quia si medicus anime complexionem quoquomodo adiuverit incantatione adiuratione sive colli suspensione, corporis quoque complexionem adiutam esse. Si autem his conveniens adiungitur medicina, velocior consequitur sanitas, cum medicina corpus incantatione anima adiuvatur, quibus coniunctis necesse est sanitatem utriusque citius consequi."

their efficacy: "Their operation is from their property and not from reasons through which we can understand them."[44]

Qūsta ibn Lūcā's treatises outlining the soul's effect on the body stand behind much of the Latin medical speculation on verbal remedies and charms.[45] Qūsta's understanding of the operation of a substance's *proprietas*, which is "not furnished to the senses," fueled theoretical speculation about the mechanics of cures that could not be explained by reason. Like Qūsta, Ibn Sīnā (Avicenna; d. 1037) explored unpredictable properties, seeking to fit unexpected effects into an otherwise universal theory of material causes.[46] For Ibn Sīnā, *forma specifica* explained how mixed substances formed new, unexpected properties. Specific forms "arise out of the divine emanation which pervades all things and makes latent energies kinetic."[47] He recognized that his theory of *forma specifica* was unsatisfactory to some physicians who yearned for material reasons, avowing that "they want to believe that every property arises out of the 'heat,' 'cold,' 'dryness,' or 'moisture' of the body."[48] Nevertheless, Ibn Sīnā sought to rationalize seemingly inexplicable phenomena such as the attraction of iron to lodestone, reasoning that "from a physical form whose constituents have become blended, there emerges a power which could not have appeared in the several separate constituents."[49]

---

44. Wilcox and Riddle, "Qūsta ibn Lūqā's *Physical Ligatures*," 39; trans., 47: "enim actio ex proprietate est non rationibus unde sic comprehendi potest."

45. Qūsta's treatise was one of the earliest of the Arabic scientific texts to be translated into Latin, probably late eleventh or early twelfth century. Wilcox and Riddle, "Qūsta ibn Lūqā's *Physical Ligatures*," 5. *De differentia spiritu et animae* established that *spiritus* formed the medium between body and soul. Qūsta distinguished between vital spirit (*spiritus vitalis*), which maintained heartbeat, pulse, and respiration, and animal spirit (*spiritus animalis*), which maintained mental faculties such as memory and reason. This idea is carried over in the *Isagoge* and *Pantegni*, which also add the *spiritus naturalis*, governing nutrition, digestion, growth, and generation.

46. McVaugh, "The Experience-Based Medicine," 115. It should be clear that *proprietas* was not used to explain verbal remedies, as verbal remedies were not complexionate. However, *proprietas* did explain material components of verbal cures such as the breath. The affects of the soul, particularly the confidence in physicians and hope for recovery, were the primary means of explaining verbal remedies, approaching something like a theory of placebo effect. Placebo effect presupposes an unknowing in the patient (or physician), but medieval physicians placed greater weight on the need for physicians to perform authority in order to garner the specific emotions, such as hope and delight, required for cure. On the history of the placebo effect, see Anne Harrington, *The Cure Within: A History of Mind-Body Medicine* (New York: Norton, 2008).

47. Avicenna, *The Canon of Medicine*, trans. Cameron Gruner (New York: AMS Press, 1973), 10.1124, 549; on specific form, see Avicenna, *Liber canonis* (Venice: Bonetum Locatellum Bergomensem, 1507), bk. 1, fen. 2, summa 1, ch. 15. On the penetration of specific form or "fourth virtue," as it was known to Arabic physicians, into Latin medical texts, see Isabelle Draelants, "The Notion of Properties: Tensions between *Scientia* and *Ars* in Medieval Natural Philosophy and Magic," in Rider and Page, *The Routledge History of Medieval Magic*, 174.

48. Avicenna, *The Canon of Medicine* 10.1126, 549.

49. Avicenna, *The Canon of Medicine* 10.1124, 549.

These Islamicate treatises entered the Latin corpus along with other translations of medical texts by Constantine the African, James of Venice, and Dominicus Gundissalinus, which made available for learned Western audiences key works on the science of the soul, such as Aristotle's *De anima* and Ibn Sīnā's *Kitāb al-nafs*.[50] These treatises generated among Latin medical theorists pressing questions and suppositions about the relationship of body or material to unseen forces. For example, Albertus Magnus explored the notion of a specific form, and transmitted the concept among his Dominican interlocuters in northern Europe. Writing of the nonelemental powers of certain stones, such as counteracting poison, driving away abscesses, attracting or repelling iron, he asserted, "The power of stones is caused by the specific substantial form of the stone. There are some powers of [mixed] bodies that are caused by the constituents [in the mixture]."[51]

Arnald of Villanova (d. 1311) also played an important role in transmitting Ibn Sīnā's notion of unexpected properties to the Western medical tradition. The translator of Ibn Sīnā's *De viribus cordis*, Arnald incorporated the idea of *proprietas* into his own medical reasoning, determining that there existed numerous substances with properties that could not derive from reasoning, but were only known from revelation and *experimenta*.[52] Arnald and his students and colleagues relied on the possibilities of hidden forces theorized in *proprietas* to license investigation of experimental remedies and to question the causes of their tested effects. Substances in their simple form, he explained, had certain qualities that affected the body in predictable ways. But composite substances occasionally produced complexions that, once mixed, could not be determined by the sum of their parts. The mixture of the substance made possible the acquisition of new properties specific to the composite.[53] The notion of *proprietas* allowed physicians to explain the effects of remedies that were not explicable according to the action of primary qualities. It also provided some latitude for them to incorporate empirical remedies into otherwise "rational" medical treatises.

---

50. Dag Nikolaus Hasse, *Avicenna's "De anima" in the Latin West: The Formation of a Peripatetic Philosophy of the Soul, 1160–1300* (London: Warburg, 2000); Damien Boquet and Piroska Nagy, "Medieval Sciences of Emotions in the 11th–13th Centuries: An Intellectual History," *Osiris* 31 (2016): 21–45.

51. Albertus Magnus, *De minerabilis* II.4; translated by Dorothy Wyckoff as *The Book of Minerals* (Oxford: Clarendon Press, 1967), 65. Albertus cites Constantine the African's translation of Qūstā ibn Lūcā's *Physical Ligatures*.

52. Joseph Ziegler, *Medicine and Religion c. 1300: The Case of Arnau of Vilanova* (Oxford: Clarendon Press, 1998), 120; from *Medicationis parabole* vi.I.31, no. 16: "Proprietas incognita ratione vel sillogismo, revelatione vel experimento iuvantium et nocentium innotescit."

53. McVaugh, "The Experience-Based Medicine," 116.

For Urso of Salerno (d. 1225), efficacious verbal remedies raised questions about the relationship of the bodies, souls, and affective states of practitioners and patients.[54] Urso understood incantations to work, but posited that their efficacy hinged on the affective state of the person to whom they were directed, "[who] believes in the power of incantation and already imagines its effect."[55] Like Qūsṭā, Urso encouraged physicians to include verbal remedies as an enhancement to material ones. They were efficacious insofar as they worked on the patient's affects and made the practitioner appear competent. He asserted: "Some people simulate incantations while administering a drug, not because [they believe that] a simulated incantation has any effect, but only to administer the efficacious object competently. And sometimes when one thing is joined to another, it enhances the effect of the other."[56] Urso recognized that material remedies were sometimes not sufficient to bring about cure. In Urso's phrasing, words mixed with material cures rendered a new, more efficacious prescription, "just like the conjunction of a formula and a material substance effects a sacrament."[57] For Urso, these verbal remedies required theatrics, appeals to the patient's imagination that positioned them to expect bodily transformation, that instilled their hope. Verbal remedies "joined to" material ones potentially engendered composite substances with unexpected effects. In direct parallel to the verbal formulae that, when uttered by a consecrated priest, substantially altered the materials of the sacraments, Urso positioned incantations as possessing the power to alter the physical body.

Urso based his understanding of the causal power of verbal remedies in material, rational processes. For him, the physician was the true agent of the incantation. His superior virtue induced the recovery of a patient's health through his performance of words and gestures. The power of words in an incantation, Urso argued, was not inherent in the words. Rather, their power relied on the merit of the practitioner pronouncing them, a material cause. When speaking incantatory words, the practitioner exhaled his own pure

54. On Urso's rationale for incantations, see Maaike van der Lugt, "The Learned Physician as a Charismatic Healer: Urso of Salerno on Incantations in Medicine, Magic, and Religion," *Bulletin of the History of Medicine* 87.3 (2013): 307–46.

55. Van der Lugt's Appendix includes an edition and translation of Urso's *Commentary on Aphorism 39*, 335–46.

56. Urso, *Commentary on Aphorism 39*, 336; trans., 341: "Quidam tamen in medicinae exhibitione quandoque simulant incantationes, non quia simulata incantatio effectum habeat, sed tantum res exhibita competenter. Et aliquotiens unum alteri iunctum alterius auget effectum."

57. Urso, *Commentary on Aphorism 39*, 336; trans., 341: "cum verbum additum elemento faciat sacramentum."

spirits, which purified the air shared by the speaker and his patient.[58] "The diffusion of [this spirit]," he stated, "boosts the power that governs the body to such an extent that it brings on a perfect crisis."[59] When the patient thus inhaled the breath of the physician, their body underwent a process of purification that enabled the humors to improve.[60] For this process to work, of course, the physician's spirit must be pure. Were he to exhale ill spirits, the patient's condition would further deteriorate.[61]

Ultimately, the physician's breath in uttering the words of incantation aroused in the patient the passion of delight "so the spirits, purified by the movement and then directed toward the [parts] in need of the incantation, put the incantation into effect."[62] The patient received bodily comfort from these words, and began to imagine their own healing process, calling away the spirit from the site of bodily pain. Urso asserted that this very process explains how the martyrs were able to patiently endure torment: "The more they yearned for celestial joys through the attentive contemplation of their mind—their spirits withdrawn from managing the body—the less they felt the pain of torture. Hence, confirmed of being in God's grace by their suffering, so that God's miracles would be shown to both the torturers and the spectators when they escaped unscathed."[63] In this passage, Urso expressed medical interest in the miraculous bodies of saints. He applied medical theory to rationalize saintly bodies, the corporeal manifestations of divine grace. Just as the saints contemplated divine bliss in order to endure the pain of persecution, so the sick patient could imbibe the pure spirits emitted from

---

58. Van der Lugt, "The Learned Physician," argues that Urso had adopted the Galenic notion of spirits, likening them to invisible material substances that flow through the body animating functions such as digestion, growth, pulse, heartbeat, and emotions, imagination, reason, and memory. Avicenna proffered a similar theory of the salubrious effects distributed by "the breath."

59. Urso, *Commentary on Aphorism 39*, 339; trans., 345: "cuius diffusione per membra virtus regitiva confortata ad crisim perfectam faciendam potenter assurgit."

60. Urso's theory of breath resembles that of Avicenna, who stated that "the breath is that which emerges from mixture of first principles, and approaches toward the likeness of celestial beings." The breathed words of incantations operated on the emotional interior of a patient: "Joy and sadness, fear and anger, and passions [are] peculiarly related to the breath of the heart." Avicenna, *De viribus cordis*, in *The Canon of Medicine*, trans. Gruner, 353.

61. Van der Lugt, "The Learned Physician," 314. Urso also posited that the patient and healer must have conformity of spirit. By breathing the same local air, eating the same local food, a person absorbs the spirits of their surroundings and is conformed to the other inhabitants. Such conformity of spirit is required for the incantation to work.

62. Urso, *Commentary on Aphorism 39*, 335; trans., 340: "sicque spiritus depurati per motum et ad incantanda inde deducti effectum incantationis prosecuntur."

63. Urso, *Commentary on Aphorism 39*, 340; trans., 345 (I adjusted the translation slightly): "Unde etiam martyres in principio passionis tanto minus flagella sentiebant, quanto magis a corporis regimine sublatis spiritibus per contemplationem attentiori mente caelesita gaudia suspirabant. Deinde in Dei gratia per patientiam confirmati, ut flagellantibus et videntibus Dei miracula monstrarentur."

the physician's words to replace suffering with delight. In this way, for Urso, the physician possessed a saintly body of his own.

The importance of the physician's affective performance can be found in a script that was designed for recitation over a patient suffering from brain injury, which is recorded in Teodorico Borgognoni's *Surgery*. Such cases are usually hopeless, Teodorico stated, so that "our hope must be placed in him who does not desert those who have hope."[64] Teodorico advised that when a doctor confronts a patient with such a severe brain injury he should invest his own hope in the treatment. Note that it was not the patient's hope that Teodorico urged, but the physician's. The physician's hope, Teodorico explained, cannot be placed in his own skill, as his skill is hopeless in reversing the damage caused by such injuries. He must instead place his hope in God, "and in nature which proceeds from him." For such brain injuries, Teodorico recommended a powder of mouse-ear, pimpernel, caryophyllata, gentian, and valerian, held together under a headdress, a remedy that his own teacher, Master Hugo, had conveyed to him. The powder should be administered to the patient in the form of a cross, while stating,

> In the name of the Father and of the Son and of the Holy Ghost, in the name of the Holy and Indivisible Trinity; the right hand of the Lord hath done valiantly, the right hand of the Lord hath exalted me; I shall not die but live and I shall narrate the works of the Lord.[65]

Teodorico explained that the entire remedy should be preceded by the physician's prayer to God, asking him to cure the patient by means of the powder. In a positively counterintuitive formulation, Teodorico's prayer actually took effect on the *physician*, not the patient. The prayer encouraged *him* to summon internal hope in the cure. His hope, in turn, mixed with the material agent of the powder, was transferred to the patient who heard the words of prayer that he would not die. Hearing the physician's confident prayer, the patient would be inspired to believe, and thereby the patient would receive from the physician a means of remedy: hope of recovery. The prayer demonstrates the physician's affective responsibility for a patient. He must perform the proper affective states in order to ensure a cure's efficacy.

---

64. Teodorico Borgognoni, *Chirurgia*, Bk. II, ch. 3, 145v: "in illo qui sperentes in se non deserit, spes nostra ponenda est"; trans. *The Surgery of Theodoric*, 112.

65. Teodorico Borgognoni, *Chirurgia*, Bk. II, ch. 3, 145v: "In nomine patris, et filii et spiritus sancti. In nomine sanctae et individuae trinitatis. Dextera domini fecit virtutem: dextera domini exaltavit me: non moriar, sed vivam, et narrabo opera domini"; trans. *The Surgery of Theodoric*, bk. II, 112 (I adjusted the translation slightly).

The Italian physician Pietro d'Abano (d. c. 1315) posited an even more pronounced role for the physician in bringing about the patient's bodily health through verbal, affective, and performative means.[66] His *Conciliator* asserted that the patient's confidence in cure contained an intentional species, and he connected this confidence to material effect. Because confidence existed in the intellect, it would exert some sort of agency (*confidentia existens in intellectu modo aliquo habebit agere*).[67] For Pietro, confidence in the physician was a passion of the soul and bore the same bodily effects. Just as humans may tremble from thoughts alone, he reasoned according to an Aristotelian logic, so the confidence existing as a species of the soul alters the body.[68] For Pietro, it has "agency" within the body.[69] This agency worked to effect material change.

Like Urso and Qūsta, Pietro maintained that the crucial element of cure was the patient's hope for health and confidence in the physician. He urged that the patient should be "extremely hopeful" so that the action taken by the physician may be more likely to take effect. He argued that physicians must give great attention to the soul, because "even as the doctor may not directly consider the soul, in fact it is his true subject."[70] The physician's ability to convince the patient, to enact the patient's faith and hope in cure, depended on the purity of his soul, which should be "believable" (*credulator*, fol. 213). Although the patient's affective state was critical to the healing process, for Pietro, as for Urso, the person of the physician was the real agent of efficacy in the mechanics of affective cure. Pietro posited that it was the superior status of the physician's soul that wielded causal power over the bodies of others.[71] The physician's verbal remedy worked not because of a certain power

---

66. On Pietro's biography, see Lynn Thorndike, *A History of Magic and Experimental Science* (New York: Columbia University Press, 1923), 874–939; and Eugenia Paschetto, *Pietro d'Abano, medico e filosofo* (Florence: E. Vallecchi, 1984). On his contribution to medicine, medical astrology, and medical alchemy, see the essays in Jean-Patrice Boudot, Franck Collard, Nicolas Weill-Parot, eds., *Médecine, astrologie, et magie entre Moyen Âge et Renaissance: Autour de Pietro d'Abano* (Florence: Sismel, 2013).

67. Pietro d'Abano, *Conciliator differentiarum philosophorum* (Venice: Luca Giunta, 1520).

68. Peter of Abano's *Conciliator* is largely an attempt to reconcile differences between Galen and Aristotle on the relationship between the body and soul. See Matthew Klemm, "A Medieval Perspective on the Soul as Substantial Form of the Body: Peter of Abano on the Reconciliation of Aristotle and Galen," in *Psychology and the Other Disciplines: A Case of Cross-Disciplinary Interaction*, ed. Paul Bakker, Sander de Boer, and Cees Leijenhorst (Leiden: Brill, 2012), 275–95.

69. On the powers of the soul according to Peter of Abano, my thinking is shaped largely by Matthew Klemm, "Les complexions vertueuses: La physiologie des vertues dans l'anthropologie médicale de Pietro d'Abano," *Médiévales* 63 (2012): 59–74.

70. *Conciliator*, dif. 5, fol. 7v: "Et si medicus animam non consideret directe, verum eius amplius subiectum."

71. *Conciliator*, dif. 135, fol. 188v: "Quaedam enim sic sunt elevatae nobiles et tam gradium et mirabilium operationum, ut non modo operentur in corpore proprio factis alterationibus et transmutationibus, verum etiam alieno et absque medio quale opus oculis fascinātis."

of words, but because of a certain power reserved in the soul of the physician that was able to arouse confidence in his patients. He also cautioned that words uttered by illicit practitioners, such as unlearned *vetulae*, opened the door for demonic intervention.[72] Similar to a saint, the properly trained physician reserved discretionary persuasion over the bodies of others.[73]

Arnald of Villanova also explored this idea that physicians retained heightened powers to effect somatic transformation by working on the soul of the patient.[74] In his *De simplicibus*, Arnald asserted that physicians possessed a secret, divine knowledge that assisted them in influencing the equilibrium of the blood in their patients and in stimulating their patients' passions by arousing their confidence. In this way, for Arnald, belief in the physician's superior status was a component of the therapeutic process, a requirement for cure.[75] The physician's foremost task in achieving health was to win the patient's confidence so much that even if the physician was uncertain about the appropriate remedy, he should nevertheless feign knowledge of a salubrious treatment by prescribing a neutral regimen and harmless drugs. This way, the patient would believe they were on the path to cure.[76] Furthermore, Arnald advised his readers to supplement these prescriptions with words of hope, thereby mixing the physician's words and performance with the material remedy he prescribed.[77]

---

72. *Conciliator*, dif. 156. See Beatrice Delaurenti, "Pietro d'Abano et les incantations: Présentations, édition et traduction de la *differentia* 156 du *Conciliator*," in Boudot, Collard, and Weill-Parot, *Médecine, astrologie, et magie*, 39–105.

73. As Beatrice Delaurenti has noted, it was not the soul of the physician alone that retained the power to wield physical change via incantations. As possible causes he also included God, the angels, demons, and astral influences.

74. On Arnald's nearly mystical understanding of the physician, and his engagement with Christian theology more generally, see Ziegler, *Medicine and Religion c. 1300*.

75. Ziegler argues that this need for confidence in the physician was quasi-religious. Ziegler, *Medicine and Religion c. 1300*, 123. Taddeo Alderotti in the 1280s also relied on Ibn Sīnā to assert that the faith of the patient in the capacity of physicians was more important to recovery of health than all of the instruments and medicines at his disposal. Henri of Mondeville and Pietro d'Abano repeated this idea. See Salmón, "The Physician as Cure," 205. Guy de Chauliac argued that "potions and amulets . . . have been proven to work—it may perhaps be the confidence they encourage rather than their actual properties that does this." In Michael McVaugh, "*Incantationes* in Late Medieval Surgery," in *Ratio et superstitio: Essays in Honor of Graziella Federici Vescovini*, ed. G. Marchetti and Valeria Sorge (Turnhout: Brepols, 2003), 344.

76. The treatise was translated by Henry Sigerist, "Bedside Manners in the Middle Ages: The Treatise *De Cautelis Medicorum* Attributed to Arnald of Villanova," *Quarterly Bulletin of the Northwestern University Medical School* 20 (1936): 135–43. The section on "bland" regimen is discussed by Michael McVaugh, "Bedside Manners in the Middle Ages," *Bulletin of the History of Medicine* 71 (1997): 213.

77. Salmón, "The Physician as Cure," 210 referring to Arnald of Villanova, *Repetitio super Vita brevis*, ed. Michael McVaugh, Munich, MS Clm 14245, fol. 30r: "verbis excitantibus spem et confidenciam in animo eius et promittendo quod diligenter ordinabit pro eo salubria."

Scholastic physicians thus theorized the causality of efficacious verbal and performative remedies as residing in the learned and virtuous person of the physician. They often understood physicians' performance of authority to enhance material prescriptions. Other members of the thirteenth-century intellectual elite shared this understanding of the efficacy of personal presence and authoritative performance. In his treatise *On the Nullity of Magic*, Roger Bacon argued that physicians should be permitted to employ "symbols and characters," not because they were efficacious in themselves, "but in order that the medicine may be taken more *faithfully*."[78] The physician's performance of ritualistic gesture, their recitation of verbal charms and prayers, and the wielding of amulets and ligatures assisted the patient's spirit "to bring about many renovations in the body which properly appertains to it—so that by gladness and confidence it convalesces from infirmity to health."[79] Verbal remedies were performative acts, a way to make believe within the patient, for them to imagine the physician's power and to hope for cure. Bacon would later assert in his *Opus maius* (1266 or 1267) that words uttered with the correct intentions of mind retained a certain power on account of the rational soul that formed them. He postulated that because words [*verbi*; or "the word"] are generated from the natural interior parts of the human and are formed by thought and careful oversight, and because words cause humans delight, they have the greatest efficacy of all human products, particularly when they are uttered with firm intention, great desire, and unflinching confidence.[80] Delight, confidence, intention, and desire all shaped the process of forming the word itself, imbuing it with its unique power. For Bacon, words were the "form" or "species" of the rational soul, the medium through which its power was contained.[81] Through words, the soul could act on objects in the world as causal agents of change.[82] Drawing

---

78. Roger Bacon, "Epistola Fratris Rogerii Baconis De secretis operibus artis et naturae, et De nullitate magiae," in *Fratris Rogeri Bacon Opera quaedam hactenus inedita*, vol. 1, ed. John Brewer (London: Longman, 1859), App. 1, 527 (emphasis added); translated by Tenney Davis as *On the Nullity of Magic* (New York: AMS Press, 1982), 20: "sed ut devotius et avidius medicina recipiatur."

79. Bacon, *De nullitate magiae*, 527; trans., 20: "et animus patientis excitetur, et confidat uberius, et speret, et congaudeat; quoniam anima excitata potest in corpore proprio et multa renovare, ut de infirmitate ad sanitatem convalescat, ex gaudio et confidentia."

80. Roger Bacon, *Opus maius* IV, Treatise on Astrology, in *The Opus Maius of Roger Bacon*, ed. Henry Bridges (London: Williams and Norgate, 1900), 1:399.

81. Steven P. Marrone, "Thomas Aquinas, Roger Bacon, and the Magicians on the Power of Words," in *Contemplation and Philosophy: Scholastic and Metaphysical Modes of Medieval Philosophical Thought; A Tribute to Kent Emery*, ed. Andreas Speer (Leiden: Brill, 2018), 226.

82. His theory unfolds in the treatise on astronomy and stipulates that moments of efficacious utterance would have to align with astronomical and astrological configurations. See Bridges, *The Opus Maius of Roger Bacon*, 1:395–97.

on the same theories as Urso and Qūsta, Bacon had explained that the person uttering words was critical to the effective execution of an incantation. The physician required a superior inner virtue in order for his words to take effect. When words were uttered by a person of "a clean and healthy body of sound constitution" they produced "certain natural effects."[83] Explaining how one person can affect the body of another through words alone, Bacon stated that all actors "bring their extrinsic idea to bear on Nature; they impart certain sensible properties to things. Thus an object can have an active quality and idea beyond itself, particularly when it is nobler than other corporeal things."[84] Human agents with a superior rational soul possessed the ability to emit an idea, a virtue, that could alter bodies outside themselves.

For Bacon, those with the power to heal the bodies of others by the virtue of their soul were in possession of superior spirits. Such people tended, according to humoral theory, to be young men: "Healthy persons of good complexion, especially young men, comfort others and delight them by their mere presence. This is because of their soothing spirit and delectable and salubrious vapors, and because of their good natural warmth, and because of the idea and the virtues which they emanate, as Galen teaches in his Techne."[85] Like Qūsta ibn Lūcā before him, Bacon asserted the power of certain men to affect bodily change through incantation, placing an emphasis on their superior humoral constitution. Qūsta had also argued that only *certain* individuals possessed this power, individuals with ideal complexions. Women, the elderly, children, and people of excessively warm and cold mixtures, such as "Black Africans, the Slavs, and their likes," were inclined toward disequilibrium of the soul.[86] Their bodies, Qūsta informed his readers, were thus imperfectly functional, and their words lacked the necessary virtue to affect others. Here, we witness a textual authorization and rationalization that normalized learned, male, and nonblack bodies as the sole practitioners who were constitutionally equipped and authorized to effect transformation

---

83. Bacon, *De nullitate magiae*, 531; trans., 24–25: "quum a corpore mundo, et sano, et bonae complexionis producuntur."

84. Bacon, *De nullitate magiae*, 528; trans, 21: "et fiunt virtutes a rebus, aliquae sensibiles, aliquae insensibiles. Et ideo homo potest facere virtutem et speciem extra se, maxime quum sit nobilior omnibus rebus corporalibus."

85. Bacon, *De nullitate magiae*, 529–30; trans., 22–23: "Et e converso homines bonae complexionis et sani, et maxime juvenes, confortant alios, et homines gaudent de eorum praesentia; et hoc est propter spiritus suaves, et vapores salubres et delectabiles, et naturalem calorem bonum, et propter species et virtutes quae fiunt ab eis, sicut Galenus docet in Techni."

86. *A Philosophy Reader*, 199.

over the bodies of others.[87] In this figuring, it was their perfectly balanced internal complexions and superior virtue that enhanced their spirit, enabling them to wield physical change over others. According to scholastic medical theory, then, race and gender were crucial to the proper use of affective and verbal remedies. Only a man of virtue could possess the strong spirits to move another person, to inspire their confidence and stir their blood. It is for this reason that, on the occasions that physicians like Teodorico, Gilbertus, or Thomas Fayreford included charms or prayers in their treatises, they distinguished *their* prescriptions from the frivolous words of *vetulae* and the unlettered. In order to emerge as authoritative, they had to erase any suggestion of feminine and thus unbookish association with their approach to healing. While physicians created moderate space in their treatises for unexpected properties and affective therapies, they exerted great effort to restrict to learned male physicians the power to successfully execute such remedies.

Healing charms and other empirical medical practices proliferated outside of formal medical treatises, too. They could be found in an array of texts that were widely accessible through several media in the form of oral narrative, performance, and as kinesthetic knowledge.[88] *Erec et Enide, Yvain, Cligés,* and Marie de France's lais, *Le deus amanz* and *Eliduc,* feature women— and not men—as sources of empirical medical knowledge and practice who engaged in wound care, herbal preparations, and verbal charms.[89] *Erec et*

---

87. Although it is not stated in these terms in their treatises, one can presume that *pace* Qūsta, they also mean nonblack. On the construction of racial markers in Islamicate texts, see Kristina Richardson, "Blue and Green Eyes in the Islamicate Middle Ages," *Annales Islamologiques* 48.1 (2014): 13–30. By the fifteenth century, as Jean Dangler has shown, Jewish and Muslim men in Iberia were also being excluded from licit medical practice, showing that "gender alone was insufficient in limiting the healing duties of unwanted healers." Jean Dangler, *Mediating Fictions: Literature, Women Healers, and the Go-Between in Medieval and Early Modern Iberia* (Lewisburg: Bucknell University Press, 2001), 6. On the process of race-making through religious restriction and identification, see Geraldine Heng, *The Invention of Race in the European Middle Ages* (Cambridge: Cambridge University Press, 2018). On the restriction of non-Christian medical practitioners, see Luis García-Ballester, Michael R. McVaugh, and Agustía Rubio-Vela, *Medical Licensing and Learning in Fourteenth-Century Valencia* (Philadelphia: Transactions of the American Philosophical Society, 1989), 25–29.

88. By "kinesthetic knowledge" I refer to knowledge acquired through habitual practice, learned by doing in imitation. On this form of body knowledge, see Pamela Long, who discusses it in terms of "oral transmission of craft knowledge within apprenticeship systems." Pamela Long, *Openness, Secrecy, Authorship: Technical Arts and the Culture of Knowledge from Antiquity to the Renaissance* (Baltimore: Johns Hopkins University Press, 2001), 6.

89. See Peggy McCracken, "Women and Medicine in Medieval French Narrative," *Exemplaria* 5.2 (1993): 239–62; Kathy Krause, "Guérisseuses et sorcières: La médecine feminine dans les romans des XIIe et XIIIe siècles," *Equinoxe* 8 (1992): 161–73. As McCracken argues, the women who appear in these tales as empirical practitioners of medicine are denied the authoritative representation of occupational titles like *miresse.* McCracken shows that "the effect of women's drugs is attributed to magic not through a description of the drug's magical components nor through an account of

Enide, for example, features two sisters who oversee a chamber with health-ful air; there, they nurse Erec's wounds with knowledge and skill, carefully removing the dead skin, washing his sores, and applying a medicinal oint-ment before prescribing a recuperative regimen that eschewed garlic and pepper.[90] Jean Dangler has shown, similarly, that women appear in Iberian hagiographic texts and Marian miracles as *medianeras*, or intermediaries who facilitated healthcare.[91] And as we have seen, saints' *Lives* in the *liégeois* cor-pus also feature women—and not men—as managers of hospices, bedside nurses, and hospital staff who enjoyed therapeutic success and garnered a modest following who pursued their bodywork, prayer, and affective care. Throughout the thirteenth century, these poetic, literary, hagiographic, and other orally conveyed stories positioned female practitioners as authoritative and effective agents of care. The efforts of learned physicians were intellec-tually laborious, expensive, and time-consuming, and yet they continued to rely on many of the same methods of wound repair, herbal preparations, and verbal charms as the mothers, sisters, nuns, lovers, and saints that featured in these stories. Scholastic physicians' claim to textual transmission differen-tiated their therapeutic authority from those practitioners they considered less learned.

Mixing and Medical Anxiety

Just like their colleagues in the medical arts, hagiographers and theologians worked through the Greco-Arabic corpus of medical texts, considering the bodily effects of grace and somatic impressions on the soul.[92] Writing in the

---

actions or effects that might be characterized as necromantic, but through the naming of the woman who makes it" (242). In other words, it is her being in a gendered body, a woman, that erases her skills and therapeutic efficacy in a denial of medical knowledge and associates them with supernatural or magical power.

90. Chrétien de Troyes, *Erec and Enide*, trans. Dorothy Gilbert (Los Angeles: University of California Press, 1992), 198–99.

91. Dangler, *Mediating Fictions*.

92. On the absorption of medical translations among theologians in the thirteenth century, see Joel Kaye, *A History of Balance: The Emergence of a New Model of Equilibrium and Its Impact on Thought* (Cambridge: Cambridge University Press, 2014), in which he demonstrates the pervasive reception of Galen in scholastic thought in many different genres and disciplines. See also Joseph Ziegler, "Ut dicunt medici: Medical Knowledge and Theological Debates in the Second Half of the Thirteenth Century," *Bulletin of the History of Medicine* 73 (1999): 208–37. On the resistance of medical knowl-edge, see Mark D. Jordan, "The Disappearance of Galen in Thirteenth-Century Philosophy and The-ology," in *Mensch und Natur im Mittelalter*, ed. Albert Zimmermann and Andreas Speer, Miscellanea Mediaevalia 21 (Berlin: Walter de Gruyter, 1992), 703–13; Jordan, "Medicine and Natural Philosophy in Aquinas," in *Thomas von Aquin: Werk und Wirkung im Licht neuerer Forschungen*, ed. Albert Zimmer-mann, Miscellanea Mediaevalia 19 (Berlin: Walter de Gruyter, 1988), 233–46.

1140s, William of St. Thierry (d. 1148) was one of the earliest theologians to incorporate the Islamicate medical corpus into his presentation of a distinctly Christian understanding of the soul's effects on the body. William, a Benedictine abbot who later transferred to the Cistercian order at Signy, closely read translations of Greek and Arabic medical texts and declared his intellectual debt to "philosophers and physicians" (*philosophorum vel physicorum*). William's *On the Nature of the Body and Soul* hailed humoral balance as the key to bodily health: "When nature is in balance, it is impossible for the human body to be infected with any disease."[93] The aim in maintaining health, for William, was to preserve humoral balance, which required the action of the soul.

William's treatise on the body and soul was not simply an absorption and translation of prior medical theory into Christian theological terminology. It also sought to overcome what he considered to be an error in medical practice within western Europe. He railed against the limited scope of physicians who "fail most absurdly" in penetrating the true dignity of humanity because "by reason and experience" they limited themselves to the physical trappings of the human: "They simply commend and salute the beauty of the human, how he stands naturally erect above other living things, showing that he has something in common with heaven; how throughout the length of his body there exists a balanced unit in the distinction of his members, with a beautiful equality of members on right and left; how the whole body is ordered by weight and measure and number."[94] What medical theorists lacked, according to William, was an appreciation of the divine imprint that sustained physiological balance.

The second part of his treatise, then, was dedicated to elucidating the soul's role in determining overall health. The "author of nature" (*auctor naturis*), he argued, designed humanity so that "the bond between the intellectual substance and the corporeal" is so complete that the soul is permeated by the body's nature while still able to effect its own operations.[95] The soul, according to William, governed material life through four powers—the appetitive, retentive, digestive, and expulsive—and administered rational life in four passions—hope, joy, fear, and sadness. For William, passions were the gateway to true health. Joy and hope, in particular, facilitated a salutary life and

---

93. William of St. Thierry, *De natura corporis et animae*, PL 180:697; trans. Benjamin Clark, in *Three Treatises on Man: A Cistercian Anthropology*, ed. Bernard McGinn (Kalamazoo, MI: Cistercian Publications, 1977), 105: "Rebus enim naturalibus in temperamento manentibus, impossibile est humanum corpus ab aliquo morbo infestari."

94. *De natura corporis et animae*, 708; trans., 123.

95. *De natura corporis et animae*, 712: "intellectualis substantiae ad corporalem societatem."

enabled a good death, even eternal life after death. But fear and sadness invited suffering and created turmoil, eventually killing the body while weakening the soul.[96] William was not alone in centering the soul in discussions of bodily health. His contemporary, Hildegard of Bingen, also incorporated humoral theory into cosmic history in order to posit that human disease emerged with the origin of sin.[97] Human bodies therefore had no hope of lasting recovery without the aid of divine grace.

By the following century, those concerns about care for the ensouled body were expressed in anxieties about the diminished role of divine grace in formal medical practice. Some authors reacted to what they perceived as an overdetermination of material causality, a denial of divine providence in theories of physiological transformation. Nicholas of Poland, a Dominican friar and student at the University of Montpellier sometime between 1250 and 1270, issued perhaps the most poignant critique of the emerging scholastic medical establishment. Nicholas may not have earned a medical degree, but he demonstrates deep familiarity with the premises of scholastic medicine.[98] Nicholas framed his treatise, *Antipocras*, as a trial against Hippocratic-Galenic medicine in which he presented himself as the plaintiff. He asserted that a cure can be effected without "knowledge of the cause."[99] By focusing on the external qualities of substances, rather than heeding their hidden divine properties, Nicholas claimed that scholastic physicians failed to recognize God's role in rendering elements capable of restoring human health. He wondered, Why would physicians neglect to teach this empirical knowledge so that more people had access to it? "Perhaps [they] want[ed] to ensure," Nicholas reasoned, "that there would not be many like Hippocrates."[100] Physicians had purposefully obscured their craft, wishing to limit their competition. Throughout his treatise, Nicholas lambasted Hippocrates, declaring that natural remedies became corrupt when physicians, following Hippocrates, started to use *sermones*. By *sermones* Nicholas posed a distinction

96. *De natura corporis et animae*, 718: "spe scilicet et gaudio, timore et tristitia."

97. See Hildegard of Bingen, *Causae et curae*, ed. Paulus Kaiser (Leipzig: B.G. Teubneri, 1903). Hildegard posits that Adam's transgression led to the overproduction of black bile, resulting in despair, then disease. Participation in the liturgy was one remedy for this condition, inherited by all humans.

98. On Nicholas of Poland, see William Eamon and Gundolf Keil, "Plebs amat empirica: Nicholas of Poland and His Critique of the Medical Establishment," *Sudhoffs Archiv* 50.1 (1987): 183.

99. The treatise can be found in Karl Sudhoff, ed., "Antipocras, Streitschrift für mystische Heilkunde in Versen des Magisters Nikolaus von Polen," *Sudhoffs Archiv für Geschichte der Medizin* 9 H ½ (1915): 31–52. See William Eamon, *Antipocras: Composed and So Named by Brother Nicholas of the Preaching Friars; Also Called by Another Name, The Book of Empirical Things* (PDF file, history.nmsu.edu/people/faculty/eamon, 2014). *Antipocras*, 41: "Seu cause cognitione."

100. *Antipocras* 47, line 249; trans. 7: "ne multi sint Ypocrates."

between elegant textuality and common orality. For him, Hippocrates signified the textual tradition, the corpus of ancient medical knowledge studied in universities. Nicholas bemoaned the loss of orality in experimental medicine; he regretted that orally transmitted prayers and charms no longer awarded practitioners therapeutic authority in performative and poetic processes. Emphasizing this loss, he composed his own treatise in rhymed verse.

According to Nicholas, God created the elements of the natural world in a manner that retained hidden properties that could be known only by experience or revelation, not by reason. Like the saints, whose material relics were scattered across the earth in powerful fragments, the objects of the natural world contained numerous wondrous properties: "The same magnet pulls huge quantities of iron over to itself and yet the power of the magnet is not diminished or infracted in any way. Break it into endless pieces, yet even that won't cause the magnet to lose its strength, just like Anne or Agnes."[101] Using the same example of the magnetic lodestone that scholastic physicians puzzled over in their discussion of *proprietas*, he rendered *proprietas* as the result of another kind of mixing, the divine *virtus* inlaid in the elements through the work of divine incarnation. Nicholas compared the power of empirical things (*vis empiricorum*) to the power of the saints, who healed inexplicably: "This power, like the saint, lets people be healthy, live long, and die piously; and it also saves them from diseases."[102] *Proprietas* was akin to sanctity, with its healing grace. Saints were just like empirica; you knew their therapeutic power when you experienced it.

Nicholas's critique of scholastic medicine was explicitly gendered. Anne and Agnes, as female saints, represented for him what was excised from scholastic medicine, a feminized form of healing. In referring to the properties of the magnet, Nicholas cited common debates among scholastic physicians who engaged in logistical gymnastics in order to rationalize the efficacy of such empirica as the magnetic lodestone, coral, or theriac.[103] For them, only a concept like *proprietas* could explain these substances, only astral attributes endowed during the "mixing" or combination of substances. But for Nicholas, every object in the world was a product of cosmic mixing, and thus

---

101. *Antipocras* 43, lines 100–101; trans., 4: "Hunc adiens tangas in frustaque plurima frangas / Ex hoc non magnes vim perdet ut agna vel agnes."

102. *Antipocras* 46, lines 206–7; trans., 6: "Fortes ulternos eademque pie morituros / eripit a morbis."

103. On theriac as an empiricum, see Nicole Oresme, *Contra divinatores*, in British Library MS Lat. 15126, fol. 30v. This discussion is found in Arnald of Villanova, *Opera medica omnia*, ed. Michael McVaugh, Luis García-Ballester, and Juan Paniagua (Barcelona: Universitat de Barcelona, 1996), introduction to vol. 3, 58.

capable of retaining divine properties. Through a woman, Mary, God had implanted healing properties, divine properties, into the earth itself, into its mud (*limo*), stone (*lapidi*), forest (*silvis*), and seas (*mari*). He lauded even the most abject elements, such as excrement and menstrual blood (*in fece, in fimo*), for their hidden powers. In his praise of the power latent in menstrual blood, for example, Nicholas explained that Christ emerged from "the poison remaining in the divine veins from the ejected obscene fluid."[104] Praising the abject, he continued, "Eternal daughter of light, you give life to an enormous thing, from the simplicity that has two forms you produce one action, from two things you make one."[105] According to Nicholas, two substances, the divine and human, were "mixed" in the womb of Mary. "No one can explain how," but as a result, "all things are full of goodness and the strength contained in them gains a victory over Eve's crime."[106] As in *proprietas*, Nicholas offers as explanation only the assertion that the "mixing" of elements— here the divine and human—resulted in the acquisition of powerful qualities in the material of the earth. The incarnation had reversed the insalubrious effects of sin ("Eve's crime"), rendering "all things" full of goodness, mixing all things to generate uncanny properties.

Nicholas's concern over the erosion of divine properties in medical theory was shared by another thirteenth-century author, the Cistercian Caesarius of Heisterbach. Caesarius expressed anxiety about the course of scholastic medicine, about the role of *physici* in positing strictly material causes for bodily transformation.[107] For example, his *Dialogue on Miracles* reported a tale about an unnamed physician-monk who spent excessive time outside of the monastery tending to the sick. One day, when Mary, "the electuary," appeared to the monks during the psalmody she spooned medicine into each of their mouths, omitting only the physician. Caesarius explained his punishment by stating that Mary's medicine:

> Is understood to be the grace of devotion by whose virtue psalm-singers are comforted, and by whose sweetness the labor of vigils is

---

104. *Antipocras* 44, lines 127–28; trans., 16: "Divinis venis virus manes ab emenis. / Influis obscenis apud hoc remanes."

105. *Antipocras* 44, lines 131–32; trans., 16: "Rempis enormem de simplicitate biformen / actum producis eterne filia lucis."

106. *Antipocras* 44, lines 139, 136; trans., 16: "Nemo potest fari . . . Sicque sit ut per te, sicut res bonitate referte."

107. We could also add Roger Bacon, who chastised scholastic physicians for their preoccupation with "useless argumentation," "dialectic arguments," and "countless sophistries," so that physicians had no remaining time for experimentation, which revealed the hidden properties of substances. See Mary Catherine Welborn, "The Errors of the Doctors According to Friar Roger Bacon," *Isis* 18 (1932): 31–33.

changed into delight. The components of this medicine are remorse-ful memories of the Lord's conception, nativity, and of all the sacred relics of Christ, which are flavored with the mellifluous hope of future reward.[108]

Here, Caesarius promoted the healing effects of meditation and the perfor-mance of the Psalms, without which material remedies would not entirely take effect. Delight and hope appear in Caesarius's tale as the prelude to bodily medicine, made available through devotional and liturgical means. There is a distinct whiff of anxiety in this exemplum, an apprehension about the claims of eminence among scholastic physicians, concern that, in their focus on material causality and the physical composition of the human body, they threatened to neglect the divine origin of all remedies and the soul's role in protecting bodily well-being.

That whiff intensifies into the stench of pronounced disgust when Cae-sarius addresses the distinctions he perceived between scholastic medi-cine and spiritual therapies. He relays the tale of a young monk, Adam of Locheim, who suffered grievously from a skin condition in his scalp (*scabies capita*). Adam consulted physicians and scholars, but could not seem to find a cure for his affliction. One day, during his daily devotions, the Virgin Mary appeared to him offering an untested remedy: "Take the fruit of the *ligni fusilis* and have your head washed with it three times before mass in the name of the Father, Son, and Holy Ghost, and immediately you will be cured."[109] Thereupon, Adam followed this regimen and received immediate cure. If Adam encountered Mary, why could she not have simply reversed his condition, providing a miraculous cure? Why did she work through the ele-ments? The material remedies that Adam had tested previously were ineffec-tual because they were not administered with the essential ingredients of the words of prayer uttered in faith. Mary did not offer a spiritual remedy alone, but a *mixed* remedy. The material remedy of the *ligni fusilis* was combined

---

108. Caesarius of Heisterbach, *Dialogus miraculorum*, bk. VII, ch. xlvii, 1468: "electuarium istud gratia devotionis intelligitur, cuius virtute psallentes confortantur, cuius dulcedine labor vigiliarum vertitur in delicias. Huius species aromaticae sunt memoria compunctiva Dominicae conceptionis, nativitatis, et reliquorum sacramentorum Christi, quae omnia melliflua spe futurae retributionis condiuntur et meritis beatae Virginis psallentibus infunduntur."

109. I have not been able to track down "ligni fusilis." The "fruit of the molten wood"? Although it is possible that it is a reference to the tree of life, Mary directs Adam on where to find it on a nearby mountain. Furthermore, directing Adam to wash his head with the fruit of the tree of life (Christ) seems downright odd, even for Caesarius. Caesarius of Heisterbach, *Dialogus miraculorum*, bk. VII, ch. xxiv, 1370: "Accipe fructus ligni fusilis, et fac tibi hodie ex eo lavari caput tribus vicibus ante mis-sam, in nomine Patris et Filii et Spiritus sancti, statimque curaberis."

with the spiritual remedy of devout prayer.[110] Caesarius proceeded to explain Mary's efficacy according to the logic of incarnational mixing. "[Mary] produced the medicine of the whole human race," he asserted. Mary was the very vehicle for grace in the earth. She was the matrix in which humanity and divinity were mixed, the peculiar blend through which new elemental properties bloomed.[111] After declaring that the product of Mary's womb, Jesus, was indeed a medicine, Caesarius then launched into a pointed critique of the physicians at the center of medical learning, Montpellier. Montpellier, Caesarius explained, was the "source" of the healing arts (*ubi fons est artis physicae*). And yet, he reminded his readers, healings occurred in greater abundance at Mary's shrine, not at the hands of schoolmasters. The doctors at Montpellier sent away the poor, scoffing at them, and instructing them to go to Rocamadour, where they could be cured for free. Despite the physicians' professional contempt, Caesarius asserted, the "fever-stricken are cured."[112] His brief characterization of Montpellier lambastes scholastic physicians for their lack of charity. Not only do they charge "the poor" high prices for God's natural medicine, but they send them to Mary "in flocks." They lacked the quality of care that this feminine agent of healing offered. They lacked the charity that truly healed the wounds of the poor, sick, and indigent.

The drive to materialize and universalize the causes of physiological transformation, resorting to such concepts as the doctor's special *virtus* or the *proprietas* of complexionate objects, clearly concerned some thirteenth-century theological and hagiographic authors. To them, materialization threatened to alienate the role of divine grace in the therapeutic process. Thomas Aquinas asserted that grace was necessary as a means of curing the infirmity unleashed on the human body and soul by original sin. "In the state of corrupt nature," he maintained, humans required grace "in order to be healed."[113] Grace emitted physical effects on the human by altering

---

110. Caesarius's logic is similar to scholastic arguments for the necessity of a material vehicle of grace in the sacrament. Sacramental agency is unleashed—that is, their transformation from ordinary materials such as water, wafer, or oil into conveyers of grace took place with the intentions of words uttered by a specialized authority, a priest. The element in the sacrament is essential, as it allowed the human to sensibly apprehend the sacrament. By uttering the words of the transubstantiating ritual over the Host, the priest's words altered the substance of the Host. Thomas Aquinas, for example, understood that when Christ said the words "This is my body," he actually effected what they signified.

111. Caesarius of Heisterbach, *Dialogus miraculorum*, bk. VII, ch. xxiv, 1372: "id est ex carne virginis salvatorem. Jesus interpretatur salvator sive salutare. Quia salvator, medicus est, quia salutare, medicina est."

112. Caesarius of Heisterbach, *Dialogus miraculorum*, bk. VII, ch. xxiv, 1374: "numquid non vides quam celerem sanitatem consequantur febricitantes."

113. *Summa Theologica*, II.1.

the sense appetites, reordering psychology, and modulating the passions. Aquinas interpreted the mechanics of grace in the human body, as he did with all substances, in the Aristotelian vocabulary of qualities. Grace, according to Aquinas, was an intentional or spiritual quality.[114] The qualities were "the cause of generation and corruption and alteration in all other bodies."[115] Aquinas regarded grace as a spiritual quality within the sacramental action taken by a priest with the co-operation of God. And grace was also a spiritual quality within the saints who transformed sick into healthy bodies.[116] According to Aquinas, grace was required for bodily balance of the passions and reason, and thus for health. Grace had transformative effects on the body and on other materialities as well. The sacraments were efficacious physical conduits of grace.[117] The effect, when one ingested grace in the Eucharist, was to "flow from the soul to the body."[118] The canon lawyer Huguccio postulated in his *De consecratione* that the elements of the Mass—bread, wine, and water—were transubstantiated into Christ's body, blood, and other aqueous humors (*aquaticum humorem*). When ingesting these consecrated elements, the body of the individual communicant was conformed to the perfect humoral balance of Christ.[119]

---

114. Grace was a quality of the soul; it acted on the soul in the manner of a formal cause, "just as whiteness makes a thing white." *Summa Theologica*, II.1.

115. Thomas Aquinas, *Sententia super libros De generatione et coruptione expositione* (Salamanca: Leonardo Hutz, 1496), prooem. N. 2. "Alteration" refers to changes in accidents; "generation" and "corruption" refer to changes in substance. Secondary qualities included tactile qualities such as roughness or smoothness; sensible qualities such as color, sound, and taste; occult qualities such as magnetism; spiritual or intentional qualities such as light; and immaterial qualities such as thoughts or volitions. On this taxonomy, see Robert Pasnau, "Scholastic Qualities, Primary and Secondary," in *Primary and Secondary Qualities: The Historical and Ongoing Debate*, ed. Lawrence Nolan (Oxford: Oxford Scholarship Online, 2011), 41–61.

116. On the grace within saints, see also Albertus Magnus, *On Animals*, 1445: "Only the human is a point of union between God and the world. For the human has in himself the divine intellect and through this he is sometimes elevated about the world to the extent that even the material of the world follows upon his thoughts. We see this in the best born men who use their souls to bring about a transmutation of worldly bodies."

117. Matthew Milner discusses Aquinas's understanding of grace as qualitative in "The Physics of Holy Oats: Vernacular Knowledge, Qualities, and Remedy in Fifteenth-Century England," *Journal of Medieval and Early Modern Studies* 43.2 (2013): 228.

118. *Summa Theologica*, III.11.

119. Thomas Izbicki, *The Eucharist in Medieval Canon Law* (Cambridge: Cambridge University Press, 2013), 34. This perception of the Eucharist is also seen in anecdotes such as one in which Lutgard diagnosed her own symptoms, deciding not to go to Mass. Christ provided her with an alternative source for the sacrament, the blood flowing from his side wound. Thomas tells readers that this was a regular part of Lutgard's health regimen. Once she endured a fever that had reached its "critical point," so she sucked blood from his wound and was instantly ready for choir; Marie of Oignies also was said to receive soothing from her wounds after calling to mind those of Christ.

This understanding of the Eucharist as a medicine that distributed salutary grace throughout the individual is reflected in hagiographic depictions of the sacrament. Jacques de Vitry characterized Marie of Oignies as so routinely sick during her final illness that she could eat nothing but the Host, which "immediately alleviated her bodily illness."[120] Thomas of Cantimpré also portrayed Margaret of Ypres in her final sickness as ingesting the Eucharist as a medicine that, when consumed, provided remedy for an entire day.[121] When Alice suffered from leprosy, she ingested the body of Christ and felt "healed by a spread of aromatic herbs."[122] Hugh of Floreffe attributed to the Eucharist a "remedy" with a specialized power to "renew" life.[123] And the hagiographer of Beatrice of Nazareth predicated nearly every use of the term Eucharist or "sacrament" with salubrious adjectives, such as "life-giving" (*vivificum*), "health-giving" (*salutifero*), and "salutary and life-giving" (*saluberrimum, vivificum*).[124] This "medicinal nourishment" and "supreme remedy" generated strength within Beatrice and allowed her to "quickly recover from all sickness."[125]

According to these hagiographers, certain religious women experienced an abundance of grace, just like the medicinal sacrament. "For I know very well and know truly," Hugh of Floreffe asserted confidently, "that many people doubt these things and see evil where good is and thence incur a loss to their salvation whence they might have had matter of power. For if they do not make a mockery of the spirit of grace itself, they are seen to derogate those vessels of grace in whom the spirit makes his works manifest."[126] Those "vessels of grace" (*vasis gratiae*) were the religious women who showed remarkable charity and penance on behalf of their neighbors. Hugh contended that skeptics sought to explain the special abilities of religious women as caused not by grace but by other natural means or by trickery. These doubters denied the power of God to manifest grace in "vetulae or poor little women" (*vetulae aut mulierculae pauperes*). He chastised natural philosophers for their derision of such women. These learned men, according to Hugh, relied solely on human logic and reason because they thought

---

120. *VMO* II.12, 157; trans., 123: "corporalem infirmitatem absque mora alleviabat."

121. *VMY*, ch. XL.

122. *VAS* II.13, 479: "quasi aromatibus odorantissimis in circuitu resarciri."

123. *VBJ* XXXVI.99; XL.105.

124. *VBN* II.iii.95; II.xi.126.

125. *VBN* I.xviii.81; II.xvi.160; II.xv.151–54.

126. *VYH* XLI.109, 883; trans, 131: "scio equidem et vere scio multos exercitatos magis habere sensus in rebus dubiis ad interpretationem mali quasi boni, et inde sibi efficere dispendium salutis unde materiam virtutis habere possent, si non Spiritui gratiae facerent contumeliam in eo quod vasis gratiae derogare videntur in quibus ipsum operari Spiritum prout vult."

that "nothing can be unless he knows how it can be."[127] But Hugh asserted that humans *can* know the reasons for such manifestations of grace, arguing that "the examination and proof of spiritual things must be undertaken spiritually."[128] For him, Yvette of Huy was "a mediatrix between heaven and earth, visible and invisible."[129] She was like a rare stone with hidden properties or like a sacrament, a material vehicle for inner grace. Either way, her powers required mastery, authorization; and thus both clerics and physicians sought to control stories about who could heal, and why.

The Body of the Saint

Thomas of Cantimpré's encyclopedic *Liber de natura rerum*, book 2, displays a hagiographer's rationalization of physiological transformation in the nexus between body, spirit, and soul.[130] Although Thomas imagined that the book was based on a treatise by Augustine, the treatise he copied has actually been identified as *De spiritu et anima*, which was possibly written by Alcher of Clairvaux (d. 1183).[131] Thomas's book reveals his abiding interest in explaining the soul's role in human physiology and its co-operation with the body; it also suggests his indirect knowledge of Qūstā ibn Lūcā's *De differentia spiritus et animae*.[132] Thomas constructs the relationship between soul, body, and spirit as one in which the spirit is the soul on behalf of its spiritual nature, or "on behalf of that which breathes in the body."[133] This relationship is for him a true wonder (*mira*), which he describes in a language of mixing similar to

---

127. *VYH* XLI.109, 883; trans., 132: "nihil aestimat posse fieri, nisi quod novit quomodo fiat."

128. *VYH* XLI.109, 883; trans., 132: "examinatio et comprobatio fit eorumdem spiritualium tantum spiritualiter, id est, a spirituali."

129. *VYH* XLI.107, 883; trans., 131: "Mediatrix . . . inter caelestia et terrestria, visibilia et invisibilia"

130. The treatise *De spiritu et anima* circulated widely in the twelfth century and was attributed to Augustine, though scholars have argued that it was actually written by Alcher of Clairvaux (d. 1183). Both Thomas Aquinas and Albertus Magnus rejected it. See Constant Mews, "Debating the Authority of Pseudo-Augustine's *De spiritu et anima*," *Przeglad Tomistyczny* 24 (2018): 321–48.

131. Constant Mews, "The Diffusion of the *De spiritu et anima* and Cistercian Reflection on the Soul," *Viator* 49.3 (2018): 297–330. Leo Norpoth published an extensive study of the treatise but did not come to a certain conclusion about its authorship. See Leo Norpoth, *Der pseudo-augustinische Traktat "De Spiritu et anima"* (Würzburg: Institut für Geschichte de Medizin, 1971), 63–67. On authorship, see also Gaetano Raciti, "L'autore del *De spiritu et anima*," *Rivista di Filosofia Neo Scolastica* 53 (1961): 385–401.

132. Mews, "Debating the Authority," 336.

133. *Liber de natura rerum* (Berlin: De Gruyter, 1973), II.vi, 85: "Spiritus ipsa est anima pro spirituali natura, vel pro eo quod spiret in corpore appellatus est spiritus."

Nicholas of Poland's, pronouncing as a fulsome miracle the unity between humanity and divinity that wed "the sublime" with "slime."[134]

This wonder of conjunction was perpetuated through the spirit, which mediated between body and soul. For Thomas, the soul made a distinct impression on the physical appearance of the body, "informing the body" (*corporalem informans*). He describes a "certain fiery power" (*Quedam vis ignea*) that rises from the heart to the brain, where it is then cleansed and purified, and then proceeds out of the body through "the eyes, ears, nostrils, and other instruments of the senses."[135] This power takes shape as sense impressions (*visum, auditum, odoratum, gustum, tactum*), which move in and out of the body, informing the imagination. In other words, the imagination is formed externally when the "fiery power" emitted from the sensoria makes contact with corporeal things. It then returns into the self as imagination, which, when refined, becomes a "corporeal spirit" (*spiritum corporeum*). When this spirit moves into the brain, the content of the imagination is joined to the spirit without mediation, "truly retaining the nature and *proprietatem* of a body."[136] Through the exercise of the imagination, the properties of other bodies might arise within one's own. Thomas concludes his book on the soul with this discussion of the corporeal spirit, citing the ancient book of occult medicine, the *Kyranides*, and shifting into the second person to warn his reader that the heavens exist precisely for the labor of the body without which "you will be afflicted" (*affligeris*).

Although Thomas does not here connect the imaginative powers to the bodies of the saints about whom he wrote, throughout the book he relies on physiological processes to explain the natural origins of visions, phantasms, communications among the living and the dead, and other spiritual feats. In other words, he was invested in developing natural justifications for the kinds of hagiographic phenomena he chronicled.[137] In hagiographic terms, this imaginative process might look something like Lutgard of Aywières's physiological changes during moments of intense contemplation, which arose from her interior state: "From the intellectual consideration of her mind

---

134. *Liber de natura rerum* II.10, 90: "Plenum fuit miraculo, quod tam diversa et tam divisa ab invicem ad invicem potuerunt coniungi. Nec minus mirabile fuit . . . nichil deo sublimius, nichil limo vilius."

135. *Liber de natura rerum* II.15, 95: "ibique purificata et colata per oculos, aures, nares ceteraque instrumenta sensuum foris progreditur."

136. *Liber de natura rerum* II.15, 95: "veraciter naturam corporis retinens et proprietatem."

137. Zachary Matus has also worked through the *Life* of Christina the Astonishing, correlating her paramystical feats with Thomas's natural philosophy. Zachary Matus, "Resurrected Bodies and Roger Bacon's Elixir," *Ambix* 60.4 (2013): 323–40.

inwardly, her bodily outwardly drew its likeness."[138] The portrayal of this outward bodily manifestation of inner spirit is evident in other hagiographic constructions from the corpus as well. For example, the author of the *Life* of Alice of Schaerbeek clarifies his commitment to revealing, from his subject's external comportment, her inner virtues:

> She was concerned to experience the range of affectivity to which so grave an understanding had been leading her. . . . inwardly, there was tribulation, by this she made herself companion to God. Outwardly, there was labor; by this she brought her body under the yoke. Inwardly, there was the shower of tears, as she wakefully recalled her infirmities and the long delay ahead before seeing the divine glory. . . . Outwardly, there were her neighbors' needs.[139]

Here, Alice's hagiographer makes his method plain. For him, outward characteristics, including her outward concern to care for her neighbors' needs, denote his subject's inward state of grace. Jacques de Vitry applied the same logic to Marie's physical state. "Her external behavior and appearance," he determined, "manifested the inward state of her mind."[140] According to this hagiographic logic, the bodies of female subjects expressed their unique interior gifts, such as prophecy, healing, or the ability to detect the presence of God in natural forms or in the Eucharist.[141] In the *Life* of Juliana of Mont-Cornillon, the saint's inner grace dominated external matter so powerfully that, not only her own body, but even the surrounding elements registered change in her presence. A cloud of smoke above Juliana's head, for example, indicated the fire of love said to be burning in her heart, while similar atmospheric incidents proximate to Lutgard "signified the desire of fervid prayer."[142]

Such descriptions of the outward effects of spiritual states were rooted in a specific saintly physiology. Some powerful bodies were premised on a perfectly balanced complexion. As Zachary Matus has shown, Roger Bacon,

---

138. *VLA* II.23, 249; trans., 257: "ex intellectuali enim consideratione mentis interius, similitudinem traxit corpus exterius."

139. *VAS* 4, 478; trans., 4 (my alterations): "jam per affectum sentire conabatur quo intellectu prius gravida ferebatur . . . intus, tribulationibus se Deo sociavit; foris cum laboribus corpus subjugavit; intus imbre lacrymarum et vigili recordatione propriae infirmitatis, ac dilatione visionis divinae gloriae jugiter manavit . . . Foris proximorum cunctorum necessitas."

140. *VMO* I.13, 87; trans., 74: "Interiorem mentis eius compositionem gestus exterior extrinsecarumque partium ostendebat compositio."

141. For examples of living saints made to detect the presence of Christ in the host, see, Ida of Léau (Gorsleeuw) 35b; Ida of Leuven V.II7a.

142. *VJM* II.vii.39; *VLA* II.18, 248; trans., 253: "fervidae orationis desiderium figurasse."

following theories articulated by William of St. Thierry's treatise on the body and soul, proposed to craft a perfect medicine that would balance the complexion with exactitude.[143] This perfectly balanced complexion, in turn, would hold the power to restore humans to a prelapsarian state, sharing the corporeal forms of Adam and Eve that had been nurtured by the fruit of the tree of life. These forms depended on the continuity of the saint's body and soul, and emphasized the spiritual origin of their bodily transformations. When Ida of Léau injured her head, for example, she experienced no physical pain. According to her hagiographer, this response was no marvel. "Let the hearers not wonder at this," he exclaimed, "for it is nothing to wonder at!" The entirety of Ida's body was absorbed by grace, filled by sweetness, and thus undistracted by worldly affliction: "What part of the bosom, what cell of the brain, what sector of the sense is not seething and swelling over with the sweetness of love and joys of heaven?"[144] Her distraction from pain corresponds to Urso of Salerno's explanation of the endurance of martyrs, whose lofty cogitations drew spirits away from afflicted limbs.

The interior grace lurking powerfully just beneath the surface of a saint's body might be known, just as in *proprietas*, by experience. Jacques de Vitry, for example, commented on the intellectual hesitation any rational person might experience when hearing such wondrous stories about the mulieres religiosae. "Had you not known [them] by experience," he explains, one could not possibly understand or accept their power.[145] Jacques provides the example of a "certain amiable man," who had accompanied Guido, the cantor of the cathedral chapter at Cambrai, to visit Marie of Oignies. The amiable man scoffed at Guido, mocking him for his wish to visit the living saint. Such a reaction, Jacques apologized, was perfectly reasonable, as the stories of Marie's wondrous power were quite beyond reason. But when the man met her personally, he was immediately transformed and began weeping incessantly. He had not known "from experience" until then.[146] It was his personal experience of Marie that finally allowed him to relinquish his rational doubt, to trust and know her power. Other men came to believe in Marie's

143. Matus, "Resurrected Bodies," 337. Matus refers here to Bacon's *Liber sex scientiarum*. He also notes that Thomas of Cantimpré dedicates part of *Liber de natura rerum* to metallurgical alchemy that would produce this medicine.

144. *Vita B. Ida Lewensi* (*BHL* 4144), in *AASS* October XXIX, 120–21; *Ida the Gentle of Léau*, trans. Martinus Cawley (Lafayette, OR: Guadelupe Translations, 1998), 47; hereafter *VILeau*: "Non mirentur qui audiunt. Non est enim mirabile . . . ex plenitudine mentis dulcedinem amoris, gaudia coeli, delicias ebulliat et eructet, qua parte pectoris, qua cella cerebri, quo sensus climate."

145. *VMO*, prol., 45; trans., 42: "itaque vix posses credere, nisi fide oculata per experientiam cognovisses."

146. *VMO* I.13, 88; trans., 74: "nunc autem in hac sancta muliere virtutem dei per experientiam percepi."

special properties, too, as they "read the unction of the spirit in her face as if they were reading a book."[147] Jacques's *Life* of Marie, in this way, served as the book that would enable readers and auditors to know her power, to experience it just as they might experience the previously unknown powers of a rare stone.

While the saint's inner grace might only be known through experience, like an object's *proprietas*, her body nevertheless provided observers with copious signs of its presence. After all, part of the hagiographers' task was to assure readers that visions and other spiritual proclivities of their protégés were indeed divinely inspired, rather than demonic. Hagiographers provided the virtuous context for saints' ecstasies and charisms, instructing readers and auditors in the process of discernment.[148] For example, when Ida of Léau became rosy and pale in the face every time she passed the sanctuary near the ciborium, her hagiographer interpreted these physiological changes for his audience. He asserted that the ciborium "transmitted" to her a spiritual consolation that caused "movement inside of her."[149] Each time she experienced an infusion of grace she reacted with a physiological change. When she attended Mass, for example, she was so consumed by divine sweetness that she had to rest while her face became red and luminous. One of Ida's sisters found her complexion's alterations odd, and demanded an explanation. Ida replied that when she contemplated the Trinity, her face turned pale, but when she shifted to contemplating Christ's humanity, it reddened. This alternating physiology reflected in her outer appearance the saint's inner composition. It can also be observed in descriptions of Lutgard's visage, which, according to Thomas, blushed when she contemplated Christ's humanity, particularly his passion. He provided the example of a monk who doubted reports of Lutgard's physiological transformation. The skeptical monk once plotted to sneak up on Lutgard during her prayers so that he could test and experience for himself the supposed powers of the saint. Observing her body gleaming bright red as if sprinkled with blood, the monk was finally converted to belief.

147. *VMO* I.13, 87; trans., 74: "in vultu eius quasi in libro unctionem Spiritus sancti legentes."

148. Thomas of Cantimpré writes about discernment of evil and good spirits in book 2 of the *Liber de natura rerum*, section 26. On discernment, see Renate Blumenfeld-Kosinski, *The Strange Case of Ermine of Rheims: A Medieval Woman between Demons and Saints* (Philadelphia: University of Pennsylvania Press, 2015); on discernment in Liège, see Walter Simons, "Reading a Saint's Body: Rapture and Bodily Movement in the *Vitae* of Thirteenth-Century Beguines," in *Framing Medieval Bodies*, ed. Sarah Kay and Miri Rubin (Manchester: Manchester University Press, 1994), 10–23.

149. *VILeau* 32, col. 117; trans., 34: "transmeabat . . . motum sequens intrinsecus."

In the hagiographic portraits of the religious women of the thirteenth-century Low Countries, we find reverberations of the cultural understanding of grace as a qualitative substance. Divine grace was understood to course through the bodies of saintly women, illuminating them from within and causing physiological transformations that, in turn, ensured viewers of their distinct spiritual status. Goswin of Bossut's depiction of Ida of Nivelles's face is exemplary. He described it as turning "aflame" and her eyes becoming radiant after a divine visitation in which she saw Christ dripping white fluid into her heart. Goswin insisted that, since this visitation, Ida had no need for candles in the dark because she illuminated rooms by brandishing her radiant hands and bright face like some kind of organic flashlight.[150] In the *Life* of Arnulf of Villers, Goswin imagines a woman's infusion of grace in similarly physical terms. He reports that Theophania, a mulier religiosa and "magistra hospitalis" who ran the Hôtel-Dieu in Paris, desired to see Arnulf face-to-face and asked one of the traveling clerics through whom she relayed messages to convey this wish to Arnulf on his journey home to Brabant.[151] Arnulf, in turn, replied to the woman via the cleric that she should expect to receive an "overflow of grace," and designated the exact date and time of its arrival. Goswin then added this little note, emphasizing the anatomical equipment through which such an overflow would greet her, "unless some neglect on her part blocks the aqueduct through which the stream of grace should flow into her heart."[152] Grace not only had bodily effects; the channels through which it poured were also conceived physiologically.

If grace caused physiological transformation, then medieval authors did not always conceive of the "medicine of grace" in strictly metaphorical terms. In fact, the metaphorical dimension of medical language can reveal the instability of the category of thirteenth-century medicine itself, the range of interdependent connotations conveyed by *salus*. Metaphor shapes social experience.[153] When authors used medical terminology to describe the effects of prayer and grace, they were reporting on real experiences. When Juliana prescribed a "stronger medicine" (*medicamine fortiori*) for her

---

150. *VIN* xxii.

151. *VAV* II.16. Walter Simons identifies Theophania as the prioress of the hôtel-dieu in "Beginnings: Naming Beguines in the Southern Low Countries, 1200–50," in *Labels and Libels: Naming Beguines in Northern Medieval Europe*, ed. Letha Böhringer, Jennifer Kolpacoff Deane, and Hildo van Engen (Turnhout: Brepols, 2014), 34.

152. *VAV* II.16.45b, 626; trans., 183: "nisi obstaculo negligentiae suae obstructus fuerit aquaeductus per quem rivulus gratiae debet influere in cor ejus."

153. Charlotte Furth, *A Flourishing Yin: Gender in China's Medical History, 960–1665* (Los Angeles: University of California Press, 1999), 56. Furth states that metaphor is not just adornment but an essential aspect of linguistic meaning structures.

community at Mont-Cornillon, her hagiographer may have been thinking in terms of therapeutic treatments designed to rid the body of vice, lift the affects to joy and hope, and finally render the body and soul more health-ful.[154] Similarly, when Ida of Nivelles convinced her sister to make confession, Goswin conveyed the prescription in medical terms. She "vomited forth" her sins in a purgation and "in this way received healing for her ailing soul."[155] Goswin also described Arnulf as "a new physician" who applied a medicine to his body in undergoing ascetic practice.[156] And Jacques de Vitry called the Mass "the medicine of salvation" and bewailed those who, like an unnamed Cistercian monk he knew, became overwhelmed by melancholy so that "he thrust aside the yoke of obedience and became sick, even fleeing medicine."[157] Marie's own fasting practices were, according to Jacques, a medicine that tempered the grace within her.[158]

Hagiographers and their audiences perceived the behavior of the muli-eres religiosae of the southern Low Countries according to a logic in which grace exerted transformative powers. The presence of grace not only altered the bodies of extraordinary individuals; it also retained the potential to effect change in the bodies of others. Like a rare *empiricum*, certain women enjoyed a grace that conveyed unpredictable powers. Those who experienced that power personally, like their devotees and even skeptics, claimed extraordinary transformation in their presence. They sought to tell their stories, to transmit knowledge about them, because, like stumbling upon an unknown stone with special *proprietas*, these women, touched by grace, bore unusual powers.

Meanwhile, proponents of learned medicine and natural philosophy were faced with the task of devising explanations for inexplicable remedies. They did not wish to jettison those remedies; after all, according to certain authoritative texts and widespread contemporary practice, they worked. In order to distinguish their bona fides, and thus to wrest authority over the use of empirical remedies and unseen forces, these authors had to present themselves as offering a distinct form of knowledge about the body and the causes of material change, one that could be accessed only through book learning. Their explanations encompassed the male body itself, the virtues of learned practitioners, the purity of their spirits, and the intentions of

---

154. *VJM* II.i.3.

155. *VIN* XIII; trans., 50: "evomuit . . . sic animae suae egrotantis sanitatem recepit."

156. *VAV* I.31; trans., 145: "novus iste physicus." See also *VAV* I.2.

157. *VMO* II.3, 115; trans., 95: "quae infirma fugiebat medicinam, et quae propriae voluntati semel renuntiaverat."

158. *VMO* I.8.

their soul. Their increasingly materialized explanations of verbal efficacy, in particular, situated the masculine body as capable of healing by natural means. As long-standing medical precedent held, women's bodies were just physiologically different. Because of their cooler conditions, women's bodies required a monthly purgation of menstruation, which ideally maintained balanced humors. But there were so many opportunities for a woman's body to disfunction, resorting to its inherent defectiveness. Menstruation often failed; it was irregular. Pregnancy, infertility, and contraception threw all kinds of unexpected twists into what should have been a balanced physiology. In these common instances, women's internal mishap threatened to cause humoral corruption, a toxic condition. By the fifteenth century, physicians would begin developing a framework for figuring women's bodies as in fact venomous and *harmful* to others.[159] Women could not heal naturally, like men, through their virtuous spirits. They could only harm naturally. Women could, however, heal supernaturally, aided by divine grace and mediated by clerical authority.

Many varieties of thirteenth-century authority thus weighed in to suggest how the soul and its affective powers might alter the bodies of self and other. Physicians, theologians, clerics, and spiritual directors employed a shifting vocabulary to rationalize and explain physiological transformations that seemed impossible. For all, there was a certain logic of the soul's power to render bodily change. That is, in all of the explanations examined in this chapter, none revert to the category of miracle. The body cooperated with the soul, but, as Hugh of Floreffe had explained to his readers, it required a spiritual hermeneutic in order to understand physiological change, in order to see spiritual imprints on material bodies. Theologians and physicians agreed that something quasi-physical was emitted from the souls of their subjects. Either by the intensity of the spiritual imagination, by the pure *virtus* of the breath, by grace and the reparation of sin, or the affective arousal that occurred in their presence, both saints and physicians held the potential for enacting bodily change.

---

159. For example, in 1499 Diego Álvarez Chanca published the *Tractatus de fascinatione*. Chanca was a learned physician and an avid explorer who accompanied Columbus on his second trip to the Indies. The disease of *fascination* explained that postmenopausal women sometimes retained trapped blood within their bodies, which became poisonous. Since according to the humoral economy, it had to go *somewhere*, Chanca reasoned that it was released as noxious vapors through their eyes. People in weakened conditions who looked upon these women became ill. See Fernando Salmón and Montserrat Cabré, "Fascinating Women: The Evil Eye in Medical Scholasticism," in *Medicine from the Black Death to the French Disease*, ed. Roger French (Aldershot: Ashgate, 1998), 53–84.

PART III

Therapeutic Practice

CHAPTER 4

Rhythmic Medicine

The Psalter as a Therapeutic Technology in Beguine Communities

The *Life* of Odilia of Liège recounts the widow's use of her psalter as a physiological exercise. Through meditation on images in the psalter, she wished to transform her bodily sensorium. Such a practice, she hoped, would reverse the embodied experiences she accumulated in her former secular life, restoring her to a state of purity. In this process of reconditioning, her hagiographer explained that she had "an image of a crucifix depicted in her psalter: trembling, she meditated with intent acuity of mind on the scars caused by his wounds and the cuts caused by the lashes of the needles of the thorns and the very wound in his side."[1] In order to transform her bodily sensoria so that she would experience the world as a chaste virgin, a bride of Christ, Odilia read the psalter while meditating on Christ's wounds. Thus, in the hands of Odilia, the psalter was a therapeutic technology. It spurred a salutary transformation within her. In the following two chapters, I examine books that circulated within women's religious communities in the southern Low Countries. I ask what those books can tell us about their healthcare knowledge and practice. While their books shared certain therapeutic principles—a "common tradition"—with scholastic

---

1. *VOL* 214–15: "habebat enim in suo psaltcrio crucifixi depictam imaginem, cuius cum intenta mentis acie cicatrices vulnerum scissurasque verberum, spinarum aculeos et ipsum vulnus lateris."

physicians, they also reveal religious women's distinctive approach to care, one characterized by affective performance and prayer.

Women like Odilia performed the psalter in order to practice acts of bodily and spiritual care: to heal themselves, to heal others, and to heal their communities.[2] Psalters could serve as therapeutic tools that assisted in the promotion of bodily health and the reversal of the effects of sin, a means to a good death and ultimate salvation. When used in women's religious communities, they promoted acts of both patient care and self-care; often the practitioner was also the patient, or performed the psalter in the voice of and on behalf of the patient. Although we have access only to the material trace of the psalters, I seek to resituate the performance of the psalter within the context of charitable caregiving in which, as we have seen, mulieres religiosae operated. By the "performance" of the psalter, I intend to call attention to the sonority, gesture, and "communicative space" opened up by women's acts of chanting its words, gazing on its vibrant images, enacting its poems, meditations, and prayers, and experiencing its embrace.[3] By performing the work of the psalter, women in this region engaged in salutary acts.

While the typical psalter would contain the full run of 150 psalms plus a few other formulaic materials, such as a liturgical calendar and litany, the psalters used in beguine communities in thirteenth-century Liège demonstrate some idiosyncrasies particular to their caregiving interests.[4] Through several mechanisms copied within them, I show, the psalters made for women's communities in this region constructed women's prayer as efficacious in bodily and spiritual healing. Those mechanisms, in short, include Mass prayers, health tables, and health prayers, as well as French poems and meditations designed to goad salubrious affects. The health tables and vernacular poems, in particular, are found only in this corpus of Mosan psalters. The contextual arrangement of these elements demonstrates the salutary function of the psalters as a whole. These improvisations signal their use in the

---

2. Odilia died in the 1220s. The psalters that I examine in this chapter were primarily produced in the later thirteenth century, around 1280. My argument is not that Odilia, or the other "living" female saints of Liège, used *these* psalters. Instead, my suggestion is that the first generation of religious women who provided charitable healthcare set a pattern of therapeutic prayer that is reflected, if distantly, in this corpus of psalters. The women who used these psalters would have their hagiographic models of prayer and care to follow.

3. On reconstructing the sonority of musical books, see Emma Dillon, *The Sense of Sound: Musical Meaning in France, 1260–1330* (Oxford: Oxford University Press, 2012); she discusses the "communicative space" of musical experiences (30).

4. Judith Oliver has comprehensively examined forty-one extant thirteenth- and fourteenth-century Mosan psalters, many of which were owned by beguines. See her *Gothic Manuscript Illumination in the Diocese of Liège, 1250–1350*, 2 vols. (Leuven: Peeters, 1988).

therapeutic activities of their owners and project an understanding of the body, illness, and health that elicits our imaginative rehybridization of the theoretical and practical meanings of premodern European medicine and Christian liturgy. That is, these psalters help us to imagine what healthcare looked like from within a women's religious community.

The Psalter in Women's Religious Communities

A number of hagiographic narratives reveal how psalters brought religious women into contact with others in need of comfort. Though we often consider psalters for the personal prayer work they helped their users to perform, the psalters created for mulieres religiosae in the late medieval lowlands demonstrate their use in mutual assistance and communal healing.[5] The work of the psalter was not only self-oriented. As a therapeutic technology, the psalter also worked on others. Psalm sequences, such as the Office of the Dead, were performed explicitly for others. For example, Marie of Oignies, who dedicated part of her life to the care of people suffering from leprosy, recited psalms while spinning: "While she worked with her hands and put her hand to the test and her fingers clasped the spindle, she had her psalter placed before her from which she would sweetly belch forth psalms to the Lord."[6] Jacques de Vitry described Marie's suave purgation (her sweet vomiting, *suaviter eructabat*) of the psalter as a therapeutic skill that she exercised not only on her own body, but also on the souls and bodies of others. He characterized her prayers as a kind of medicine for the sick of body and soul in her community; her prayers "soothed their sufferings as with a precious ointment."[7] Ida of Léau and Beatrice of Nazareth recited the psalter of the Virgin every day at La Ramée, and Juliana of Mont-Cornillon, also a caretaker of lepers, was taught the psalter by nurses at the leprosarium and committed the Psalms to memory from a young age.[8] Meanwhile, Margaret of Ypres apparently combined her recital of the Psalms with unceasing genuflections. This she did, according to her hagiographer, in order to relieve the effects of

---

5. Monika Otter has advocated for a similar disruption of the dichotomy separating personal from public or communal forms of devotion in her "Entrances and Exits: Performing the Psalms in Goscelin's *Liber confortatorius*," *Speculum* 83 (2008): 283–302.

6. *VMO* I.9, 70; trans., 63: "quod etiam dum operaretur manibus, dum manum suam mitteret ad fortia, et digiti eius apprehenderent fusum, psalterium ante se positum habebat, ex quo Psalmos domino suaviter eructabat."

7. *VMO* I.9, 71; trans., 64: "pretioso unguento dolores earum mulcebantur."

8. *VJM* I.iii; *Vita Beatricis*, ed. and trans. Roger de Ganck (Kalamazoo, MI: Cistercian Publications, 1991), I.xxvi; hereafter *VBN*.

sin in her peers.[9] Ida of Leuven recited the Psalms nightly, despite demonic visitations during this time; in fact, her hagiographer likened her voice to the psaltery, her words so mellifluous and abundant with divine praise.[10] In doing so, he called attention to the sonority of the Psalms, their experience as sound rather than their meaning as text. As a sonorous performance, I show, the recitation of the psalter could be directed to therapeutic practice.

Even when religious women were not literate readers of the Psalms, many of them maintained a relationship with the psalter that brought them into contact with the sick and dying. In this way, the performance of the Psalms was an effort at communal salvation, or communal health. Thomas of Cantimpré, for example, insisted that "it is holy and devout to assist the dying and to aid them with their prayers."[11] He explained that Lutgard did not understand the Psalms, yet experienced a certain efficacious power when uttering their words.[12] Their sonority and performance outstripped the textual vestiges of their words. Lutgard's facility with the psalter was so great that when she recited certain verses demons scattered away in fear, "by the strength of the words, even when she did not understand them."[13] Her relationship to the efficacy of words points beyond the text to the significance of performance and the oral transmission of knowledge in textual communities.[14] In Lutgard's hands, the psalter became an instrument to promote the "salvific effects" of her prayer.[15] Thomas portrayed Lutgard as requesting the ability to understand "the psalter through which I pray."[16] He indicated that she often ruminated on the psalter, during which she learned the power and meaning of the verses while remaining an "unlettered," "uneducated" nun.[17] Lutgard derived power from the psalter, from reciting its verses, because she

9. *VMY* 20. Thomas asserts that she would recite fifty psalms along with the four hundred *Our Fathers* and four hundred *Hail Marys*. Judith Oliver discusses these examples of beguines and recluses using the psalter in "Devotional Psalters and the Study of Beguine Spirituality," *Vox Benedictina* 9.2 (1992): 199–225.

10. *VIL* IV.I-7b; V.I-10d-11a.

11. *VLA* II.xv, 247; trans., 251: "Sanctum ergo et pium est assistere morientibus et eos . . . precibus adjuvare."

12. *VLA* II.xvi. Thomas asserts that demons scattered when she uttered Psalm 69, "deus in adiutorium meum intende."

13. *VLA* II.XVI, 247; trans., 251: "et aliorum quorumdam versuum in Psalterio . . . Unde intelligebat virtute verborum etiam a se non intellectorum praesentias daemonum propulsari."

14. Brian Stock, *The Implications of Literacy: Written Language and Models of Interpretation in the 11th and 12th Centuries* (Princeton: Princeton University Press, 1987).

15. Susan Boynton discusses the "salvific effects" of psalm performance and the "instrumentality" of the psalter in "Prayer as Liturgical Performance in 11th- and 12th-Century Monastic Psalters," *Speculum* 82 (2007): 892–931.

16. *VLA* I.xii, 239; trans., 226: "Psalterium per quod orem."

17. *VLA* I.xii: *idiotae, laicae*.

was immersed in a culture that imbued the words of the psalter with salvific effects. The weight of cultural tradition and authority conditioned her to regard the psalter as an efficacious tool. Cassian, for example, wrote of the communal effects of psalm work:

> I chant a psalm. A verse of the psalm inflames my heart. And when I listen to the music in the voice of one of my brethren, chanting a psalm, our souls are moved together. They arise, as if from sleep, and ascend, united in ardent prayer. I know, as well, that the singularity and seriousness of someone chanting the psalms can inspire great fervor in the minds of the bystanders, who are only listening.[18]

The mulieres religiosae of Liège participated in this long tradition of inciting others through recitation of the Psalms, and they further adapted this practice to care for the sick and dying. Their psalters reflect this adaptation. The performance of the Psalms enriched mutually beneficial and reciprocal relationships among religious women in Liège and the communities in which they were embedded.

This cultural appreciation of the salutary effects of the psalter is reflected in other hagiographic *Lives,* other genres, and other regions of western Europe. For example, an episode reported in the *Life* of Walter of Bierbeek indicates that, when overseeing the infirmary in his community, the saint found himself caring for a man who was possessed by a demon. Walter treated the man by reading him prayers and verses about Mary and flaunting her image while adjuring the demon to flee. The therapy that proved to be ultimately efficacious, however, was his application of the psalter. Placing the psalter on the man's head, Walter finally cast out the demon, at which point the man dropped to the ground for an hour before rising, completely healed.[19] Other instances of the psalter's therapeutic use can be found in medical and pastoral literature. For example, Bartholomaeus da Montagnana counseled patients with cold complexions to pray or sing the Psalms in a high pitch, explaining that this exercise of the soul enhanced delight.[20] The priest Danielis de Craffoldo made the same recommendation, though he may have regarded the

---

18. *Collationes patrum in scetica eremo* 9.1.26, PL 49:477–1328, at 802; trans., Stock, *The Integrated Self,* 25: "Nonnumquam etenim psalmi cuiuscumque versiculis occasionem orationis ignitae decantantibus nobis praebuit. Interdum canora fraternae vocis modulatio ad intentam supplicantionem stupentium animos excitavit. Novimus quoque distinctionem gravitatemque psallentis etiam adstantibus plurimum contulisse fervoris."

19. *De B. Waltero de Birbeke,* in *AASS* January II, 448: "dum psalterium super caput obsessi posuisset."

20. Glending Olson discusses this *consilium* among Bartholomaeus's other recommendations in *Literature as Recreation in the Middle Ages* (Ithaca: Cornell University Press, 1982), 61–63.

act of singing more generally, rather than psalter chant specifically, as therapeutically efficacious.[21] Although psalter prayer was broadly embraced as a remedy for various afflictions, the beguines of Liège appear to have adapted this practice to their specific therapeutic expertise.

Mosan Psalters

The typical monastic psalter served as a support for the divine office, so that at each canonical hour the monk or nun recited a number of psalms, along with antiphons, responses, versicles, hymns, and canticles.[22] Over the course of the week, each of the 150 psalms were recited.[23] By the twelfth century, after a long period of development, the form of the psalter had more or less stabilized so that, in addition to the Latin text of the Psalms, it included a calendar, litany, canticles, collects, and the Office of the Dead.[24] By the mid-thirteenth century, members of the laity began acquiring similar prayerbooks with a different pattern of psalms and prayers, including the Hours of the Virgin, the Hours of the Cross and of the Holy Spirit, the prayers *Obsecro Te* and *O intemerata*, the Penitential Psalms and Litany, the Office of the Dead, and Suffrages. These books were known as books of hours because the prayers within them were to be recited throughout the course of the day.[25]

The art historian Judith Oliver has identified a corpus of forty-one "Mosan" (from the Meuse valley) psalters from the thirteenth and early

21. Cohen-Hanegbi elaborates on Danielis's prescription in *Caring for the Living Soul: Emotions, Medicine, and Penance in the Late Medieval Mediterranean* (Leuven: Brill, 2017), 129n88.

22. The Psalms were arranged into daily reading so that by the end of the week the practitioner would have recited all 150 psalms. Virginia Reinberg, *French Books of Hours: Making an Archive of Prayer, 1400–1600* (Cambridge: Cambridge University Press, 2012), 16. Psalters for the laity appeared as early as the eleventh century, and included special offices like the Office of the Dead and the Little Office of the Blessed Virgin Mary. On the development of the psalter and books of hours, see also Roger Wieck, *Time Sanctified: The Book of Hours in Medieval Art and Life* (New York: George Braziller, 1988); Eamon Duffy, *Marking the Hours: The English People and Their Prayers, 1240–1570* (New Haven: Yale University Press, 2010); Anne Rudloff Stanton, *Queen Mary Psalter: A Study of Affect and Audience* (Philadelphia: American Philosophical Society, 2011); Andrew Hughes, *Medieval Manuscripts for Mass and Office: A Guide to Their Organization and Terminology* (Toronto: University of Toronto Press, 1982).

23. The distribution could vary according to monastic order or cathedral use. On the development of the psalter throughout the Middle Ages, see Chanoine Leroquais, *Les psautiers manuscrits latins des bibliothèques publiques de France* (Mâcon: Protat, 1940).

24. Eric Palazzo, *A History of Liturgical Books from the Beginning to the Thirteenth Century* (Collegeville, MN: Liturgical Press, 1998), 130–32.

25. Roger Wieck, *Painted Prayers: The Book of Hours in Medieval and Renaissance Art* (New York: George Braziller, 1997), 9–10.

fourteenth centuries, many of which were owned and used by beguines or other religious women in the region.[26] This corpus of Mosan psalters bears some distinctions. As Paul Meyer first noted, the psalters demonstrate a remarkable interest in local saints, both in their feast days and in their rich illuminations.[27] Although typical in their liturgical ordering, the psalters are also distinctive in their inclusion, among some examples, of features such as the Lambertum Easter table, personal prayers and other incidental scribbles, calendars of health rules, and a series of French devotional poems with corresponding full-page illustrations.[28] The Lambertum table was a verse used to determine the date of Easter.[29] While thirteenth-century psalters often included Easter tables, the Lambertum verse appears only in the Mosan corpus. Its prominence here can be explained in part by reference to Saint Lambert of Liège. In some instances, however, the table conflates the patron saint of Liège with Lambert le Bègue, the mythical founder of the beguines.[30] Another additional distinction of this corpus is that eight of the samples include Mass prayers at the beginning or end of the psalter, some with historiated initials featuring women engaged in confession and communion. The Mass prayers alternate between Latin and French, or sometimes appear exclusively in French. They include the prayers of confession (*Confiteor*), and petition (*Misereatur*), and a few psalters also feature the *Perceptio corporis tui* and the *Indulgentium*. The prayer texts often employ feminine endings and terms (*mulierem, famule, pecherise*) that place this corpus of psalters squarely in the hands of women. Given these additional texts and images, it might be more appropriate to describe these books as psalter-hours, falling somewhere in between a psalter from a religious community and a lay book of hours. In sum, women's psalters in the region display a highly elastic quality. Their inclusion of a varied array of prayers as forms of speech and guides for action opens a window onto therapeutic practice in feminine space, such as beguinages and their affiliated hospitals.[31]

---

26. Oliver, *Gothic Manuscript Illumination*, 1:112–19. The term "Mosan" here refers to the region around the Meuse valley in Liège, Namur, Huy. Oliver's exquisite catalog and her essay "Devotional Psalters and the Study of Beguine Spirituality" have been fundamental to my thinking in this chapter.

27. Although Oliver subsequently identified more psalters in the corpus, Paul Meyer first described the unique character of psalters in the region in his article "Rapport sur d'anciennes poésies religieuses en dialecte liégois," *Revue des Sociétés Savants des Départements* 6 (1873): 236–49.

28. Oliver, *Gothic Manuscript Illumination*, 1:34–38.

29. *Lambertum talem qui nobis ingerit artem ad paradisiaci perducat lumina regni magnus celorum factor*. On the phrase, see Paul Meyer, "Le Psautier Lambert le Bègue," *Romania* 29 (1900): 536–40.

30. See Oliver, *Gothic Manuscript Illumination*, 1:33–34.

31. On the grammar and practice of prayer as a form of speech, see Peter Metcalf, *Where Are You/Spirits: Style and Theme in Berawan Prayer* (Washington, DC: Smithsonian Press, 1989).

The French poems occurring throughout many of these psalters (or psalter-hours) are particularly striking. Several books in the corpus include a series of twenty-one French poems that either precede or follow the Psalms, and in some cases they manifest in both positions. The poems appear in various combinations, with some psalters including as many as eight, and others only a single poem.[32] They occur in two forms: either a *historia* narrating Gospel events, such as the visit of the three Marys or the presentation in the temple, or in the form of a long series of impassioned Aves. All of them conclude with a supplication for the intercession of the Virgin and the forgiveness of Christ.[33] Reflecting the structure of the psalter itself, the poems consist of 150 stanzas in which each four-line Ave paraphrases a verse from the 150 psalms, and the poems unfold as three sets of fifty quatrains.[34] Although the poems are not attributed to a single author, their feminine associations are visible in their language, which includes petitions from *ton ancelle, vostre ancelle, la toie ancelle, a filhe et a amie.*[35]

These supplications are also a hallmark of the poems' vocality. They read like scripts for performance, and may have functioned in that manner as well. Together, the poems align in a narrative of the life and passion of Christ, suggesting their use as a form of paraliturgical performance. Such performances were encouraged by the famous *liégeois* preacher, Lambert le Begue, who taught his parishioners to engage in recitations of versified vernacular translations of the Acts of the Apostles, the letters of Paul, and scenes from the lives of Christ and Mary.[36] The narrative poems may have functioned as *historia*,

---

32. Keith Sinclair identified the poems and the manuscripts in which they appear. Oliver's investigation of Mosan psalters added additional manuscripts to Sinclair's list, bringing the total to fourteen. See Keith Sinclair, "Les manuscrits du psautier de Lambert le Bègue," *Romania* 86 (1965): 22–47; Oliver, *Gothic Manuscript Illumination*, 1:38–39. Paul Meyer discusses the poems in "Rapport sur d'anciennes poésies."

33. The Aves, as Judith Oliver has noted, draw on a Cistercian tradition of transforming the Psalms into praises of the Virgin, which developed into the Marian Psalter. Oliver, *Gothic Manuscript Illumination*, 1:39. The earliest version was *Ave porta paradysi*, c. 1130. Gerard Meersseman argues that the Marian Aves originated at Pontigny, perhaps with Hugh or Peter. See his *Der Hymnos Akathistos im Abendland* (Freiburg: Universitätsverlag, 1958), 2:12–14.

34. Oliver, *Gothic Manuscript Illumination*, 1:39.

35. Oliver, *Gothic Manuscript Illumination*, 1:41. Oliver notes that these supplications occur in every copy of the poems and may refer either to the author or to the manuscript's owner. In one of the psalters in which the petition occurs (New York, The Morgan Library, MS 183), male patronage is certain.

36. Lambert of Liège, "L'Antigraphum Petri et les lettres concernant Lambert le Bègue, conservés dans le manuscrit de Glasgow," ed. Arnold Fayen, *Compte-Rendu des Séances de la Commission Royale d'Histoire* 68 (1899): 255–356. A narrative enactment of this emotive form of theater can be found in Thomas of Cantimpré's *Life* of John of Cantimpré, which features the priest directing penitents in a melodramatic spectacle of their own contrition, one even performing ritual suicide and

a paraliturgical form that became increasingly popular in the later Middle Ages when office compositions with antiphons and responsories in modal order were being composed in celebration of living saints.[37] The poems are also striking for their adaptability as *contrafacta* to existing melodies, a characteristic that would have fit comfortably in Liège as a center of office production and development.[38] As Catherine Saucier has shown, polyphonic sound rang from the cathedrals and indoor and outdoor processions of Liège as the prince-bishopric forged a civic identity through the performance of offices celebrating local bishop saints.[39] The poems, as well as the psalters in which they are inscribed, gained significance within this broader culture of performance in thirteenth-century Liège. It seems that they were not only prayer texts that were read privately; they were also performed publicly by beguines and other mulieres religiosae in processions, at wakes and funerals, and in other dramatic devotional recitations. Beguine devotional readings were so common, so public, and so theatrical, in fact, that they were the source of mockery at a 1298 carnival in Huy in which a group of boys (*juvenes masculini sexus*) processed two by two in beguine garb while clutching books in their arms from which they sang (*canendo*) and read.[40]

Finally, each of the poems is illustrated with full-page, facing miniatures that depict the Gospel events referenced therein, as well as images of saints

---

resurrection in front of a crowd to demonstrate his rebirth as a forgiven man. On this spectacle, see Rachel Smith, *Excessive Saints: Gender, Narrative, and Theological Invention in Thomas of Cantimpré's Mystical Hagiographies* (New York: Columbia University Press, 2019), 88. The ritual suicide is in the *Life* of John of Cantimpré at II.13.

37. Barbara Walters considers the narrative poems as *historia*: "One might think of these as liturgical-musical versions of saints' *vitae*." Walters, "Introduction to the Mosan Psalters," in *The Feast of Corpus Christi*, ed. Barbara Walters, Vincent Corrigan, and Peter Ricketts (University Park: Pennsylvania State University Press, 2006), 434. On the *historia* of liturgical offices, see Margot Fassler and Rebecca Baltzer, *The Divine Office in the Latin Middle Ages: Methodology and Source Studies, Regional Developments, Hagiography* (Oxford: Oxford University Press, 2000), 430–62.

38. Walters, "Introduction to the Mosan Psalters," 436.

39. Catherine Saucier, *A Paradise of Priests: Singing the Civic and Episcopal Hagiography of Liège* (Rochester: University of Rochester Press, 2014). The performance of song in celebration of local saints is visible at the microlevel of the abbeys in this region as well. For example, an early thirteenth-century manuscript from Villers features liturgical offices created for Marie of Oignies and Arnulf of Villers, Brussels, KBR, MS II–1658. The offices were most likely written by Goswin of Bossut, who served as the cantor at Villers. Even though these saints were not canonized, their offices show that they were endorsed by the Cistercians at Villers. On the Office of Marie, see Hugh Feiss, "Introduction to the Texts for the Mass and Divine Office in Honour of Mary of Oignies," in *Mary of Oignies: Mother of Salvation* (Turnhout: Brepols, 2006), 177–83. On the *historia* of Marie in the context of the musical and literary culture of Villers, see Pieter Mannaerts, "An Exception to the Rule? The Thirteenth-Century Historia for Mary of Oignies," *Journal for the Alamire Foundation* 2 (2010): 233–69.

40. *Chroniques liégeoises*, ed. Sylvain Balau (Brussels: P. Imbreghts, 1915), I:47–48 (1298).

and biblical figures. Some of the more common images include the Tree of Jesse, Christ among the Doctors, and the Three Magi. In some manuscripts, only the full-page illustrations appear, without poems, suggesting a mode of oral transmission beyond the poems' text. This imagetext quality of the psalter poems indicates their polyvalence, weaving together Gospel events, psalms, images, lyric, and supplications in an intertextual performance.[41] The psalter supported this multimodal performance, guiding its users in gesture, voice, and affect. These unique features of Mosan psalters, I will argue, reveal how the mulieres religiosae of Liège integrated prayer with bodily care in a distinct form of therapeutic performance. They demonstrate how mulieres religiosae created and constructed therapeutic knowledge specific to their communities.

These psalters circulated in women's hands in a rather informal manner. They were not mass-produced books, but, as the textual distinctions discussed above suggest, were instead personalized with selections of text and images.[42] A woman with the wealth to do so could have such a book made to spec at a stationery shop. Writing in 1273, Guibert of Tournai complained of beguines who read together "in their little convents, in workhouses, in the streets" from books that were readily available for purchase at such shops (*stationarii*); and, as Walter Simons has noted, the details of his invective seem directly addressed to the beguines of Flanders, Hainaut, and Liège.[43] Beguines who could not afford to purchase their own personalized psalters might share one in a network of ad hoc borrowing. For example, a will from 1264 indicates that a man from Ypres left his psalter to the beguinage of St. Christine so that the mistress could oversee its lending out to beguines who might need one.[44] On another occasion, the will of Helvide Blandine, a

---

41. By imagetext, I mean to indicate that the images and texts have a synthetic quality. For example, even in the absence of the text, the images in these psalters still communicate the content and musical rhythms of the poem. On imagetexts and their distinction from image/text or imagetext, see W. J. T. Mitchell, *Iconology: Image, Text, Ideology* (Chicago: University of Chicago Press, 1987). On medieval imagetexts, see Jessica Brantley, *Reading in the Wilderness: Private Devotion and Public Performance in Late Medieval England* (Chicago: University of Chicago Press, 2007).

42. Judith Oliver, "Reflections on Beguines and Psalters," *Ons Geestelijk Erf* 66.4 (1992): 249.

43. Guibert of Tournai, "Collectio de scandalis ecclesiae," *Archivum Franciscanum Historicum* 24 (1931): 61–62: "Legunt ea communiter . . . in conventiculis, in ergastulis, in plateis."

44. As discussed in Walter Simons, "Staining the Speech of Things Divine: The Uses of Literacy in Medieval Beguine Communities," in *The Voice of Silence: Women's Literacy in a Men's Church*, ed. Thérèse de Hemptinne and María Eugenia Góngora (Turnhout: Brepols, 2004): 108. The will from Lauwers Brichame is dated 1264. It can be found in Guillaume Des Marez, "Le droit privé à Ypres au XIIIe siècle," *Bulletin de la Commission Royale pour la Publication des Anciennes Lois et Ordonnances de Belgique* 12 (1927): 310.

beguine from St. Christopher in Liège, made provision in 1266 for women to acquire psalters after her death.[45] Beguine psalters, then, were both personal and communal. They included specific texts and images that reflected the interests of the original owner, but they were also shared in networks that encouraged their public performance.

Orality, Performance, and Routes of Transmission

Performance as a medium of cultural transmission has often escaped the documentary, textual realm of the archive.[46] Attending to performance as a means of transmission, then, has the potential to remake our understanding of what "counts" as documentation; performance can capture traces of feminine health knowledge and practice that have escaped the record of medical acts.[47] For thirteenth-century religious women who practiced caregiving, the repertoire of their practice becomes visible only when searching beyond the written word, in the "unstable realm between writing and orality."[48] Monica Green's use of the phrase "unstable realm" points to the overlapping, co-constitutional qualities of speech and writing, a phenomenon that Ngugi wa Thiong'o calls "orature."[49] Orature's unstable realm encompasses multiple forms of communication, including gesture, dance, procession, storytelling, prayer, song, and ritual.

We can begin to grasp the orature through which medical knowledge was transmitted in women's communities in a variety of sources, but it is particularly visible in practice-oriented literature such as regimens of health, penitential manuals, meditational guides, and sermons. For example, when Conrad of Marburg began to outline the treatment that Elizabeth of Thuringia provided to patients in the hospital she founded, he remarked in the case of a "poor little boy" that "by bathing and treating him—from whom she learned this, I do not know—she succeeded

---

45. See Oliver, *Gothic Manuscript Illumination*, 1:206. The will is preserved in Liège, Archives de l'État, Dominicains, chartes, no. 22 July 1266.

46. Diana Taylor, *The Archive and the Repertoire: Performing Cultural Memory in the Americas* (Durham: Duke University Press, 2003).

47. Diana Taylor, "Remapping Genre through Performance: From 'American' to 'Hemispheric' Studies," *PMLA* 122 (2007): 1417.

48. Monica Green, "Books as a Source of Medical Education for Women in the Middle Ages," *Dynamis* 20 (2000): 360.

49. *Critical Perspectives on Ngugi Wa Thiong'o*, ed. G. D. Killam (Washington, DC: Three Continents, 1984), 58–66.

in curing him."[50] Conrad here acknowledged the therapeutic skill and success that Elizabeth possessed, while also recognizing the unstable source of her knowledge, knowledge that was not derived from formal means of medical reading or apprenticeship. Or take the example of the Cistercian nun Gertrud of Helfta, whose *Legatus* recounts an experience of seeing Christ wounded on the cross. While envisioning her care for Christ's wounds, Gertrud explained her process of spreading an ointment and bandage and related, "I had *heard it said* that wounds have to be bathed, anointed, and bandaged."[51] By asserting an oral source for the transmission of knowledge about wound care, Gertrud applied therapeutic concepts to her prayer practice. Without identifying the exact medical source to which she refers, her claim to have heard it and appropriated it in her meditational experiences indicates some of the ways in which religious women constructed their own therapeutic epistemologies from medical information delivered orally in sermons and daily conversation, as well as in confessional manuals, meditational guides, and regimens.

Some of this medical information would have been disseminated as common tradition over many decades by confessors, priests, and clerics. For example, Hugh of Folieto (d. 1172), Domenico Cavalca (d. 1342), and William of Auvergne (d. 1249) drew on medical concepts such as purgation, evacuation, humoral balance, and the bodily effects of the accidents of the soul.[52] These concepts explained the bodily bearing of sin and the means through which it could be relieved. Alan of Lille's *Art of Preaching*, for instance, invoked the language of diagnosis to train priests in their inquiry into penitents' sins, their duration, intensity, and location, even noting the patient-penitent's daily regimen, pulse, bearing, and facial expression.[53] Academic medical discourse and penitential literature were co-constitutive media and knowledge systems. They informed one another in the proper approach to care. Late medieval patients were conceived in

---

50. Kenneth Wolf, *The Life and Afterlife of St. Elizabeth of Hungary* (Oxford: Oxford University Press, 2010), 48.

51. This comment occurs in book 2, which was written by Gertrude. The remaining four books in the *Legatus divinae pietatis* were composed by other members of her community at Helfta, notably a "Sister N." Book 5 of the *Legatus* includes detailed information about the infirmary at Helfta. See Gertrude of Helfta, *Oeuvres Spirituelles*, ed. and trans. Jacques Hourlier, Pierre Doyere, and Jean-Marie Clement (Paris: Éditions du Cerf, 1967–86). Gertrude of Helfta, *Herald of Divine Love*, trans. Margaret Winkworth (New York: Paulist Press, 1993), 102 (emphasis added).

52. On the medical language of purgation, balance, and catharsis in the literature of confession, see Cohen-Hanegbi, *Caring for the Living Soul*; Winston Black, "William of Auvergne and the Rhetoric of Penance," in *Learning to Love: Schools, Law, and Pastoral Care in the Middle Ages*, ed. Tristan Sharp (Toronto: PIMS, 2017), 419–42.

53. Alan of Lille, *The Art of Preaching*, trans. Gillian Rosemary Evans (Piscataway, NJ: Gorgias Press, 2010), prologue to book 1.

hylomorphic terms, as ensouled bodies, and thus required specialists of body and soul to ensure health and well-being. Both doctors and confessors worked out healthcare methods for treating aspects of the human in which the material and spiritual were conflated, particularly in the "accidents of the soul," the sixth non-natural roughly corresponding to the emotions (also sometimes referred to as "passions" of the soul). Priests and physicians each employed meditation, psalmody, the recitation of miracles, and the exercise of faith as therapies designed to strengthen the soul and thus improve the body. Albertus Magnus, for example, fashioned confession as an attempt to conform the self to the humoral body of Christ, asserting that "the bitter humors must be vomited by confession and the antidote of penance before the food of health can be administered."[54] Peter of Blois described confession as a kind of bloodletting through which disease-causing sin is purged from the body.[55] And sermons and penitential literature adopted the language of the Fourth Lateran Council's Canon 21, which asserted the bodily effects of the Eucharist when designating the priest as a "skilled doctor" who, by facilitating the purge of sin, attended to the "wounds of the injured one," employing various salutary techniques to "heal the sick."[56]

Religious women were steadfast auditors of this literature. Take the example of the sermons of Guiard of Laon, the thirteenth-century bishop of Cambré and chancellor of the University of Paris. Guiard was a dedicated champion of the religious women of Liège, as well as a theologian with an abiding interest in the effects of the Eucharist. Guiard's sermons labeled the Eucharist with medical terminology such as *digestivum, apothece,* and *remede contra tot maladie* and adapted a Galenic typology of treatment to outline how this sacramental medicine assisted the body in manners preventative, curative, conservative, and comforting.[57] One of Guiard's sermons appears, in Latin, in a manuscript belonging to the Cistercian women's abbey of

---

54. Albertus Magnus, *On the Body of the Lord*, trans. Sr. Albert Marie Surmanski (Washington, DC: Catholic University of America Press, 2017), 311.

55. Peter of Blois, *De duodecim utilitatibus tribulationis*, PL 207:992–93, in Cohen-Hanegbi, *Caring for the Living Soul*, 103.

56. *Constitutiones Concilii quarti Lateranensis una cum commentariis glossatorum*, ed. Antonius García y García (Vatican City: Bibliotheca Apostolica Vaticana, 1981). Several scholars have remarked on the influence of Canons 21 and 22 on medieval understandings of health. See especially Jessalynn Bird, "Medicine for Body and Soul: Jacques de Vitry's Sermons to Hospitallers and Their Charges," in *Religion and Medicine in the Middle Ages*, ed. Joseph Ziegler and Peter Biller (York: York Medieval Press, 2001); Marcia Kupfer, *The Art of Healing: Painting for the Sick and the Sinner in a Medieval Town* (University Park: Pennsylvania State University Press, 2003), 133–35; Naoë Kukita Yoshikawa, "Holy Medicine and Diseases of the Soul: Henry of Lancaster and the *Le livre de seyntz medicines*," *Medical History* 53 (2009): 397–414.

57. P. C. Boeren, *La vie et les oeuvres de Guiard de Laon* (The Hague: Njhoff, 1956), 252–53.

La Cambre, KBR MS 8609–20, which will be discussed in detail in the following chapter. This sermon also appears, in a vernacular translation, in British Library, Harley MS 2930, a Mosan psalter from 1280 belonging to a thirteenth-century woman, most likely a beguine. Its multiform appearances in these codices suggest the multiple avenues through which medical discourse and concepts permeated women's religious communities. Confession and penance were understood in these communities as salutary modes of purgation practiced alongside bloodletting and emetics; knowledge of these practices circulated in sermon literature, meditational guides, confessional treatises, and regimens. They are part of the "common tradition" of humoral medicine, meaning that basic principles of humoral balance and the regimen and recipes required to maintain and restore balance were shared widely, not solely among learned physicians.[58] These modes of knowledge transmission operated within a culture that valued the authority of speaking and gesturing to the same degree that it valued writing.[59] In sermons, penitential literature, and regimens, therapeutic knowledge was communicated not only textually but also in musical, lyrical, vernacular, visual, and gestural forms.

Women's religious communities were not, of course, the only sites at which confession and penance were enacted medically. At the hospital of St. John in Bruges, for example, the chaplain was mandated, beginning in the thirteenth century, to confess each new patient upon arrival lest any new sin infect the entire ward.[60] This requirement was replicated in thirteenth-century French hôtels-Dieu.[61] But women took on new roles within this penitential context. Following Lateran IV's canonical ordinance that all Christians wishing to achieve salvation make annual confession, religious women in Liège assumed roles in proselytizing the urgency of confession and penance.[62] The mulieres religiosae's association with confession and penance was integral to a larger concern for the bodily and spiritual well-being of

---

58. On the "common tradition" of knowledge systems, see Richard Kieckhefer, *Magic in the Middle Ages* (Cambridge: Cambridge University Press, 1989), 56–94.

59. David Gentilcore, *Medical Charlatanism in Early Modern Italy* (Oxford: Oxford University Press, 2006), 302. In fact, women's communities likely valued oral, gestural, and visual forms of knowledge over written ones.

60. Peregrine Horden, "Religion as Medicine: Music in Medieval Hospitals," in *Religion and Medicine in the Middle Ages*, ed. Peter Biller and Joseph Ziegler (York: York University Press, 2001), 139; see also Emmanuel Van Der Elst, *L'Hôpital Saint-Jean de Bruges de 1188 à 1500* (Bruges: Vercruysse-Vanhove, 1975), 61–62.

61. James Brodman, "Religion and Discipline in the Hospitals of Thirteenth-Century France," in *The Medieval Hospital and Medical Practice*, ed. Barbara Bowers (New York: Routledge, 2007), 123–32.

62. Dyan Elliott, *Proving Woman: Female Spirituality and Inquisitional Culture in the Later Middle Ages* (Princeton: Princeton University Press, 2004), 47–84.

their neighbors, for the health of the Christian community.[63] For example, Ida of Nivelles once encouraged a nun's confession in explicitly therapeutic terms when she sensed a sister's sin. Her hagiographer, Goswin of Bossut, compared the experience to "imbibing a salubrious potion. Thanks to this potion she could completely vomit up all the filth she had been heaping up in the bottom of her heart."[64] Goswin presented the effects of Ida's intervention in salutary terms as well, stating that "she received healing."[65] Ida facilitated a similar transformation for a canon who was wearied by an unconfessed sin. Paying a visit to Ida, he found consolation "and removed the sorrow clouding his heart."[66] In many cases, mulieres religiosae negotiated a final, therapeutic confession for their clients at the moment of their death. For example, when Lutgard perceived that Mary of Brabant had become ill, her first concern was to exhort the duchess to remain in bed and make confession. When she learned that Godfrey of Brussels had fallen ill, she issued the same urgent plea.[67]

Confession before death was of course tantamount to a healthy afterlife. It was a final gesture required to secure the well-being of the soul, true life, and many of the mulieres religiosae of Liège came to be regarded as specialists in encouraging this form of preventative care. Christina Mirabilis, for example, became well known for her attentiveness to deathbed confession. Thomas asserted that Christina sought out the dying to provide them the comfort of confession. She "assisted the dying most willingly and gladly exhorted them to a confession of their sins."[68] The Count of Loon, who offered Christina his dying confession, was no exception. In her eagerness to encourage confession among the dying, Thomas asserted that Christina "showed solicitude and wondrous compassion not only to dying Christians, but also to Jews."[69] Such a statement demonstrates the communal proximity of Jewish and Christian women in western Europe, particularly around

---

63. Oliver, *Gothic Manuscript Illumination*, 1:113.

64. *VIN* XIII; trans., 50: "facta confessione tamquam salubri prelibata potione, quidquid sordidum per incuriam suam in fundo cordis . . . vi eiusdam potionis perfecte evomuit" (I altered the translation slightly).

65. *VIN* XIII; trans., 50: "sanitatem recepit."

66. *VIN* XVI: "amovens a corde suo tristitiae nubilum."

67. *VLA* II.36.

68. *VCM* I.27, 655; trans., 142: "Libentissime ac benignissime morientibus assistebat, exhortans ad peccatorum confessionem." Scholars have long commented on the excessive melodrama, even the "horror," of Christina's lamentations for the souls of sinners. This exuberant mourning was not specific to her, or to Christianity. The trope of women's excessive mourning is found in contemporaneous Islamic traditions; see Nadia Maria El Cheikh, *Women, Islam, and Abbasid Identity* (Cambridge, MA: Harvard University Press, 2015), 38–58.

69. *VCM* I.27, 655; trans., 142: "Nec hoc solum in Christianos morientes, verum etiam in Judaeos."

domestic topographies such as wells and ovens, two sites Christina was said to frequent.[70] One wonders how Christina would have been perceived by the Jewish community to whom she offered compassion as they died. Portrayed as solicitude by Thomas, her outreach, linked to exhortations to conversion and warnings of divine punishment, seem more exasperating than therapeutic. But Christina—or a woman very like her—appears as a kind of helpmate to the dead in Jewish tradition as well. As Elisheva Baumgarten has shown, Christina appears in a text shared among women in nearby Jewish communities.[71] *Sefer Hasidim* (The Book of the Pious), a thirteenth-century halakhic (legal), moral, and narrative composition written by three German pietists (Hasidei Ashkenaz), features the story of a "gentile mistress" (*sarit*) who died and then sprung from her coffin at her funeral.[72] When she returned from the dead, this woman provided postmortem reports on the status of the souls of her neighbors whom she saw in heaven and hell, including the Jewish people she spotted in the garden of Eden.[73]

These hagiographic portraits affirm that religious women played important roles in communicating and facilitating a "good death," which, among Christians, required confession.[74] In a faith that was premised on resurrection of the body and achievement of everlasting life, prayer for the dead was crucial to communal well-being, and skilled practitioners were essential to ensuring the circumstances of a good death. Religious women prayed for the sick and dying, tended to their comfort, elicited their final confessions, called priests to administer sacraments, and finally cleaned, wrapped, and escorted

---

70. On the cooperation of Christian and Jewish women in caregiving, see Elisheva Baumgarten, *Mothers and Children: Jewish Family Life in Medieval Europe* (Philadelphia: University of Pennsylvania Press, 2007). On Thomas's efforts to convert via hagiographic production, see Barbara Newman, *Thomas of Cantimpré: The Collected Saints' Lives* (Turnhout: Brepols, 2008), 16. John of Cantimpré played a role in the death of a Cathar; *VJC* I.19. Thomas says that the Jewish community of St. Trond was "a very large company in the town," suggesting perhaps his concern as a preacher to eradicate religious minorities, a concern exemplified in his enthusiasm for the anti-Cathar campaign and for the Crusades.

71. Elisheva Baumgarten, "A Separate People: Some Directions for Comparative Research on Medieval Women," *Journal of Medieval History* 34.2 (2008): 212–28. Baumgarten makes it clear that this woman is very much like Christina in the circumstances of her death, resurrection, and postresurrection visions, if she was not actually Christina herself.

72. On *Sefer Hasidim*, see David Shyovitz, *A Remembrance of His Wonders: Nature and the Supernatural in Medieval Ashkenaz* (Philadelphia: University of Pennsylvania Press, 2017).

73. Baumgarten, "A Separate People," 224.

74. On making preparations for a good death, see Anu Lahtinen and Mia Korpiola, eds., *Dying Prepared in Medieval and Early Modern Europe* (Turnhout: Brill, 2017).

cadavers to burial and sang psalms at their funeral services.[75] As they did so, a psalter was often in their hands.

Regimental Advice

While medical concepts were transmitted into women's religious communities through sermons and penitential literature, we also have evidence of therapeutic knowledge circulating in the form of health regimens, or books of routine medical advice. These regimens provide another example of the "unstable realm" through which medical information was transmitted into women's communities. Take the example of a vernacular regimen created for the nuns of the Cistercian abbey of Maubuisson (figure 2). In 1281, a doctor named Thomas of Thonon had retired to the nearby Benedictine abbey of St. Martin de Pontoise in northern France, where he claims to have come into frequent contact with the women of Maubuisson, taking advantage of being familiar with "their home."[76] Thomas wrote a regimen addressed to the nuns, though his work also mentions lay subjects of care. He either intended his treatise for broader circulation than the nuns of Maubuisson or he expected that the nuns occasionally provided advice to patients from outside their walls. Maubuisson had amassed an array of granges and housed pensioners and underaged girls, among them at least one beguine, so it is possible that these residents were among the nuns' patients.[77]

The treatise is written as a "simple book" that will impart knowledge on "how to preserve health and cure [God's] diseases."[78] This "simple book" referred both to its modest goals and the fact that it provided "simples," or remedies composed of a single substance. Although offering only a "little education" (un petitet d'ensaignement), Thomas sought to authorize his knowledge in the study of classical medical texts, citing Ibn Sīnā, al-Rāzī (Rhazes), Isaac of Israel, and Constantine the African. But even though he authorized

75. R. C. Finucane, "Sacred Corpse, Profane Carrion: Social Ideals and Death Rituals in the Later Middle Ages," in *Mirrors of Mortality: Studies in the Social History of Death*, ed. Joachim Whaley (New York: Routledge, 1981), 40–60.

76. An edition with brief introduction can be found in Alain Collet, "Traité d'Hygiène de Thomas le Bourguignon (1286)," *Romania* 112 (1991): 450–87. Lines 62–63: "[Aü]sé ai en leur maison / [Main]te foez en oi grant profit."

77. On the development of Maubuisson under patronage of Blanche of Castille, see Constance Berman, *The White Nuns: Cistercian Abbeys for Women in Medieval France* (Philadelphia: University of Pennsylvania Press, 2018), 114–30.

78. Collet, "Traité d'hygiène," line 50: "petit d'avisemenz"; lines 75–76: "[Conm]ent l'en doit garder santé / [Et g]uerir son enfermeté."

il qui fist tout le monde
Si come il fist a la ronde
Si me dont cele chose enprendre
Que je puisse a boine fin rendre
a loneur et a tuilite
De toute la communite
Des cles et de lais de pontoise
Ou jai este maintes foiz acte
Leur voudroie bailler briement
Son petites ensaignement
Qui est estrait de la racine
De noz livres de medecine
De touz les plus anciens
Ypocras et de Galiens
Et des autres a mon auis
A inerne ysaac rasis
Costentin ni oublige mie
Car il fu plain de grant clergie
Si fu moigne religieus
Et de servir dieu convoiteus
De touz ceus que jai devant dit
Si com lensaigne li escrit
Viaire prendre mon fondement
A gon gaillour ausement
Si come vous ooroiz retraire
Et sil ia cuer debonnaire

Je pri a dieu quil voille entendre
Si e me amal ta reprendre
Les annueus non pas je me
Car ce seroit agoille grant folie
Pour ma pere non forvient
Amours agon dit plus blasme sont
Car ce quil aiment il leur plest
ages de je deus blasme estoie
Ales plus loer enserne
Car leur blasme ce mest auis
Vaut j bon los par saint denis
agel ce nest mie mentente
Retourner voudrai en la sente
Dont je conte cest huimi afaire
Qui nest pas de maul grant afaire
ages son proufit faire ipoura
Qui bien entendre voura
Ce di bien et nai pas doutance
Que nul ne poura la sentence
Ensi peute home desarme
Que ni ait alez a bedme
ages ce nest que i ensaignement
Et j petit dauisement
Comment en chascune saison
Doit len pris diuer t pur parir
Chascun puisse son cors deffendre
Que ne puisse ensemble pas
ages estre thomas nez de thonone
Que len apele le bourgaigne

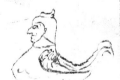

FIGURE 2. Thomas of Thonon, *Cil qui fist tout le monde*. Paris, Bibliothèque nationale de France, Nouvelles acquisitions françaises, MS 6539, fol. 99r.

the information he conveyed in the Latin medical tradition, at the heart of his treatise, texts were wholly absent. Of humoral medicine, he related, "I desire to sit down to the best of my reflection, *as you will hear it.*"[79] That is, he conveyed that he was working not from medical texts, but from memory, from embodied medical knowledge that he was recalling, not transcribing.[80]

Most striking, however, is the form Thomas's regimen takes, vernacular poetry. Throughout his poem, Thomas calls attention to its oral transmission and affective command, to the necessity of hearing the words of his poem and adapting to the passions it advises. Thomas introduces his audience to the basic principles of the four elements, qualities, and humors and their characteristics. He runs through his description somewhat curtly, asserting, "You have heard me about the four humors; you know their qualities and how they are necessary to the body that is worth little without them. I come to the four periods of the year."[81] The remainder of the treatise, the following six hundred lines, is focused on how to adapt the regimen appropriately to each of the four seasons. That is, what truly concerned him were the non-naturals. His treatise centers on the regulation of the environment, the six external factors that influenced health: air, food and drink, diet and rest, sleeping and waking, evacuation and retention, and the passions of the soul.[82]

Throughout the treatise Thomas calls attention to the acoustic register of the regimen he imparts. After reminding his audience that they have "heard" him discuss the humors, he continues to describe the seasons, stating, "I will *say* their characters and when they begin."[83] And again, "I will say their nature and also what I believe about it and know."[84] In these four sections, Thomas lays out basic precepts on diet, cleanliness, moderate exercise, and the principles of phlebotomy. The oral character of the treatise comes through especially in his intermittent interjections, such as "Shut up and listen!" a command he

79. Collet, "Traité d'hygiène," lines 24–25: "A mon meilleur avisement, Si conme vous m'orroiz retraire" (emphasis added).

80. It should be noted, in terms of the oral circulation of this regimen, that there is only one extant manuscript copy of the treatise, Paris, Bibliothèque nationale de France, Nouvelles acquisitions françaises, MS 6539. This manuscript is described by Collet, "Traité d'hygiène," 450–55. It is a fourteenth-century manuscript containing four medical treatises: *Régime du corps* of Aldebrandino of Siena, medical recipes in French and Latin, Thomas's regimen, and an anonymous medical treatise.

81. Collet, "Traité d'hygiène," lines 207–12: "Des IIII humeurs oï avez / Et leur proprieté savez / Et com au cors sont necessaires / Sanz ces IIII ne valt il gaires. / As IIII tems de l'an m'en vai."

82. For example, after listing the elements, he asserts, "Des elemenz plus ne diray" at line 137.

83. Collet, "Traité d'hygiène," lines 212–14: "Et leur proprieté dirai / et en quel point chascun conmence" (emphasis added).

84. Collet, lines 287–89: "Leur nature je te dirai / Einsi com je la croi et sai."

delivers before explaining in detail the proper diet to resume after the Lenten fast.[85] He reiterates his clarity of language, calling attention to its vernacularity: "I do not speak in Latin."[86] The sonic quality of the lesson, he asserts, should arouse pleasure so that the text is embodied. To this end, he reminds his auditors that for proper health they must possess joy (*esjoïssables asez*, line 70). That is, one learns by embodying the principles laid out in the regimen, but also by the experience of listening to its poetic form. To be known, the text itself required performance. Through the poetic form, he imparts an awareness of the quality of air, the need for regular exercise, proper rest, bodily temperature, and the passions of the soul. He concludes: "Whoever follows these precepts and keeps to them wisely, I do not believe that they will be surprised by illness their whole life long."[87]

The acoustic index of Thomas's verse regimen informs our understanding of how religious women would have encountered fragments of learned medicine, and how, in a social and intellectual realm removed from Latinity and scholastic medicine, they may have reformulated it.[88] A vestige of a Mosan psalter that once belonged to a thirteenth-century beguine provides an example of feminine encounter with such regimental health principles. Oxford, Bodleian Library, MS Douce 381, fol. 64v is a cutting showing a health calendar from a psalter made for a woman, as indicated by the appearance of feminine forms, *peccatrix* and *pecherise* (figure 3).[89] The health calendar provides a set of rules, a regimen adapted to each month of the year. Although not lyrical, as in Thomas's formulation, the regimen here is presented graphically, in twelve medallions bearing vernacular advice on diet, purgation, and bleeding.[90] Each month offers a brief lesson on regimen, such as July's recommendation to avoid fish and consume sage and rue.[91]

---

85. Collet, line 386: "Or escoutes, et si te tai."

86. Collet, line 394: "Je ne parle mie en latin."

87. Collet, lines 797–800: "Qui cest enseignement fera / [E]t sagement le gardera / [J]e ne croi que de maladie / [S]oit seurpris en toute sa vie."

88. On marginal or oral encounters with literate epistemologies, see Pablo Gómez, *The Experiential Caribbean: Creating Knowledge and Healing in the Early Modern Atlantic* (Chapel Hill: University of North Carolina Press, 2017). On the acoustic register of knowledge and affective expression, see Nancy Rose Hunt, "An Acoustic Register, Tenacious Images, and Congolese Scenes of Rape and Repetition," *Cultural Anthropology* 23 (2008): 220–53.

89. On the cuttings in the group, see Oliver, *Gothic Manuscript Illumination*, 2:285–86. The feminine forms are found on fols. 63 and 65, which surround the health table.

90. Faith Wallis has discussed the transition from seasonal to monthly hygienic systems in her "Medicine in Medieval Calendar Manuscripts," in *Manuscript Sources of Medieval Medicine*, ed. Margaret Schleissner (New York: Garland, 1995), 105–44. Wallis argues that the reorganization of seasonal regimens into monthly formats was a result of their incorporation into computus manuscripts.

91. Oxford, Bodleian Library, MS Douce 381, fol. 64v: "El mois de Jule, ne te saine pas a la vaine, ne pren poisons. Manjue sauge et ruele et rue et fort et flors d'aipe destrempreit abonfort vin." The

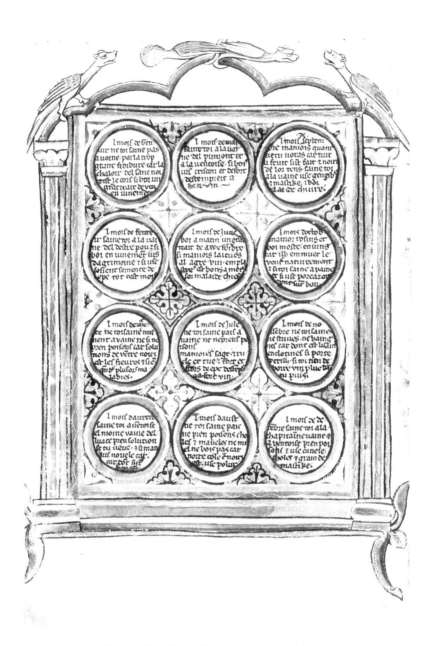

FIGURE 3. Health Table. Oxford, Bodleian Library, MS Douce 381, fol. 64v.

In women's religious communities, it seems, this kind of salutary advice was finely integrated into liturgical and devotional codices. The 1154 Guta-Sintram codex, for example, was a compilation of liturgical and devotional texts undertaken by the Augustinian canoness Guta of Schwarzenthann. It features a hygienic text inscribed alongside the martyrology.[92] Similarly, we see that in MS Douce 381, the health calendar follows the Easter table and precedes Latin and French Mass prayers. These manuscripts suggest that the search for the construction of feminine therapeutic knowledge might begin not in standard academic texts, but in the liturgico-devotional compilations used in women's communities.

This mediation of health knowledge was consistent with other regimens circulating in women's communities in the region. For example, Aldobrandino of Siena's *Régime du corps* was composed in French sometime before 1257.[93] As the physician to the Countess of Provence, Béatrix of Savoy, Aldobrandino directed his regime to noble women and men.[94] Examining the circulation of early manuscripts of the *Régime*, Jennifer Borland has exposed the book's itineraries through feminine spheres in Artois, Flanders, and Hainaut in the 1260s–1280s.[95] The illustrations decorating early manuscripts of the *Régime* feature women as practitioners of domestic forms of intimate care: washing babies, tending births, inspecting breasts, cupping, and facilitating

---

calendar is adapted from Pseudo-Bede's *Ephemeris*, an early medieval Latin treatise in which monthly health rules follow verses for the Egyptian Days; Oliver, *Gothic Manuscript Illumination*, 1:34–35. On the Egyptian Days, see H. Stuart, "A Ninth-Century Account of Diets and Dies Aegyptiaci," *Scriptorium* 33 (1979): 237–44. On medical calendars more generally, see Jean Barboud and Pierre Gillon, "Cinq calendriers diététiques provenant de manuscrits de la Bibliothèque nationale de Paris: Réflexions sur l'origine et la destination de ces calendriers," in *XXX Congrès international d'histoire de la médecine (Düsseldorf 31 sept.–5 oct. 1986)*, ed. Hans Schadewaldt and K. H. Leven (Düsseldorf: Organisationskommittee des XXX. Int. Kongresses, 1988), 179–87. Wallis, note 19 also includes an extensive bibliography.

92. On the manuscript, see Fiona Griffiths, "Brides and Dominae: Abelard's *Cura monialium* at the Augustinian Monastery of Marbach," *Viator* 34 (2003): 57–88.

93. There are seventy-one extant copies. See Françoise Féry-Hue, "Le régime du corps d'Aldobrandin de Sienne: Tradition manuscrite et diffusion," in *Santé, médecine et assistance au Moyen Âge* (Paris: Actes du Congrès national des Sociétés Savantes, 1987), 110; Marilyn Nicoud, *Les régimes de santé au Moyen Age: Naissance et diffusion d'une écriture médicale (XIIIe–XVe siècles)* (Rome: École française, 2007).

94. Monica Green, "The Possibilities of Literacy and the Limits of Reading: Women and the Gendering of Medical Literacy," in *Women's Healthcare in the Medieval West: Texts and Contexts*, ed. Monica Green (Aldershot: Ashgate, 2000), 26.

95. Borland uses the notion of "object itineraries" to envision the manuscripts' movements among royal households affiliated with Beatrice's daughters, who would become queens of England, France, Germany, and Sicily. See Jennifer Borland, "Female Networks and the Circulation of a Late Medieval Health Guide," in *Moving Women, Moving Objects*, ed. Tracy Hamilton and Mariah Proctor-Tiffany (Leiden: Brill, 2019), 108–36.

with purgation.[96] A fourteenth-century adaptation of Aldobrandino's regimen translated the physician's health advice into devotional vocabularies. *Lyen du corps a l'ame et de l'ame au corps* (The Bond of Body to Soul and the Soul to Body) sought to connect the health of the body to that of the soul.[97] As with Thomas of Thonon's regimen, the audience of *Lyen du corps* was likely mixed. The Vatican copy of the *Lyen du corps* asserts that the book holds "le secret de medicine" in its very title. The "secret de medicine" in this treatise is the *Lyen* itself, that is, the bond between body and soul. By the time of its circulation, as we saw in the previous chapter, that link had clearly become a matter of some medical and theological importance. The maintenance of this salutary link between body and soul, these manuscript itineraries suggest, often fell to religious women.

The mingling of liturgical and hagiographic conveyances of medical knowledge is found in British Library, Sloane MS 1611, which conveys regimental advice within liturgical rhythms. A fourteenth-century manuscript of uncertain provenance, Sloane 1611 opens with a psalter and a series of canticles to saints as well as the offices of two saints, Augustine and Eligius (Eloi). An addition that was incorporated in the fourteenth century binds the liturgical material to vernacular medical texts. Here, a series of verses was added to address the need for joy and avoidance of sin in this life, in service to Christ and Mary.[98] The second part of the codex, then, introduces medical material in French. A French regime follows the heading "Ci commence Avicennes selonc fisique" (fol. 69), and advises on general rules for diet, rest, purgation, clean air, and seasonal health.

The notes penned in the margins of this treatise are also of interest, as they point to likely female readership or access to this manuscript. At fols. 136v–137r, notes about Saint Anne's holy progeny are included under a lesson on the properties of mother's milk.[99] The regime is followed by the *Lettre de Hippocrates*, which includes a series of recipes of particular interest to women, such as the peperit charm for childbirth (fol. 147r). Additional notes on Saint Anne and Mary appear across the bottom margins.[100] These notes indicate that the community that used this volume was interested in

---

96. On the presence of female practitioners in the illustrations, see Borland, "Female Networks," 122.

97. It appears in three extant manuscripts, the earliest of which is Brussels, KBR, MS 11130–32; the other two are Valenciennes, Bibliothèque municipale, MS 329; and Rome, Biblioteca Apostolica, MS Pal. Lat. 1990. See Féry-Hue, "Le régime du corps d'Aldebrandin de Sienne," 114.

98. They are transcribed in Paul Meyer, "Notice du MS Sloane 1611," *Romania* 40.160 (1911): 532–58.

99. Monica Green, "Women and the Gendering of Medical Literacy," 27.

100. On fols. 146v, 147r, and 147v.

childbirth, and linked biblical, liturgical, and medical knowledge with obstetric care. It is no small coincidence that these notes continue from the recipes to the opening folio of the manuscript's copy of an Anglo-Norman verse *Life* of Saint Margaret, the textual "relic" often used to ease childbirth.[101] Since at least the twelfth century, the *Life* of Margaret had been used in obstetric practices in which a birth attendant would assume the voice of Margaret, who exclaimed that "in the house where a woman is lying in labor, as soon as one reads my passion, or in the place where my life is inscribed, Lord, make haste to help her and hear the prayer and let her deliver without peril."[102] In this way, narrative hagiographic texts might work, when reappropriated in the context of parturience, as healing charms and contact relics that assume the voice, or the very body, of the saint whose life was inscribed, transferring her therapeutic power to the laboring woman. In MS Sloane 1611, Margaret's *Life* is followed, in the same hand, by additional psalms and a litany.[103] Although we do not know with certainty that this manuscript circulated in women's religious communities, the recipes for infant and maternal health are striking in the way that they blend delivery of information on the regulation of the non-naturals with liturgical and hagiographic knowledge. Depending on context, regimens could adopt religious significance, a means of altering the body to enhance the perception and clarity of the soul and, ultimately, to preserve health in life and after death. The manuscript thus alerts us to conveyances of therapeutic knowledge in poetic, liturgical, and performative registers.

---

101. Margaret's *Life* had been used in childbirth practices since at least the twelfth century, when Wace's legend invoked her as a protector of mothers. On the evolution of the legend and its use as a textual amulet in childbirth, see Wendy Larson, "Who Is the Master of This Narrative? Maternal Patronage of the Cult of Saint Margaret," in *Gendering the Master Narrative: Women and Power in the Middle Ages*, ed. Mary Erler and Maryanne Kowaleski (Ithaca: Cornell University Press, 2003), 94–104.

102. Several versions are extant. See Meyer, "Notice du MS Sloane 1611," 556: "Ou feme ençainte ait en moi fiance, / Sire Dieu, dones li delivrance / Que son enfant por nul forfait." Another version can be found in Léon de Herckenrode, "Une amulette: Légende en vers de Sainte Marguerite, tirée d'un ancien manuscrit," *Bulletin de Bibliophile Belge* 4 (1847): 2–23: "Qui naquira en la maison / Ou lon lira ma passion / Ja le deable ny ait pouoir / Ne ou pourprinz ne ou manoir / Ou ma vie sera escripte / Dieu tu moctroys ceste merite . . . Dieu tu sans peril la delivre." For yet other versions, see Wace, *La vie de St. Marguerite, poème*, ed. Aristide Joly (Paris: Vieweg, 1879).

103. On this manuscript, see Jocelyn Wogan-Browne, "Clerc u lai, muïne u dame: Women and Anglo-Norman Hagiography in the Twelfth and Thirteenth Centuries," in *Women and Literature in Britain, 1150–1500*, ed. Carol Meale (Cambridge: Cambridge University Press, 2009), 61–85.

The Psalter as a Therapeutic Technology

The act of locating female healthcare practitioners and their constructions of therapeutic knowledge necessitates a profound shift in the conceptualization of the kinds of reading, writing, and performance that constitute medical history.[104] The embodied therapeutic behavior represented in the MS Douce health calendar has long been forgotten as a *medical* practice largely because it was recorded in a psalter, which we have come to think of as a "religious" book. In order to make this fragment of the psalter legible as a medical technology, we might remap the genres of medicine and religion, unbounding each of them so that ritual, regimen, prayer, prognosis, liturgy, and ligature communicate the fullness of their thirteenth-century significations.

A trace of past therapeutic practice within a women's religious community can be found in Cambridge, Fitzwilliam Museum, MS 288, a psalter-hours from thirteenth-century Liège (for the purpose of rhetorical ease I will refer to this book as "the Fitzwilliam psalter"). While the provenance of this particular psalter is not entirely certain, Judith Oliver places its production in Liège around 1280 and suggests beguine ownership.[105] Even if it was not owned by a beguine, the manuscript was certainly intended for use by semi-religious women, as indicated by the feminine forms (i.e., *pecherise, peccatrix,* fol. 2r) and elaborate observances. The book opens with a Mass prayer, the *Confiteor,* or the form of prayer for confessing sins prior to Mass.[106] Mass prayers were somewhat unusual in thirteenth-century psalters.[107] Thus, the presence of the *Confiteor,* along with two other Mass prayers in Latin and French, distinguishes this codex and raises questions about its function.[108] These features of the Fitzwilliam psalter reflect the importance of religious women's roles in this region as participants in and facilitators of confession, as we have seen in the case of Christina Mirabilis. Beguine statutes from the region stipulated that women attend Mass daily, praying the *Confiteor* prior to confession and the *Misereatur* at confession.[109] Additionally, within hospitals, patients made regular confession as part of the therapeutic process, a

---

104. Hunt, "An Acoustic Register."

105. Oliver, *Gothic Manuscript Illumination,* 2:252.

106. For a complete catalog description of the manuscript, see Oliver, *Gothic Manuscript Illumina-tion,* 2:250–51.

107. Oliver, *Gothic Manuscript Illumination,* 1:36.

108. Reinberg, *French Books of Hours,* 13–17.

109. Oliver, *Gothic Manuscript Illumination,* 1:37–38; Ernest McDonnell, *The Beguines and Beghards in Medieval Culture: With a Special Emphasis on the Belgian Scene* (New Brunswick: Rutgers University Press, 1954), 135.

washing away of the filth of sin.[110] Illustrations accompanying each of the Mass prayers depict women performing the inscribed words and actions, fulfilling their roles as religious women. For example, a woman first confesses to a gray-robed priest at the opening of the book (fol. 1r); in the initial of the *Misereatur*, a group of women pray at the altar as a priest celebrates the Mass (fol. 2r); and painted into the Mass prayer, *Panis angelorum*, is a group of women kneeling in prayer at their reception of the Eucharist (fol. 2v). The illustrations serve as a visual instruction manual, reflecting the bodily and ritualistic comportment expected of the book's users.

These prayers restructured a person's internal affects by delving into their consciousness and memory. This process readied them for confession by launching the introspection that was necessary for reception of the Eucharist. The process was also corporeal, purging the body of toxic sin. The reader thus encountered the text of the confession and each of the Mass prayers that followed as a means of searching the self, arousing the proper interior affective state that would enable the Eucharist to take maximum effect, conforming the body to Christ's. The prayers themselves focus on the body of Christ as a means of eternal life, "vitam eternam" (fol. 2r). By arousing contrition and uttering the words of prayer, the votary began the process of purging sin from her soul; by undertaking penance and ingesting the Eucharist she, in turn, conformed her body to Christ's humoral state. The prescribed affects are reflected in the text of the Mass prayers. The *Misereatur*, for example, localized the user's prayers, specifically calling on martyrs, Saint Lambert and Saint Katherine, as intercessors for her plea (fol. 2r). The Mass prayers single out the body and blood of Christ, recognizing the Eucharist as a means of salvation. In the prayer *Panis angelorum*, for example, the user beseeches the sacrament to dispel her misery, naming the Eucharist as the "remedy" (*remedium*, fol. 2v) for her ailments. In this formulation, sin was pathological, a cause of illness and a hindrance to *salus*, to health. Christ's body and blood, another Mass prayer states, "remain within me" for health and promote "eternal life."[111]

While it might be tempting to explain such language as strict metaphor, the following entry in the prayer book suggests that we might not write off literal possibilities quite so hastily. On fol. 6v, written in French, the makers of this book have included a health table matching the content of the one

---

110. On regular confession in hospitals, see Carole Rawcliffe, *Medicine for the Soul: The Life, Death, and Resurrection of an English Medieval Hospital; St. Giles's Norwich, 1249–1550* (Stroud: Sutton, 1999), 104–6.

111. Fol. 3r: "maneat in me ad salute et proficiat michi in vitam eternam."

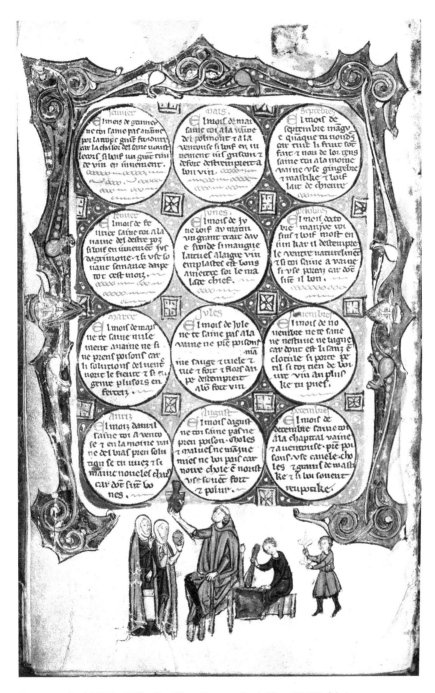

FIGURE 4. Health Table. © The Fitzwilliam Museum, Cambridge, MS 288, fol. 6v.

produced in MS Douce 381 (figure 4). Under the table, a marginal illustration features two women visiting an apothecary, presumably gathering the "potions" recommended above. The table suggests the proper months to practice bleeding, and it recommends salubrious food and drink and the necessary potions and herbs for the environmental conditions of each month. Lettuce, vinegar, and cold water, for example, are appropriate in June, while goat's milk, along with ginger and mastic, is recommended as a salubrious beverage for September.[112]

As in MS Douce 381, the health table in Fitzwilliam MS 288 is part of a calendrical series. On its recto is copied a table for calculating the date of Easter, the time at which, following Lateran IV, each Christian should make annual confession and receive the Eucharist.[113] On the facing recto is a calendar listing by month the saints' feast days. That the health calendar is embedded among these liturgical computations points to an understanding of bodily health embraced by its users as one that linked purgation, bloodletting, and diet to penitential and liturgical efficacy. Medical practices, according to the Fitzwilliam psalter, were effective to the extent that they were integrated within a liturgical regimen, a regimen of hourly prayer maintained by the users of this book.

The Fitzwilliam psalter also includes a copy of the Office of the Dead for Liège use, reflecting women's roles as mourners and caretakers of the dead and dying and providing further suggestion that this book belonged to a local beguine.[114] As discussed in chapter 2, wills and bequests appointed beguine women as caretakers of corpses and performers of prayer at funerals. The position of women's prayers in death ritual is represented in the Fitzwilliam psalter by an historiated initial depicting lay mourners at a funeral service (figure 5). Women appear below the bier with open books, presumably chanting the words of the Psalms written in this very book. The reflexive illustration, featuring the book itself in the hands of its users as they performed the central

---

112. See Oliver's discussion, *Gothic Manuscript Illumination*, 1:35. As Oliver notes, the rules dictating bloodletting and purgation are simultaneously related to body and soul. Some communities of beguines and Cistercian nuns in Liège legislated the times during which women should be bled. Rodolphe Hoornaert, "La plus ancienne règle du béguinage de Bruges," *Annales de la Société d'Émulation de Bruges* 72 (1930): 32–33.

113. The Easter table is copied on 6r; it uses Lambertum verse.

114. Fols. 189r-209v; on women's roles as mourners in Islam, see Leor Halevi, "Wailing for the Dead: The Role of Women in Early Islamic Funerals," *Past & Present* 183 (2004): 3–39. Halevi shows that women in medieval Islam fulfilled similarly vital roles as mourners. Uncovering the fragments of their practice presents similar challenges as well. In medieval Islam, dramatic expressions were a kind of poetry of lament that constituted a public memory of the deceased. But the poems they composed were not transmitted in literary form or even as history; they were regarded as spontaneous, improvised utterances.

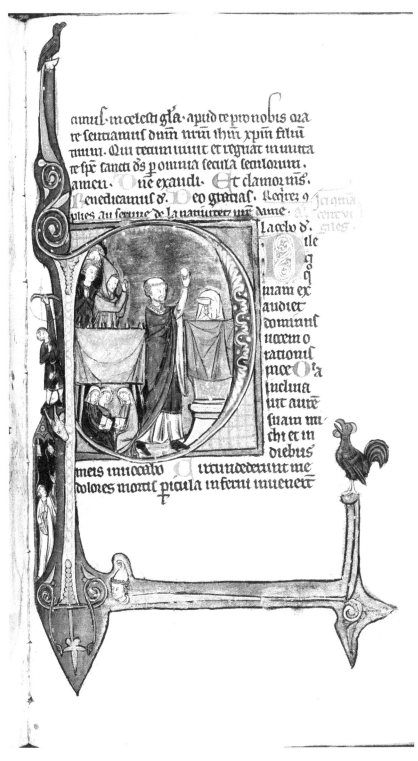

amuſ·in celeſti gľa· apud te pro nobis ora
re ſentiamuſ dñm nrm ihm xpm filiu
tuum. Qui tecum uiuit et regnat in unita
te ſpe ſancti dſ p omnia ſecula ſeculorum.
amen. ᴐne exaudi. Et clamor mis.
Benedicamuſ dˀ. Deo gratias. Legitur q
pfues au ſerme de la natiuitez mˀ dame.
Lacelo dˀ·
tle
g.
q.
niam ex
audiet
dominuſ
uocem o
rationiſ
mee O'a
inclina
uit aure
ſuam mi
chi et in
diebus
meis inuocabo. ᴐ ircumdederunt me
dolores mortis periculā inferni inuenere

FIGURE 5. Women mourning at funeral service. © The Fitzwilliam Museum, Cambridge, MS 288, fol. 189r.

prayers it provided, stresses the importance of care of the dead in beguine communities and the role played by such books in delivering that care.

Just as in the image of women visiting the apothecary, the funeral scene represents the women who use this book in their specialized roles and functions. The psalter was thus converted via its own image-making into an object, a tool. The women who were responsible for performing prayers are figured as part of the book's work, its effects; they were the engineers who activated this therapeutic tool. Like the prayers contained within, they possessed the power to alter penitents' affects, to transform bodies and souls, to accomplish *salus*.

The Fitzwilliam psalter also contains four French meditational poems on the life of Mary and Christ.[115] Some of the poems guide the reader or listener through a lyric meditation fixed on the emotional tenor of the lives of Christ and Mary and based on the retelling of Gospel scenes. Others weave together an incantatory string of Aves focused on the love and joy experienced by Mary. Each poem in the series concludes, after having taken the audience on a profound affective journey, by calling on Christ or Mary to forgive her sins. The recitation of the poems is fashioned as a therapeutic process through which performers and audience recognize Mary's conception of Christ as a remedy. The poems praise Mary's body as that which manufactured "the sweet theriac that destroyed the deadly venom which Adam our father had drunk."[116] The reader salutes her "from whom came forth the holy theriac by which humankind was reborn."[117] The poems' interpellations cue the reader to call out, "Hail, gentle medicine,"[118] reiterating, "Hail, you who are the health of all illnesses."[119] In this formulation, Mary's body is the vessel in which she brewed the remedy for sin, the origin of human disease. Mary concocted a potion within her, Christ, whose blood, "heal[s] all pain" and whom she created to "heal the sick man."[120] It is significant that, despite the long and pervasive tradition, beginning with Augustine, of figuring Christ as a doctor, *Christus medicus*, that is not the imagery on which this poem

---

115. I will refer to the critical edition of the poems and the numbering system in Peter T. Ricketts, "Critical Edition of the Poems of the Mosan Psalters," in Walters, Corrigan, and Ricketts, *The Feast of Corpus Christi*, 445–532, noting scribal aberration from the critical edition in parentheses. Fols. 210r-219v (Ricketts XVII, XVIII, XX); also at fol. 14r, *Sire donez nostre orisons* (Ricketts XVI).

116. The poems are edited and translated by Ricketts, "Critical Edition of the Poems of the Mosan Psalters." *Ave, ree de grant dulchor* (Ricketts XX), lines 208–210: "u fut gardez li duz triacles / ki le mortel venin destruit / k'Adans nos peres avoit buit."

117. *Ave, ree de grant dulchor*, lines 200–201: "de cui eisit li sains triacles / dont li hom fut rasoagiez."

118. *Ave, ree de grant dulchor*, line 203: "ave, debonaire mecine."

119. *Ave, rose florie* (Ricketts XVIII), lines 77–78: "ave, qui es santeiz / de totes enferteiz."

120. *Ave, ree de grant dulchor*, line 234: "ki sanat toutes nos dolors"; line 213: "kant le malade vint saner."

draws.[121] Rather, Christ and Mary are remedies, not doctors. The practitioner is she who performs this prayer, making the healing remedy of Christ and Mary available through her potent intercession.

The poems in the Fitzwilliam psalter not only recognize Mary and Christ as agents of healing, but also offer *themselves*, the performance of their rhyme, as the means of activating healing agency. The poems' effects were not accessible simply as content, as text, but also in the form of an embodied performance. Such rhymed rhetorical performances had a recognized place in medical therapy. The Parisian master John of Garland praised the thera-peutic effects of poetic rhyme, which he understood as a branch of music. His *Parisiana poetria* claimed that rhymed poetry served to "embrace the har-mony and concord of the humors" in the human body.[122] Ibn Sīnā prescribed repetitive chants (*cantilenis*) to dispel melancholy.[123] And Arnald of Villanova recommended music as the chief means to produce the cheerful and glad-dened mind (*laetus et gaudens*) that prolongs life.[124] The poems are just one component of the psalter's comprehensive sonority, which positioned it as an effective technology for assisting caregivers in modulating the rhythms of body and the affects of soul.

Musicality was built into the very conceptualization of internal harmony.[125] In addition to recommending music as a means to enhance the salubri-ous passion of delight, Arnald of Villanova used harmonic proportions to describe the theory of medicinal degrees.[126] And Ibn Sīnā developed an index for describing the sensation of the pulse according to its meter, rhythm, har-mony, measure, and accent.[127] He asserted that the proportions of the pulse

121. Darrel W. Amundsen and Gary B. Ferngren, "Medicine and Religion: Pre-Christian Antiq-uity," in *Health/Medicine and the Faith Traditions*, ed. Martin Marty and Kenneth Vaux (Philadelphia: Fortress, 1982), 53–92.

122. *The Parisiana Poetria of John of Garland*, ed. and trans. Traugott Lawler (New Haven: Yale University Press, 1974), 158–61: "in humanam, que constat in proportione et concordia humorum." William of Auvergne (*De universo* II.3.20) also attested that "musical sounds" could cure melancholy and other mental disturbances.

123. Avicenna, Canon 3.i.4.21: "Cantilenis et letificantibus."

124. Arnald of Villanova, *Regimen salernitanum*, in *Opera omnia* (Basel, 1585), col. 1875.

125. Bruce Holsinger, *Music, Body, and Desire in Medieval Culture: Hildegard of Bingen to Chaucer* (Palo Alto: Stanford University Press, 2001) is essential reading on the broader culture of corporeal musicality.

126. Peter Murray Jones, "Music Therapy in the Later Middle Ages: The Case of Hugo van der Goes," in *Music as Medicine: The History of Music Therapy since Late Antiquity*, ed. Peregrine Horden (Aldershot: Ashgate, 2000), 134. See Arnald of Villanova, *Aphorismi de gradibus*, in *Opera medica omnia*, vol. 2 (Grenada-Barcelona: Seminarium Historiae Medicae Granatensis, 1975).

127. Avicenna, *The Canon of Medicine*, trans. Cameron Gruner (New York: AMS Press, 1973), 293–96. See Nancy Siraisi, "The Music of the Pulse in the Writings of Italian Academic Physicians (Fourteenth and Fifteenth Centuries)," *Speculum* 50 (1975): 689–710.

were "easy" to read for anyone with knowledge of music and a bit of daily practice in the touch.[128] Rhythms thumped within the body, pulsing through veins in the movement of *spiritus*.[129] This somatic music was audible in the pulse; but the body also *responded* to music, altered its rhythms in reaction to music, including the music of the Psalms, lyric poetry, and liturgical songs. Although scholastic physicians produced no treatises dedicated solely to the theorization of the rhythmic pulse or the rationale for music therapy, nevertheless practical medical advice often recommended music as a means to encourage humoral balance and psychic serenity: the most common applications of music therapy were end-of-life care, ease of labor and delivery, the rearing of infants, and the enhancement of salubrious passions of the soul.[130] In the literature of practical medical advice it was Aldobrandino of Siena's *Régime du corps* that most clearly and powerfully associated music with control over the passions of the soul. The manuscript tradition of the *Régime* features a musician decorating the capital *I* in the chapter on the passions of the soul, which, not coincidentally for a book addressed to women and transmitted in women's communities, was the first complete and separate chapter dedicated to the care of the passions in a regimen in western Europe. The placement of the musician suggests the importance, in the communities that shared this treatise, of musicality as a means of generating salutary passions.[131]

Returning to our psalter, then, it seems as if the very purpose of the poems was to generate this concord. The poems in the Fitzwilliam psalter participated in the salutary effects they described, heightening the reflexive quality of their performance. "Lord grant that our prayers be acceptable to pray to you," exhorts the poem *Sire, donez nostre orisons*, connecting the labor of the praying women with the product of their prayer.[132] That product was a transformed bodily self, God's renewal of our "physical make up" (*faiture*, line 16). The reader concludes the poem with the injunction "Lord give a

---

128. Siraisi, "The Music of the Pulse," 699. See also Charles Burnett, "European Knowledge of Arabic Texts Referring to Music: Some New Material," *Early Music History* 12 (1993): 1–17.

129. For example, Gilles of Corbeil accounted for variations in the pulse by employing a metrical and musical vocabulary that described flow in terms of discordant and consonant movements. See Siraisi, "The Music of the Pulse," 707. Siraisi discusses *musica humana* in conjunction with Qūsta ibn Lūcā's physiology of spirits.

130. Jones, "Music Therapy in the Later Middle Ages," 134–35.

131. See, for example, British Library, MS Sloane 2435, fol. 10v, where a musician plays the vielle for a person suffering from melancholy.

132. *Sire, donez nostre orisons* (Ricketts XVI), lines 1–2: "Sire, donez nostre orisons / a vos proier soit acceptable."

good end to the one who spoke and wrote this," calling attention to the poem's composition, its words, as a tool for ensuring a good death, one that required activation through speaking.[133]

The poems in the Fitzwilliam psalter request and simultaneously structure an affective experience designed to capture within the practitioner and her audience the salubrious joy of the saints. Throughout the poems, joy is pitted against the ill effects of sadness. "Lord, permit us to have that joy which is all-enduring," requests one.[134] Calling to mind Joseph and the three Marys who stood at the foot of the cross, it insists that these figures were not aggrieved by the events they witnessed, and that the poem described, and thus demands that Christ "bring us together with complete joy."[135] In summoning salutary joy, the poems enacted a long tradition of medical advice promoting the healthful qualities of delight. The "new Galen" introduced in the thirteenth century prompted diverse medical commentary on the role of pleasure and joy in basic hygiene.[136] Arnald of Villanova's *Regimen sanitates ad regem Aragonum*, for example, recommended *gaudium* and tranquility of mind as basic components of a daily regimen, a means of counteracting the cardiac constriction caused by anger and sadness.[137] The poems participated in a medical conceptualization of regulating the passions for therapeutic purposes. In their musicality, the tranquility and delight of the saints became a means of mimetic affective therapy, stimulating gaudium and thereby supporting the body.

If this psalter belonged to a beguine of Liège, as Oliver has suggested, then we can imagine the institutional circumstances in which she used it. A prayer book like the Fitzwilliam psalter would have been present in the hands of a beguine while tending to the sick and dying, guiding her prayer and her efforts to comfort the patient, to assist in easing their spirits, preparing their meals, maintaining their regimen, and perhaps transitioning their bodies and souls

---

133. *Sire, donez nostre orisons*, lines 29–30: "Sire, metez a bone fin / ki ci ditat et ce escrit."

134. *Sire, donez nostre orisons*, line 20: "icele joie qui tout jors dure."

135. *Sire, donez nostre orisons*, line 24: "nos aünent de joie entiere."

136. Luis García-Ballester, *Galen and Galenism: Theory and Medical Practice from Antiquity to the European Renaissance* (Aldershot: Ashgate, 2002). García-Ballester uses the term to refer to the new works of Galen that were translated into Latin in the thirteenth century, which had not circulated as part of the traditional medical syllabus, the *Articella*. Galen's *De morbo et accidenti*, in particular, generated extensive medical commentary on the role of the passions in health and sickness.

137. On pleasure in Arnald's regimen, see Fernando Salmón, "The Pleasures and Joys of the Humoral Body in Medieval Medicine," in *Pleasure in the Middle Ages*, ed. Naama Cohen-Hanegbi and Piroska Nagy (Turnhout: Brepols, 2018), 39–58. Arnald's regimen is edited as *Regimen sanitatis ad regem Aragonum*, in *Opera medica omnia*, vol. 10.1, ed. Michael McVaugh, Luis García-Ballester, and Juan Paniagua (Barcelona: Editions Universitat de Barcelona, 1996), 436: "Gaudio sepe vacare debent et honestis solaciis, ut animus refloreat et spiritus recreentur."

from life into death. The beguines of Liège had entered into formal relationships with the hospital of St. Christopher by 1224.[138] A document of that year refers to the "sorores" who lived near the hospital and paid an annual rent.[139] The exact nature of the relationship between the first beguines of Liège and the hospital of St. Christopher is unclear in part because of the informal and ad hoc services they provided. Comparative evidence, however, suggests that in return for their modest annual rent, the beguines would have received sacramental services from the hospital chaplains and would have exercised their charitable mission by performing nursing services to patients as needed; these services might include laundering linens, changing bandages, preparing food, entertaining patients, guiding them on walks, praying with them, and providing all the other forms of care discussed in chapter 2. At nearby Tongres, for example, beguines performed these duties as informal, unofficial hospital staff. In 1245, Thibaud, a canon of St. Denis and citizen of Tongres, allowed the beguines of Tongres to participate in services at the hospital of St. Jacques. They divided with the hospital the revenue they earned from their work in funerals and prayers for the dead.[140] Although the beguines of Tongres opened their own infirmary in 1257, their prior therapeutic history was shaped by their experience sharing a rector, income, labor, urban space, and prayer with the hospital of St. Jacques. Psalters like Cambridge, Fitzwilliam Museum, MS 288 would have played a key role in guiding their everyday actions and in building their therapeutic knowledge as they interacted with patients on a daily basis. Their psalters, then, are vital sources for uncovering constructive forms of beguine therapeutic knowledge, indeed of beguine theologies of body and soul.

Returning to Liège, it is clear that by 1241 the number of beguines relying on the liturgical services of St. Christopher had grown to overwhelming proportions, so that the archbishop, Conrad of Hochstaden, introduced an indulgence encouraging the faithful to assist with the construction of a larger church.[141]

---

138. Pierre de Spiegeler, *Les hôpitaux et l'assistance à Liège: Aspects institutionnels et sociaux* (Paris: Les Belles Lettres, 1987), 61–63. The hospital was staffed by a master, and brothers and sisters followed the Rule of Saint Augustine.

139. Walter Simons, *Cities of Ladies: Beguine Communities in the Medieval Low Countries, 1200–1565* (Philadelphia: University of Pennsylvania Press, 2001), 283; McDonnell, *Beguines and Beghards*, 44.

140. Émile Schoolmeesters, ed., *Les regestes de Robert de Thourotte* (Liège: D. Cormaux, 1906), 119.

141. The document is edited in J. De Ryckel, ed., *Vita S. Beggae, Ducissae Brabantiae Andetennensium, Begginarum et Beggardorum* (Leuven: Oorbeeck, 1631), 573–74. It refers to the women attached to St. Christopher's as "mulieres religiosae de Parochia Sancti Christophori Leodiensis nouam ecclesiam" and states that they numbered fifteen hundred. On the archaeological excavation of St. Christopher's, see Thomas Coomans, "Saint-Christophe à Liège: La plus ancienne église médiévale du movement béguinal," *Bulletin Monumental* 164 (2006): 359–76. The excavations are primarily revelatory of postmedieval construction.

With their steady increase in numbers, the beguines established their own independent hospital in 1267, the Hôpital Tirebourse.[142] Tirebourse was situated across the Rue St. Gilles from the hospital of St. Christopher, and archaeological excavations have revealed that the two institutions maintained physical connections through linked pathways that constituted a social network for service to the sick poor.[143] The excavations also uncovered the remains of Tirebourse's patient ward, showing that it was surrounded by small chapels that oriented patients to view the consecrated host, a means of specular remedy. A few decades later, the beguines of St. Christopher established a leprosarium known as Florichamps.[144] Throughout their daily lives—in burials, caregiving, and the recitation of prayer—a prayer book like the Fitzwilliam psalter would have informed their work.

We find additional dimensions of beguine care in the French poems copied into another psalter-hours, Brussels, KBR, MS IV–1013 (I will refer to this book as the "Brussels psalter"). Like the Fitzwilliam psalter, the Brussels psalter was produced in Liège in the 1280s and most likely for a beguine of St. Christopher's.[145] A poem copied here, *Sires deus ki en Jerusalem venis a passione*, provides a verbal picture narrating Christ's entry into Jerusalem.[146] The poem reflects the joyful affects of the characters it describes—for example, the crowd of children who "received [Christ] joyfully."[147] These statements of affect are accompanied by affirmations of belief such as "Sweet God, as what we say here is true."[148] Such affirmations strengthen the therapeutic goals of these poems, as many vernacular medical practices, such as pilgrimage to saints' shrines or prayer before relics, were explained as having effect

---

142. Spiegeler shows that the process of integration of the hospital was intermittent, and only completed in 1473. Next to the hospital, the beguinage also established a leprosarium sometime before 1304, called the Leproserie de Florichamps. See Madeleine Pissart, *"Tirebourse et Florichamps*: Histoire d'un hôpital resérvé aux beguines (Tirebourse) et d'une léproserie (Florichamps)," *Annuaire d'Histoire Liégeoise* 3 (1950): 285–99.

143. Guillaume Mora-Dieu, "Liège/Liège: Évaluation archéologique sur le site de l'ancien hôpital Tirebourse," *Chronique de l'Archéologie Wallonne* 15 (2008): 132–34. The excavation showed that little roads connected the hospital to the abbey of St. Laurent and to the hospital of St. Christopher.

144. The original documents are collected at the City Archives in Liège, *Inventaire des archives du béguinage de Saint-Christophe à Liège, son hôpital et sa léproserie de Florichamps.*

145. For a complete description, see Oliver, *Gothic Manuscript Illumination*, 2:247–48. Oliver suggests beguine ownership because of references to "ancelle" in one of the poems. The Collect to St. Christopher may link the book to St. Christopher's beguinage in Liège.

146. Ricketts IX. It is copied just before the psalter at fol. 8r.

147. *Deus, sire, en Jerusalem venis a passion* (Ricketts IX), line 10: "Joaument (joianment) vos receuent (rechuirent) can venistes laenz." The manuscript lines here are slightly different from the critical edition, so I've included the scribal particularities in parentheses.

148. *Deus, sire, en Jerusalem venis a passion*, line 15: "Duz Deus, si com c'est voirs ke nos ici disons."

only when accompanied by internal faithful assent.[149] As we saw in the previous chapter, this cognitive assent was considered an integral component of effective remedies according to academic physicians as well, who insisted that the patient's belief in cure, hope for recovery, and confidence or faith in their healthcare practitioner stimulated the process of cure.

After these statements of belief, the poem in the Brussels psalter proceeds to portray numerous examples of the way that God intervened in human history by protecting humans from physical harm. For example, it reminds readers that God released Daniel from the lion's den and delivered Jonah from the belly of the whale. But the manuscript copy of the poem in the Brussels psalter includes a telling aberration in this biblical enumeration. While there are at least four known copies of this poem, the Brussels psalter makes a revealing substitution.[150] Instead of describing divine assistance to *Susanna* in her *perdition*, as the other copies do, in the Brussels psalter, the words *sainte Juliane* and *predication* are substituted.[151] These words refer to Juliana of Mont-Cornillon and the preaching campaign to adopt her liturgy for the feast of Corpus Christi. Juliana, as we have seen, was a local woman who served lepers outside of Liège and managed to convince a few key clerics in the region, including Guiard of Laon, Hugh of St. Cher, and Jacques Pantaleon (who later became Pope Urban IV), to support her mission to create a liturgical feast for the Eucharist. The words demonstrate that the local community that used this book identified with the work of Juliana. In his final confirmation of the feast in 1264, Pope Urban IV likened it to a medicine with the power to heal humanity, praising it as a universal cure for all wounds, which was necessary because all humans were made sick at the fall. The *predication* of Juliana in this psalter poem supports Urban's view of the Host as a healing agent, aligning Juliana's creation of the liturgy with God's acts to save humans from disease.

The poem ends by stating that "the image of you, which we see here, brings to mind your acts, as we believe."[152] The poem is thus dependent on an image that evokes God's saving work, protecting humans from harm. As

149. Lea Olsan, "Charms and Prayers in Medieval Medical Practice and Theory," *Social History of Medicine* 16.3 (2003): 343–66.

150. On this substitution, see Ricketts, "Critical Edition," 462; and Oliver, *Gothic Manuscript Illumination*, 2:248. The three other psalters in which the poem occurs are New York, The Morgan Library, MS 440; Paris, Bibliothèque nationale de France, MS Latin 1077; and Brussels, KBR, MS IV–1066.

151. At fol. 8r. at line 17. In Brussels, KBR, MS IV–1013, the line reads: "sainte Juliane ostastes de la predication."

152. *Deus, sire, en Jerusalem venis a passion*, line 19: "et ceste vostre ymagene, ke (que) nos ici veons / ramenbre (ramenbreit) les vos (de nos) fais, si com nos le creons."

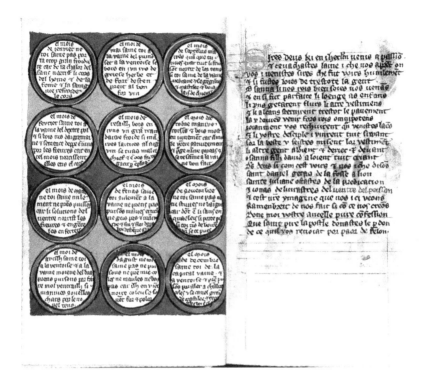

FIGURE 6.   Health Table and Poem, *Sires deus ki en Jerusalem venis a passione*. Brussels, KBR, MS IV–1013, fols. 7v–8r.

with all the full-page images attached to the French poems in the Mosan corpus, the image was to be meditated upon as the poem was performed. Unlike the iterations of this poem in the three other manuscripts, however, where the accompanying image features the holy family's entry into Jerusalem and Christ's teaching at the temple, here the poem appears opposite a table of health rules (figure 6). The health rules undergird the significance of the performance of the poem as a mode of healthcare. Although decorated differently, in a striking red-and-blue pattern, the medical advice and layout of the calendar are identical to those included in the Fitzwilliam and Douce psalters. Perhaps this is no codicological accident; perhaps the calendrical regimen of diet and purgation *is* the image designed to bring to mind God's acts of salvation.[153]

---

153. Oliver has a different interpretation; see her *Gothic Manuscript Illumination*, 1:49. While it is possible that "the image" refers to the historiated *B* in *Beatus vir* that opens the psalter on the verso of fol. 8, the other French poems also do not operate in this manner.

Another poem in the Brussels psalter, *Ave ki ains ne comenchas*, is copied just after the Office of the Dead. This one, found in seven other psalters in the corpus, leads the orant in a series of Aves dedicated to the work performed by Christ's incarnation and crucifixion. It praises the grace that entered earth as a result of the incarnation, which enables those who "drink of it" to live "all days without end."[154] The string of Aves are composed in the present tense and are designed to be experientially meditative. The auditors and performers of these poems undergo an affective process, one premised upon violence and vilification that would be replaced by its contrary, delight. For example, they position the meditant to vilify the Jews as tormentors of Christ and to sigh at the sin introduced by Adam and Eve. The evocation of these negative emotions—the use of Jewish people, especially, as affective tools—may have primed the petitioner, like a purgative. It also suggests a foundational violence in this practice, a need to purge or expel non-Christians in order to ensure a sense of communal health. Such moments remind us that the conditions of care were always situated within social hierarchies premised upon certain exclusions. Ultimately, the poem even issues gestural prescriptions, inducing the performers to supplicate themselves in a plea for divine contact. The poem is premised on a kind of medicine of opposites, of contraries, in which the "pain and sadness" (*dolour et en tristece*, line 8) of the pre-Christian world is driven out by the joy of Christ and hope for bodily reunion with an eternal "substance," Christ.[155] "Grant us true hope," the poem ends, "you who are forever a substance."[156] The hope encouraged by the poem is to partake in the substance of God, in grace. Throughout the poem, the practitioners, meaning the persons who perform it, issue pleas that their prayers be received, that the work of prayer that took place on earth is accomplished in the divine dimension, in heaven, releasing sin and ensuring life. "Receive the prayers of your servants," it commands.[157] "Receive and hear my prayer," and again, "Holy lord, receive my prayer, and accord your kindness to the

---

154. *Ave ki ains ne commenchas* (Ricketts XVII), lines 15–16: "qui (ki) ki par toi en beverat / a toz jors sain fin viverat."

155. The race-making of both Jews and Christians is evident here in the association of Christians with a "rightful heritage" (*lor droit hyretage*) wrested from the "wicked" Jews. On Jewishness in medicine, humoral theory, and complexion, see Irven Resnick, *Marks of Distinction: Christian Perception of Jews in the High Middle Ages* (Washington, DC: Catholic University of America Press, 2012). On the creation of Jews as a race in the Middle Ages and the use of religion as a basis of race-making, see Geraldine Heng, *The Invention of Race in the European Middle Ages* (Cambridge: Cambridge University Press, 2018).

156. *Ave ki ains ne commenchas*, lines 195–96: "Otroie nos vraie E(n)sperance / qui (ki) tot dis es une substance."

157. *Ave ki ains ne commenchas*, line 32: "rechoiz proieres de tes sers."

one who wrote and composed these *Aves*."[158] The performance of the poem was thus a means to convert the prayer work of its users into remediation of sin. This process was highly adaptable depending on immediate needs. It could be performed on the self, as a means of self-care; it could be performed within the entirety of the community; and it could be performed at the bedside of the sick.

The therapeutic uses of the Brussels psalter are further intensified by the presence of scattered prayers addressed to saints. The prayers were added after the codex was composed, improvisationally.[159] For example, an antiphon and collect for Saint Giles (Aegidius), who was known to provide special assistance to the leprous, the disabled, and to nursing mothers, is copied into the space remaining after the *Ave rose florie*, on fol. 248v. The prayer beseeches Giles to cure the sick, cast out demons, and restore sight to the blind.[160] Giles was a popular healing saint whose legend and miracles enjoyed wide circulation and whose relics attracted pilgrims to Bruges, Tournai, and Antwerp.[161] He was particularly associated with nursing mothers, as he was believed to have survived in the forest as a result of the milk offered by his only companion, a doe. Although Giles's legend, as told by Jacobus of Voragine, includes numerous instances of his ability to cure, when Giles himself was offered the assistance of a physician, he refused.[162] Particularly resonant in this context is the association of Giles with the confession and penance of Charlemagne. Giles's legend stated that Charlemagne was especially fond of Giles and, during their frequent conversation "about the soul and salvation, the king asked his visitor to pray for him, because he had committed an enormous crime, which he dared not confess even to the saint himself."[163] In response to Giles's prayers, an angel delivered a scroll stating that

---

158. *Ave ki ains ne commenchas* (note the use of the first person collective in this manuscript), line 176: "rechoiz ma (nos) proiere(s) et entens"; lines 178–80: "pieuz sire, rechoiz ma (no) proiere / et celui mez en tes bonteiz / qui (ki) scrit et trovat cez aveiz."

159. In addition to the prayer to Saint Gilles, which I describe below, MS IV–1013 also includes a prayer to Saint Christopher that reads, at fol. 167v: "laudabile miraculi per beatus Christoforus fecit redemptor . . . Ora pro nobis pie pater Christofore. ut digni efficiam promissione xpisti. Amen." Oliver, *Gothic Manuscript Illumination*, 2:248, speculates that this prayer may indicate ownership by a beguine of St. Christopher's in Liège. If she is right, then it is quite possible that this book was used in bedside care in St. Christopher's hospital.

160. Fol. 248v: "Iste homo ab adolescentia sua [par]im meruit infirmos curare. Dedit illi dominus claritatem magnam cecos illuminare et demones effugare."

161. On his relics, see Ernest Rembry, *Saint Gilles: Sa vie, ses reliques, son culte en Belgique et dans le nord de la France* (Bruges: Gailliard, 1881–82).

162. Iacopo da Varazze, *Legenda aurea: Edizione critica*, ed. Giovanni Paolo Maggioni (Florence: SISMEL, 2001), 2:887–90; Jacobus de Voragine, *The Golden Legend: Readings on the Saints*, trans. William Granger Ryan (Princeton: Princeton University Press, 1993), 2:147–48.

163. Jacobus, *The Golden Legend*, 147.

Charlemagne's sin was forgiven as long as he repented and confessed; "furthermore, anyone who had committed a sin and prayed to Giles to obtain pardon should have no doubt that by the saint's merits, the sin was forgiven."[164] The prayer to Saint Giles is enveloped in the psalter's therapeutic work, structuring acts of confession as a purgative process. This prayer would have been familiar locally, and likely served as an all-purpose apotropaic, a source of divine protection and healing, like the famous "Charlemagne prayer" that it evokes.[165]

Turning now to British Library, Harley MS 2930, produced in Liège around 1280, we find another example of a woman's prayer book functioning as a therapeutic technology. After a series of Mass prayers, this codex features an extensive vernacular meditation on the hours of the passion of Christ built around seven hours recalling the stations of the cross.[166] Although it captures many of the themes articulated in the French poetry, this exercise is a prose meditation.[167] The meditation describes the effects of the passion on human life—each of Christ's wounds is offered as a salve for human pain and sin. Following the meditation is a vernacular adaptation of Guiard of Laon's aforementioned sermon on the twelve fruits of the Eucharist (fols. 186v–193v), introducing the image of the cross as a fruit-bearing tree that healed injurious sin caused by the Edenic arbor. The sermon borrows heavily from Bonaventure's meditation the *Tree of Life*, which the minister general of the Franciscan order had offered as "the most effective medicine to prevent and cure every kind of sickness."[168] Guiard constructs his tree with a salutary vocabulary, one that proclaims the health effects of meditation on Christ's passion. Christ's suffering and death, according to the sermon, extinguished human death and disease. By ingesting the medicinal sacrament, the

---

164. Jacobus, 148.

165. The Charlemagne prayer was a charm that usually accompanied a measure of Christ's body or an image of his wound, and was used to assist in childbirth and protect against sudden death. It was said to have been brought to Charlemagne in battle by an angel, to protect him from harm. It is included in a few books of hours. See Reinburg, "Prayer and the Book of Hours," in Wieck, *Time Sanctified*, 40; and Eamon Duffy, "Two Healing Prayers," in *Medieval Christianity in Practice*, ed Miri Rubin (Princeton: Princeton University Press, 2009), 164–72.

166. The Mass prayers are at fols. 181v–182v. They include *Domine Jesu Christi fili dei vivi* and *Purificent nos quaesumus domine sacramenta*. The Mass prayers revisit the image of the Eucharist as a medication, naming it as "remedium anime," "sumti medicina," and "remedium sempiternum."

167. The author is unknown. Incipit: *Cilh ki ne seit dire des hores.*

168. Bonaventure, "The Tree of Life," in *The Soul's Journey into God, the Tree of Life, and the Life of St. Francis*, trans. Ewert Cousins (New York: Paulist Press, 1978), 120. Judith Oliver discusses the meditation's resonance with Bonaventure's *Lignum vitae* in her "Je pecherise renc grasces a vos: Some French Devotional Texts in Beguine Psalters," in *Medieval Codicology, Iconography, Literature, and Translation: Studies for Keith Val Sinclair* (Leiden: Brill, 1994), 248–62.

fruit of the tree of life, the supplicant pleads for its medicinal intervention. The sermon fashions the Eucharist as a medicine that reverses the bodily infirmities caused by sin.[169] It directs its audience to demand, "Heal me, Lord" (*saneix moi, sire*), as they conjure a mental image of the tree's salutary herbs (fol. 187).[170] Shifting tenses situate the listeners among the past events they conjured imaginatively and the present injunctions they directed to the cross, demanding that it take effect, that it act in the present.

The late twelfth-century influx into Liège of relics from Christ's passion helps us to map the therapeutic topography of these meditative practices.[171] The collegiate church of St. Croix in Liège housed a *staurotheca*, a reliquary containing a piece of the true cross, from roughly 1170. In the same city, the Dominicans claimed to own a thorn, given to them in 1267 by the French king Louis. The church of St. Aubin in Namur also possessed a relic of the true cross as well as drops of the blood of Christ and a thorn from the crown of thorns. And at Salzinnes, the Cistercian nuns enumerated among their passion relics sherds from the true cross, a bit of the column to which Christ was tethered and whipped, threads of his purple robe, fragments of the lance, and stone filings from the very sepulcher.[172] In the presence of such relics available in the region, the practice of meditation on the hours of the cross as found in the Harley psalter became an imaginative enactment, one equipped with props. The practice signals the multireferential space in which a therapeutic performance might occur. Real fragments of Christ's passion assisted the votary in connecting the wounds discussed in her meditation with the instruments of their making. Thorn and splinter produced the blood that healed, that provided a pathway for human salvation. While hospitals like those visited by beguines in Liège may not have possessed such precious relics, we do know that beguines and conversi engaged in the transport of saints' relics, as we saw in chapter 1, and that relics were often carried by nurses, along with portable icons, crucifixes, and other devotional

---

169. Fol. 187: "la medecine de larme qui le sanet de tote enfermeten de pechier."

170. The sermon uses a masculine ending, *pechier*, on fol. 193v, which contrasts with the feminine endings used in the Mass prayers (*peccatricem*, fol. 181v).

171. On the dispersion of relics in the Low Countries, see Nicholas Paul, *To Follow in Their Footsteps: Crusades and Family Memory in the High Middle Ages* (Ithaca: Cornell University Press, 2012), 90–133; Ferdinand Courtoy, "Les reliques de la passion dans le comte de Namur au XIII siècle," *Anciens Pays* 14 (1957): 85–98.

172. Thomas Coomans, "Moniales cistercienne et mémoire dynastique: Églises funéraires princières et abbayes cisterciennes dans les anciens pays-bas médiévaux," *Cîteaux* 56 (2005): 132. Coomans cites an inventory provided by Pierre-Lambert de Saumery in *Les délices du Païs de Liège* (Liège, 1740), 299–301.

imagery, to the beds of hospital patients.[173] By enacting these meditations in the presence of Christ's image and saints' relics, supplicants could convert words into work. The medicinal fruits of the tree of life that they imbibed through sermons and meditations became, in the presence of fragments of the true cross, real therapeutic agents.

The *Commendatio animae*, a prayer performed at the sickbeds of the dying, follows Guiard's sermon in the Harley psalter. The recitation of the *Commendatio animae* represents a communal form of care in which rhythmic and repetitive adjurations request that God liberate the soul from the body of the dying. As Frederick Paxton has noted, the rhythmic repetition of the prayer contributed to its ritualistic action, creating a sense of community among the living and dying and marking the moment at which dying became a participatory act.[174] At fol. 195r, a series of crosses appear just as the script of the petitioner requests defense against visible and invisible adversities. These signs interrupt the flow of the text right at the moment of divine petition for safety. *Christus vincit, christus regnat, christus imperat*—each phrase is separated by a cross to signify a manual blessing. Caesarius of Heisterbach recommended the use of this gesture and injunction as "medicine" protecting against "diverse demonic infections," and Jacques de Vitry advocated using it nightly before bed to prevent sudden death.[175] Here, the words posed a stark interruption in the text of the *Commendatio,* signifying a gestic animation of the prayer to stave off malfeasance as women shepherded the sick toward death. They represent a spontaneous medical improvisation, a performed therapeutic plea that added emphasis to the prayer's request. These three little crosses, tiny fragments of past practice, are easily overlooked. And yet they reveal performance-oriented forms of care in women's religious communities.

In closing this chapter, I turn to one final psalter, British Library, Additional MS 21114 (commonly referred to as "the Lambert-le-Bègue Psalter"). This psalter-hours includes a rather famous image of Lambert le Bègue, anchoring its production in Liège for the beguines of St. Christopher.[176] Although

---

173. On beguines who transported relics in Liège, see Philippe George, "À Saint-Trond, un import-export de reliques des Onze Mille Vierges au XIIIe siècle," *Bulletin de la Société Royale Le Vieux-Liège* 12 (1991): 209–228. On nurses carrying relics, see Rawcliffe, *Medicine for the Soul*, 104. Rawcliffe calls this "a practice which was almost certainly universal."

174. Frederick Paxton, *Christianizing Death: The Creation of a Ritual Process in Early Medieval Europe* (Ithaca: Cornell University Press, 1990), 119.

175. Caesarius of Heisterbach, *Dialogus miraculorum*, bk. V, ch. 47, 1110–15, 1112: "contra diversas daemonium infestationes diversas creaverit medicinas"; Don Skemer, *Binding Words: Textual Amulets in the Middle Ages* (University Park: Pennsylvania State University Press, 2006), 92.

176. On its provenance, see Oliver, *Gothic Manuscript Illumination*, 2:262–63.

the book was made sometime between 1255 and 1265, I wish to focus on a later insertion, added in the fourteenth century. These additional writings demonstrate an extemporaneous tailoring of this book to the specific needs and interests of the community that used it. A series of prayers, they suggest how the psalter could be altered to perform at the bedside in different therapeutic environments. They also indicate the ways that a psalter could retain its therapeutic function or identity, even as it changed hands and locations over time. The original portion of the psalter (fols. 1–122v) unfolds in a manner similar to the others under investigation here. It includes a calendar with Lambertum poem, an Easter table with Lambertum poem, Mass prayers, two of the French poems (*Pius deus omnipotens ki haut sies et lonc vois* and *Sire ki por nos fustes traveilhies et penez*), the Psalms, canticles, and a litany. As the psalter was created for the beguines of St. Christopher, we can imagine it functioning in a roughly corresponding manner to the three other psalters I have discussed in this chapter.

The fourteenth-century coda, then, points to a possible afterlife for the book, one that continued to resonate therapeutically. Some of the prayers in this annex section are in Catalan and Latin, providing interweaved instructions and scripts, similar to amuletic or charm texts. For example, one of them provides instructions to the reader on when to utter the prayer in Catalan. Then in Latin it offers the words of prayer that should be repeated. For example, one prayer very concisely reads, "Oh blessed Mary, mother of grace, mother of mercy, protect me from enemies and receive me at the hour of my death."[177] The following two folios (through 157r) continue in this manner, with Catalan instructions in red, for example to utter thirty-three Glorias and nine Magnificats, followed by the text of the Latin prayers. At the end of this Catalan-Latin series of directives, the final Latin prayer (*Precor te sanctissima virgo Maria*) is marked with a red cross, in the manner of a charm (figure 7). The specifically medical use of this charmlike prayer is supported by the surrounding cursive inscriptions, which include several prayers for the pregnant Mary's intervention (*virgine puerpera*), marked in the margins by red crosses, as one might designate a charm or charm-like prayer.[178]

---

177. "Aquesta oratio se deu lo yorn ho la nit de Nadal; siu dius de nits, devets dire nocte, si de dia, devets dir dies. O beata Maria, mater gracie, mater misericordie tu me ab hoste protege et hora mortis suscipe." My sincere gratitude to Montserrat Cabré and Lluís Cifuentes for their generous assistance in identifying the Catalan script.

178. On the use of marginal crosses to mark a charm, see Suzanne Parnell and Lea Olsan, "Index of Charms: Purpose, Design, and Implementation," *Literary and Linguistic Computing* 6.1 (1991): 59–63.

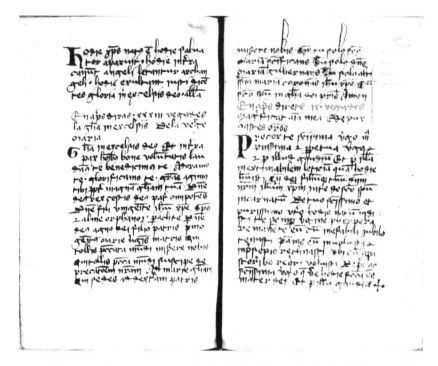

FIGURE 7. Prayer with marginal cross. © The British Library Board, MS Additional 21114, fol. 157r.

At fol. 161v a scribe has copied a prayer for relief of toothache, dedicated to Saint Apollonia, the third-century deaconess martyr who was tortured by having her teeth pulled one by one.[179] Prayers and supplications to Saint Apollonia were common sources of remedy for dental suffering, even among schooled physicians.[180] An inscription written in a separate hand offers a prayer to Saint Sebastian for relief from plague.[181] This later inscription shows that the book continued to have therapeutic resonance for later users, by which time it may have passed into a Cistercian women's abbey, as suggested by the Cistercian history inscribed in the final folios.

179. Fol. 161v: "Virgo martir egregia pro nobis appollonia funde preces ad dominum ne pro reatu criminum vexemur morbo dentium."

180. In his *Rosa medicinae,* John of Gaddesden recommended, for relief of dental pain, praying to Apollonia on her feast day. *Johannis Anglici Rosa Anglica seu Rosa Medicinae,* ed. Winifrid Wulff (London: Simkin Marshall, 1929).

181. Fol. 157v: "Beatissime Sabastiane . . . intercede pro nobis . . . ut a peste sive morbo epidemie liberemus."

In addition to these saintly injunctions for healing intercession, this adjunct section of the Lambert-le-Bègue Psalter includes a series of prayerful meditations that exhort the user to transform her affects in order to accept the wounded body of Christ, the Eucharist, as a medical unguent. The words of the prayers in this series included directions to the reader, so that, like the French poems, it required activation in order to take effect. As a whole, the meditation moves the practitioner imaginatively to each corporeal site of the passion, from head to hands to chest to feet. It begins with the form of the crucifix as an instrument, a tool for accomplishing the work of the passion, and calls attention to its material substance, wood. Each of Christ's punctured body parts is a portal through which his blood poured out a salutary tonic that the practitioner consumes through performance, by engaging the wounded body conjured textually and meditatively before her.[182] From the bleeding crown, the prayer transitioned the viewer's gaze to the wound in Christ's right hand, where nails affixed him to the cross, and then, in a separate prayer, to the wounded left hand. In these two dynamic stanzas, the practitioner envisioned the flowing blood from Christ's hands as rivers that washed away sin, refreshing the practitioner with joyfulness.[183] Although the verbal images evoke Christ's woundedness and suffering, the affects stirred by the meditation are not anguish and sorrow. Rather, the blood, which is styled as honeyed sweetness, arouses tranquility, delight, and joy. As the supplicant moved from the hands to the side wound, she imagined ingesting a nectar that served as the greatest remedy, the "medicine of all people."[184] Affixing her gaze on the right foot of Christ, the petitioner then insisted that Christ's outpouring of blood enabled humans to achieve tranquility and to prevent a regrettable death.[185] Each wounded limb was a point of contact with the medicine of a holy body, as the head, feet, hands, and side wound of Christ became active in a therapeutic performance. By conjuring in her imagination the experience of Christ's broken body, the reader rendered Christ's death as efficacious, transforming herself, or the person for whom she prayed, from a state of sin to salvation, sickness to health. Prayers to the wounds of Christ, such as this one, increased

---

182. For example, the verses on fol. 159r: "O corona preciosa quem corona tinxit rosa plasmatoris homini[um] per te fiat speciosa mens humana mens spinosa declinans in vicium."

183. Fol. 159r: "Oratione ad vulnus sinistre manus: Ave tu sinistra Christi, perforata tu fuisti, clavo perdurissimo. Velud guion efudisti, rivum tuum quo lavisiti, nos a malo. Te o vulnus adoramus tibi capud inclinamus, ut fonti dulcissimo. Per te detur ut vincamus, hostes et ut gaudeamus, in die novissimo."

184. Fol. 159v: "dulce vulnus," "tale nectar," "medicina populi."

185. Fol. 159v: "Salve vulnus dextri pedis . . . sit ergo in solamen, istud vulnus, et iuvamen, cum mors ad est flebilis."

dramatically in fourteenth-century western Europe.[186] Given that these wound prayers are bundled with the prayer to Sebastian for relief of plague, it is possible that they participated in efforts to fight disease and comfort sufferers. They were mechanisms of affective production, instruments for producing a specific affective constitution, one associated with the serenity and endurance of the body of Christ, which underwent torment for the sake of eternal life, for *salus*.[187] Indeed, the entirety of the psalter could be put to this very function.[188]

As I will discuss in the following chapter, wound meditation from women's religious communities in the region was associated with explicit forms of healthcare, such as relief from the pain of childbirth and protection from sudden death. When a meditation on Christ's wounds such as the one in the Lambert-le-Bègue Psalter is considered in the context of medical wound imagery, its therapeutic function in a hospital or leprosarium like those run by the beguines of St. Christopher becomes appreciable.[189] The wound prayers in the Lambert-le-Bègue Psalter may be a textual form of a medical practice drawing on wound prayer that, by the fifteenth century, had become widespread. The same side-wound prayer from the psalter ("aque paradysi" on fol. 159v) can also be found inscribed next to a red illustration of the side wound in a Cistercian manuscript from Vrouwenpark abbey, where it carried a medical indulgence (figure 8).

Later, such imagery could be found, for example, in an English roll belonging to Prince Henry in which the side wound promised protection from sudden death and poison.[190] In London, Wellcome Library, MS 632, a late fifteenth-century birth girdle, a drawing of the side wound appears along with instruments of the passion. The parchment roll on which it is written offers not only protection from death but also, when placed on the

---

186. Kathryn Rudy, *Rubrics, Images, and Indulgences in Late Medieval Netherlandish Manuscripts* (Leiden: Brill, 2016), 87. As Andrée Hayum has shown, patients who suffered from plague conformed their bodies to the wounded body of Christ in an effort to self-comfort. Andrée Hayum, *The Isenheim Altarpiece: God's Medicine and the Painter's Vision* (Princeton: Princeton University Press, 1993), 13–52.

187. They are similar to William Reddy's "emotives," which he considers a means of "changing, building, hiding, intensifying emotions." William Reddy, *The Navigation of Feeling: A Framework for the History of Emotion* (Cambridge: Cambridge University Press, 2001), 104–5.

188. On the physical and social work of psalter prayer, see Annie Sutherland, "Performing the Penitential Psalms in the Middle Ages," in *Aspects of the Performative in Medieval Culture*, ed. Almut Suerbam and Manuele Gragnolati (Berlin: De Gruyter, 2010), 15–37; and Michael Kuczynski, "The Psalms and Social Action in Late Medieval England," *The Place of the Psalms in the Intellectual Culture of the Middle Ages*, ed. Nancy Van Deusen (New York: SUNY Press, 1999), 191–214.

189. As I will discuss in the following chapter, on either side of the indulgenced medical wound in Brussels, KBR, MS 4459–70 are two prayers addressed to it, including precisely the same prayer that is inscribed here in British Library, MS Additional 21114, "aque paradisi."

190. Durham, Ushaw College, MS 29. See Skemer, *Binding Words*, 266.

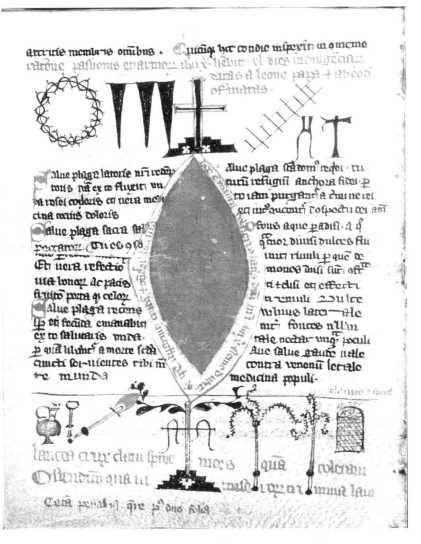

FIGURE 8. Indulgenced wound with prayers. Brussels, KBR, MS 4459–70, fol. 150v.

abdomen of a parturient woman, safe delivery of child.[191] And in Princeton University Library MS 138.44 the wound appears as part of a parchment amulet that promised parturient women an uncomplicated birth; to relieve

191. See Mary Morse, "'Thys moche more ys oure Lady Mary longe": Takamiya MS 56 and the English Birth Girdle Tradition," in *Middle English Texts in Transition: A Festschrift Dedicated to Toshiyuki Takamiya on His 70th Birthday*, ed. Simon Horobin and Linne Mooney (Woodbridge: York Medieval Press, 2014), 199–219; and Carole Rawcliffe, "Women, Childbirth, and Religion in Later Medieval England," in *Women and Religion in Medieval England*, ed. Diana Wood (Oxford: Oxbow Books, 2003), 91–117.

infertility, it instructed women to gaze upon the wound while uttering those efficacious words discussed earlier in this chapter, "spiritus vincit, christus regnat, christus imperat."[192] The wound prayers in the Lambert-le-Bègue Psalter are witness to an early tradition, forged in women's caregiving communities, of comforting patients through performative prayer and mimetic association with the salutary body of the crucified Christ.

In women's communities in the thirteenth-century southern Low Countries, health knowledge was communicated and constructed within a context of penitential practice and liturgical prayer. In this context, the psalter became a technology for constructing, transmitting, and implementing therapeutic knowledge. Other examples of psalters fulfilling this role include Liège, Bibliothèque de l'Université de Liège, MS 431, another psalter from St. Christopher's beguinage in Liège.[193] This psalter features a number of reflexive images that would have instructed the women who used it, including one featuring two midwives attending Mary's birth. Another example worthy of extended analysis is New York, The Morgan Library, MS 155, a Latin psalter from Liège (c. 1290–1305) with canticles, a litany, and two collects. Here, the *Life* of Margaret of Antioch appears in a pictographic cycle in the bottom margin under the Psalms (fols. 13c–21), a visual hagiography that beguines could have used to care for parturient women. Just as in the *Life* of Margaret discussed above (MS Sloane 1611), childbirth assistants could use Margaret's images, the recitation of her *Life*, and even the codex copy of the *Life* itself to ease labor. In Morgan Library MS 155, a veiled woman is depicted holding a folio or possibly a book in the initial *A* of Psalm 25 as below we see Margaret escorted to her execution (figure 9). Given the widespread use of Margaret's *Life* as a remedy for hastening and easing childbirth, it is possible that the graphic rendering of her *Life* in this psalter fulfilled a similar function. The veiled woman in the initial may be instructing readers and users of this book to utter the *Life* of Margaret or to place her image, illustrated within the book, on the abdomen of the parturient.[194] In a book intended to guide women in their daily work and prayer, these images may

192. Skemer, *Binding Words*, 249.

193. I have analyzed this psalter in detail in Sara Ritchey, "Caring by the Hours: The Psalter as a Gendered Healthcare Technology," in *Gender, Health, and Healing, 1250–1550*, ed. Sara Ritchey and Sharon Strocchia (Amsterdam: Amsterdam University Press, 2020), 41–66.

194. For examples of other French textual amulets of Margaret, see Jean-Pierre Albert, "La legend de sainte Marguerite un mythe maïeutique," *Razo* 8 (1988): 19–33; and M. Louis Carolus Barre, "Un nouveau parchemin amulette et la légende de sainte Marguerite patronne des femmes en couche," *Académie des Inscriptions et Belles-Lettres Comptes Rendus* 123.2 (1979): 256–75.

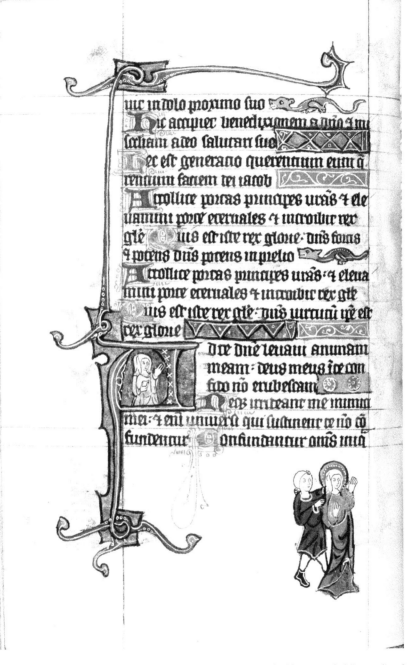

FIGURE 9. Margaret of Antioch heading to her execution; initial with woman holding a slip of parchment. The Morgan Library & Museum, MS 155, fol. 20v. Purchased by J. Pierpont Morgan (1837–1913) in 1902.

have been partly instructional and mnemonic, serving to link the work of prayer with their daily labor of bodily care while recalling the story inscribed in Margaret's *Life*.

The mulieres religiosae of Liège were certainly not unique in using prayer books to convey therapeutic data. Monica Green has assembled detailed surveys of the various forms of medical knowledge present in women's religious communities.[195] For example, she has found that a thirteenth-century psalter owned by German Benedictines features images of bloodletting (February) and a steam bath (March).[196] Such images indicated how and when this kind of practice might be safely undertaken, and may have interacted with other health tables and orally circulating regimens. In another case, a thirteenth-century psalter owned by Dominican nuns in the Rhineland contains a recipe for exorcising a diseased womb, a therapy that would certainly have been handy among religious women.[197] And a diurnal from the Cistercian house of Marienstern in Panschwitz-Kuckau features a nun performing phlebotomy on another nun, with a young girl holding a bowl to catch the blood.[198] Even beyond the psalter itself as a textual source, the Psalms played a formidable role in healing traditions, certainly predating Christian uses.[199] They could circulate as remedies orally and in miscellaneous medical or devotional manuals, such as British Library, Harley MS 2253, a fourteenth-century English miscellany that advised its readers to write out psalm 63, 72, and 73 and wear them on their arms as textual amulets in order to combat temptation and to treat particular illnesses.[200] These modes of recording hygienic knowledge are not simply happenstance. They are not marginal notations, but planned inscriptions with a therapeutic rationale of their own. They are constitutive of a regular practice that aimed to strengthen the *lyen du corps et anime*. They suggest a therapeutic rationale that linked medical

---

195. For summaries of this work, see Green's two articles, "Books as a Source of Medical Education for Women in the Middle Ages" and "The Possibilities of Literacy and the Limits of Reading: Women and the Gendering of Medical Literacy."

196. London, British Library, MS Additional 60629. This manuscript is probably from the Benedictine Abbey in Bamberg.

197. Wolfenbüttel, Herzog-August Bibliothek, MS 146.2, fol. 2r. See Green, "Books as a Source of Medical Education," Table 1, 362.

198. Green, "Books as a Source of Medical Education," 342–43. See Judith Oberste, "Zeit und Ewigkeit: 128 Tage in St. Marienstern," in *Neues Archiv für sächsische Geschichte*, ed. K. Blaschke (Stuttgart: Verlag Hermann Böhlaus, 1999), 248.

199. On Jewish uses of the Psalms for healing purposes, see Carmen Caballero-Navas, "She Will Give Birth Immediately: Pregnancy and Childbirth in Medieval Hebrew Medical Texts Produced in the Mediterranean West," *Dynamis* 2 (2014): 377–401.

200. On this practice, see Skemer, *Binding Words*, 86.

efficacy to performative prayer. These hygienic fragments nestled into prayer books from women's communities represent the many subtle and highly blended modes through which women constructed and transmitted medical knowledge.

The prayer books discussed in this chapter constitute one more item in the thirteenth-century constellation of feminine knowledge production about the body, health, and dying well. Beguine and Cistercian women's social expectation of penitential practice placed them in these gatherings proximate to the sick and dying. There, patients attributed to their combined caregiving and prayers a kind of generative immediacy. Those attributions are encoded not in academic medical texts, but in the books, objects, performances, and relationships of religious women who practiced charitable caregiving. These fragile traces of healthcare practices did not make it into the canon of Western medicine, thus they urge us to push back on a portrait of premodern healthcare framed by texts claiming masculine authority and legitimacy. They invite us to pause, to imagine alternate possibilities for what constitutes medical knowledge, for who counts as healthcare experts, and for what forces imperil health, what agents merit our attention.[201] By casting our gaze on sites of feminine bodywork and the fragile traces of therapeutic performance that linger there, we can recapture bits of healthcare knowledge and practice that never achieved authoritative status or archival substantiation. The therapeutic knowledge constructed within women's religious communities in thirteenth-century northern Europe rested on a concept of the body that was unthinkable outside of the operations of the soul, and unknowable removed from particular relationships with other human and nonhuman actors. It was exercised as embodied knowledge in the everyday behaviors required to maintain a non-natural environment: the washing of linens, the preparation of meals, insurance of access to open air and proper exercise, and the modulation of healthful affects, which were efficacious for these practitioners only within a regimen of liturgy and prayer.

---

201. Stacey Langwick, *Bodies, Politics, and African Healing: A Matter of Maladies in Tanzania* (Bloomington: Indiana University Press, 2011), 49.

CHAPTER 5

Salutary Words

Saints' Lives *as Efficacious Texts in*
Cistercian Women's Abbeys

The *Life* of Ida of Leuven reports a curious inci-
dent in which young Ida, gravely ill and convalescing in the infirmary, witnessed the sudden death of her sister. In apparent shock and grief, Ida hurled
herself over the body of the deceased sister, wailing in lamentation until a
sizable crowd had gathered in observation of the pitiable scene. Thereupon,
Ida shifted her internal disposition from lamentation to entreaty, praying for
the restoration of life to her departed sister. The unidentified hagiographer
noted the exact gestures and wording of Ida's prayer for resurrection, providing the details of how she raised one knee at a time from their clutch on the
dead sister's body, then each arm in similar succession. He described how she
prayed that the same power used by Elisha, Elijah, the daughter of Jairus, the
boy from Naim, and Lazarus be summoned immediately through her words,
infused into the corpse before her, restoring it to life as it had done in biblical times.[1] Finally, he noted that Ida touched the mouth of the deceased girl,

---

1. A version of this chapter was previously published under the title "Saints' *Lives* as Efficacious Texts: Cistercian Monks, Religious Women, and Curative Reading, c. 1250–1330," *Speculum*
92.4 (2017): 1101–43; the appendix of that article includes a complete list of the featured manuscripts'
contents and other codicological details. The powerful names that Ida cites serve as biblical precedents, suggesting a *historiale* that might have accompanied an orally circulating healing charm. Edna
Bozóky has argued that *historiales* on charms provided historical context and worked to assure self
and audience that a prayer offered real potential for efficacy. See Edna Bozóky, "Medieval Narrative

who, giving out seven breaths, quickened instantly. "Indeed these ancient miracles were renewed," pronounced the hagiographer, who then portrayed the awe of the spectators who were affectively transformed from grief to joy by the healing performance.[2]

According to this story, the performance of Ida's words yielded physiological and spiritual transformation of the deceased girl. They also generated changes in the audience who observed her ministrations. Moreover, I argue, the thirteenth- and fourteenth-century readers of Ida's *Life* would have understood the transformational power of Ida's words to extend even to themselves. In this chapter, I examine the role of the *Life*, the textual artifact, in the therapeutic process that first began with religious women's living caritative actions and the orally circulating stories of their therapeutic power. The *Life* itself, the experience of its words as well as the physical presence of its manuscript inscription, often served therapeutic purposes. The manuscript materialization of the *Life* channeled the presence of the saint and became a therapeutic tool, just like her tomb or relics, her prayer, or her touch.

Readers of the living saint's *Life* encountered it in what Judson Allen has called the reading "event."[3] The reading event established meaning through the tripartite relationship of the text, the audience (the readers and auditors), and the cultural space or circumstances in which the reading event unfolded. To capture the significations generated by the reading event, John Dagenais has proposed the study of "lecturature," by which he means that we search for literary sense "not in the fixed points of the authorial work or 'text' (as edited by the printing press and modern readers) but in the fluid (but often quite concretely documented) interstices between them."[4] Such an approach requires close scrutiny of the material support for the reading event, that is, of the manuscript. But it also requires an understanding of manuscripts in

---

Charms," in *The Power of Words: Studies on Charms and Charming in Europe*, ed. James Kapaló, Èva Pòcs, and William Frances Ryan (Budapest: Central European Press, 2013), 101–16; and *Charmes et prières apotropaïque*, Typologie des Sources du Moyen Âge Occidental, fasc. 86 (Turnhout: Brepols, 2003). Lea Olsan has considered the relationship of oral and textual (that is, manuscript) charms in "Latin Charms of Medieval England: Verbal Healing in a Christian Oral Tradition," *Oral Tradition* 7.1 (1992): 116–42. In particular, she examines the "Lazarus charm" for childbirth, showing how Latin errors and attention to sound patterns situate the charm in an oral performance.

2. *VILeuv*, 169: "Ac huius facti mirabili novitiate." The hagiographer describes their transformation as a washing over of pure serenity; their grief (*tristesse*) dissipated, and they were filled with joy (*gaudium*).

3. Judson Allen, *The Ethical Poetic of the Later Middle Ages* (Toronto: University of Toronto Press, 1982).

4. John Dagenais, *The Ethics of Reading in Manuscript Culture: Glossing the Libro de Buen Amor* (Princeton: Princeton University Press, 1994), 24.

their social setting.[5] Medieval readers understood their texts not as single, closed works, but through a multiplicity of material and cultural factors that mediated their reception of the text. These factors included the other texts within the manuscript, the readers who handled it, the formal elements of the manuscript, its emplacement in a specific library, and the lore, liturgy, relics, and other vital identity markers that were associated with its location and handlers. Taking account of the social setting of the complete codex helps to recreate the reading experience and to reevaluate the various ways that the corpus of *Lives* of religious women from the thirteenth-century southern Low Countries signified to their first generation of readers.

Viewing hagiographic texts from the vantage of their manuscript context suggests that the corpus of *Lives* were read as "efficacious texts" in the thirteenth- and early fourteenth-century Cistercian textual community. By "efficacious texts" I mean to indicate that the process of reading or hearing these *Lives* promised to precipitate physiological and spiritual transformation. The selection and arrangement of *scripta* (each individual inscription of a text) within these manuscripts shows that readers clearly associated the *Lives* with other texts that effected change, such as blessings, Mass formularies, indulgences, and charms. This association points to their significance as scripts designed for performance, all texts that promised spiritual and physical change: from affliction to grace, from bread to body, from sin to forgiveness, from illness to health. The texts with which these *Lives* were bound were largely scripts for performing or making grace present in objects in the material world. Like the audience who witnessed Ida's efficacious words resurrect a sister, the reading and audition of her *Life* generated physiological changes, stimulating healthy passions and embodying grace.

While we have no early version of the *Life* of Ida of Leuven, other late thirteenth- and early fourteenth-century *Lives* of religious women in the corpus clearly circulated together.[6] Two of the earliest extant manuscripts containing a cluster of these *Lives*—Brussels, KBR, MSS 8609–20 (mid- to late thirteenth century with some early fourteenth-century scripta) and 4459–70 (1320)—were produced within a matter of decades at the monastery of Villers and were created for use in women's communities under their

---

5. On the "social lives" of manuscripts, see Michael Johnston and Michael Van Dussen, "Introduction: Manuscripts and Cultural History," in *The Medieval Manuscript Book: Cultural Approaches*, ed. Michael Johnston and Michael Van Dussen (Cambridge: Cambridge University Press, 2015), 8.

6. The earliest extant scriptum of Ida of Leuven's *Life* is preserved in a fifteenth-century manuscript from the Rooklooster, where it was copied alongside the *Lives* of several other Brabantine saints. Vienna, Österreichische Nationalbibliothek, Series Nova, MSS 12706–12707.

patrimony.[7] They are our closest witnesses to the ways that these *Lives* were experienced by their first generation of readers. After the deaths and first posthumous miracles of the saintly mulieres religiosae of the southern Low Countries, the text of their *Lives* carried on the work of the stories about them that had circulated orally. These *Lives* continued to convince audiences that certain religious women were capable caretakers of the sick, infirm, weary, and distraught. Both manuscripts point to collaborative practices between Cistercian women and supporters and petitioners beyond their walls. Together these manuscripts demonstrate the extent to which those social networks depended on Cistercian women's intercession, and provide further indication of the kinds of therapeutic roles played by religious women in this region.

These early inscriptions of the *Lives* illuminate the ways that certain religious women continued to serve their communities in a therapeutic manner even after their deaths. While in chapter 1, I discussed postmortem access to the saint in her relics and at her tomb, here I focus on access to those women in the experience of reading her *Life*. As Rachel Smith has shown in an examination of the hagiographic writings of Thomas of Cantimpré, the goal of hagiographic reading was to "take up" (*suscipiant*) the saint's *Life*; that is, for the reader or audience to be acted upon by their encounter with the saint embodied in the text.[8] Such reading was transformational, a physical process of altering the self to reflect the ideals represented in the saint's *Life*.[9] This transformational power of the encounter with the saint of the text was promulgated in hagiographic tales that feature audiences as witnesses to the saint's life, as we read in the audience who witnessed Ida's resurrection of her sister and thus experienced delight. Readers of the *Life* replicated

---

7. I know of only one other thirteenth-century manuscript containing multiple regional lives from the corpus of thirteenth-century saints' *Lives* from the southern Low Countries. Berlin, Staatsbibliothek Preussischer Kulturbesitz, MS Theol. Lat. Qu. 195 was also produced in the thirteenth-century monastery of Villers. Unlike the two manuscripts examined in this chapter, there is no indication that this book was used outside of Villers. A colophon reads: *Liber sancte marie de villari in brabantia.* The manuscript contains only the *Lives* of Arnulf and Margaret *Contractae.* The rubrications and marginal notes, particularly on the *Vita Arnulfi*, suggest a very different kind of readership than the two with connections to women's communities. Several passages in the *Vita Arnulfi* are underlined, and notes highlight sections on different virtues and stages in the lives of both saints, suggesting that perhaps these *Lives* were used in the construction of sermons.

8. Rachel Smith, *Excessive Saints: Gender, Narrative, and Theological Invention in Thomas of Cantimpré's Mystical Hagiographies* (New York: Columbia University Press, 2019), 93–96.

9. Augustine models and theorizes this kind of transformative reading. On his method of reading, see Brian Stock, *The Integrated Self: Augustine, the Bible, and Ancient Thought* (Philadelphia: University of Pennsylvania Press, 2017); Rita Copeland, *Rhetoric, Hermeneutics, and Interpretation in the Middle Ages* (Cambridge: Cambridge University Press, 1995); Geoffrey Galt Harpham, "The Fertile Word: Augustine's Ascetics of Interpretation," *Criticism* 28.3 (1986): 237–54.

the reactions of the original witnesses to the saint's remarkable behavior. Hagiographers like Jacques de Vitry, Thomas of Cantimpré, and Goswin of Bossut worked to incorporate into their *Lives* details of the public's witness to the saints' overabundant grace, often describing a particular miracle or ecstasy in terms of precise liturgical time and communal setting, as well as providing the names and emotional reactions of the spectators. Such details emphasize the preservation and re-presentation of the living saint's performance of grace to a fresh audience, a new community, one that did *not* know her personally or witness her spiritual effects directly.[10] For example, Thomas of Cantimpré's *Life* of Christina Mirabilis cites his source for a narrative anecdote, relating that "a venerable man whom I remember, Thomas, now abbot of Sint-Truiden but then a priest of that city, told me a very edifying story about Christina." The hagiographer goes on to paraphrase the abbot's story, in which he and another companion surreptitiously observed Christina. He underscores the men's stupefaction as they saw Christina enter a trance-like state in which she sighed, wept, and alternately beat, then lovingly caressed the limbs of her body until she was so filled with grace that "one would believe her exterior body would burst."[11] Thomas describes Christina's words and gestures; he records details of the setting and time of her ecstatic performance, thereby recreating the scene for his readers, allowing them to position themselves as witnesses whereby they might reexperience Christina's performance. He remarks on the transformation to joy (*gaudium*) of Christina and her onlookers, and even himself as he experienced the story secondhand.[12] Just as the abbot and his companion, convinced of her unusual holiness, were moved to a more positive affective state, so would the readers of her *Life*, inwardly transformed by what they heard or read, ideally experience a conversion process.[13] More central than the moral or spiritual meaning of the narrative was the affective conversion it structured, the triggering of salubrious internal passions.[14] The written text encoded the audience

10. Mary Suydam has examined the *Lives* of the liégeois mulieres religiosae through the lens of performance studies. See her "Visionaries in the Public Eye: Beguine Literature as Performance," in *The Texture of Society: Medieval Women in the Southern Low Countries*, ed. Ellen Kittell and Mary Suydam (New York: Palgrave, 2004), 138; and Suydam, "Women's Texts and Performances in the Medieval Southern Low Countries," in *Visualizing Medieval Performance: Perspectives, Histories, Contexts*, ed. Elina Gertsman (Aldershot: Ashgate, 2008), 143–59.

11. VCM V.36, 659: "ut rumpi exterius un corpore crederetur"; trans., 151–52.

12. VCM III.19; V.36.

13. Giselle de Nie has noted descriptions of affective transformation said to have taken place within readers, auditors, and witnesses of early medieval miracle stories. See her *Poetics of Wonder: Testimonies of the New Christian Miracles in the Late Antique World* (Turnhout: Brepols, 2012).

14. Mary Carruthers has described how readers imbued with emotional tenor the *catena* in monastic meditative texts; see her *The Craft of Thought: Meditation, Rhetoric, and the Making of Images,*

experience of witnessing the original saintly performance; in this way, the reading process was oriented around the transformational *effects* of the *Life*. The manuscript context of the *liégeois Lives* reveals their encounter as stories that took effect in their very performance, narratives that soothed. Brussels, KBR, MSS 8609–20 and 4459–70 were framed by their makers as therapeutic books. Through close analysis of these codices, we can gather how the women whose *Lives* they transmitted continued to perform therapeutically in their communities long after their deaths, and how those who possessed and performed these books acted as their therapeutic agents.

Efficacious Words at La Cambre

Brussels, KBR, MS 8609–20 was produced at Villers in the mid- to late thirteenth century for La Cambre, a women's community located about thirty-two kilometers to their north.[15] It includes eight saints' *Lives*, seven of which were of women, three of which had Cistercian affiliation, and five of which formed part of the *liégeois* corpus.[16] In addition to the *Lives*, the manuscript includes miracles, sermons, prayers, hymns, instructions on the Eucharist, and healing charms. Despite the seeming miscellaneous quality of these assembled texts, the codex is by no means random. Each of the texts copied within it works with the others to create a medium for efficacious action, for devotional acts that anticipate the transformation of material bodies by means of an infusion of divine grace. As a whole, the manuscript conditioned its users to expect personal transformation through the reading process.

Manuscript 8609–20 opens with a cluster of hagiographic *scripta* on three saints who were *not* from Brabant, but who nevertheless held significance

---

400–1200 (Cambridge: Cambridge University Press, 2000). For the affective responses generated by meditative reading in later periods, see Sarah McNamer, *Affective Meditation and the Invention of Medieval Compassion* (Philadelphia: University of Pennsylvania Press, 2009); and Jessica Brantley, *Reading in the Wilderness: Private Devotion and Public Performance in Late Medieval England* (Chicago: University of Chicago Press, 2007).

15. The classic work on Villers is Édouard de Moreau, *L'abbaye de Villers en Brabant aux XIIᵉ et XIIIᵉ siècles: Étude d'histoire religieuse et économique, suivie d'une notice archéologique par le chanoine R. Maere* (Brussels: Dewit, 1909). For more recent work on the material construction of Villers, see Thomas Coomans, *L'abbaye de Villers-en-Brabant: Construction, configuration et signification d'une abbaye cistercienne gothique* (Brussels: Commentarii cistercienses, 2000); and Émile Brouette, "Abbaye de Villers à Tilly," in *Monasticon Belge* IV-2 (Liège: Revue Belge de Philologie et d'Histoire, 1968), 341–405; on the cultural life of the abbey, see Thomas Falmagne, *Un texte en contexte: Les "Flores Paradisi" et le milieu culturel de Villers-en-Brabant dans la première du 13e siècle* (Turnhout: Brepols 2001).

16. The saints *Lives* are Mary Magdalene (*BHL* 5439), Elizabeth of Hungary (*BHL* 2507), Lutgard of Aywières (*BHL* 4950), Christina Mirabilis (*BHL* 1746), Alice of Schaerbeek (*BHL* 264), Ida of Nivelles (*BHL* 4146), Odo (*liégeois* priest; *BHL* 6286), and Margaret *Contracta* (*BHL* 5322).

for its mulieres religiosae. These scripta include the *Life*, translation, and miracles of Mary Magdalene, a model of lay penitence for the mulieres religiosae; Caesarius of Heisterbach's *Life* of Elizabeth of Hungary (d. 1231), the royal widow who founded a hospital in Marburg, was canonized in 1235, shortly after her death, and after whom no less than thirteen beguinages were named; and a miracle cure attributed to the Virgin Mary.[17] Capping Mary's healing miracle are a few paragraphs from the Cistercian Guerric of Igny's sermon IV on Palm Sunday.[18] It is likely that the later compiler of the manuscript only wanted to include the text from Mary's miracle, as, following Guerric's sermon, there begins the hymn to Mary, *Ave sponsa insponsata*, composed by the bishop-saint Germanus, but it is cut off on the final folio in the quire.[19] The scribe has included a catchword, indicating that the hymn is not a fragment but rather, in its original inscription, would continue onto the next folio of a different quire. Instead of continuing with Germanus's hymn, however, the manuscript's compiler introduced new material. This later authority inserted into the midst of the volume a series of extended expositions that, although they are in fact four separate eucharistic texts, are labeled uniformly as "de sacramento" in the table of contents. The compiler therefore made a deliberate effort to disrupt the flow of the original assemblage with these eucharistic texts. They were not randomly chosen; I would suggest that he made an explicit association between the salutary effects of the Eucharist and the *Lives* of religious women in this region.

The texts that follow elucidate the connection between these saintly women and the Eucharist. Scholars have long associated religious women in this region with bombast piety, characterized by the frequency with which they communicated at Mass and the eucharistic content and character of their visions.[20] While substantiating that association, this manuscript also offers some nuance. It connects the mulieres religiosae with

---

17. The narrative of the discovery of Mary Magdalene's body at Vezelay is also included (*BHL* 5489).

18. On the eucharistic texts copied in MS 8609–20, see Albert Ampe, "Een oud *Florilegium eucharisticum* in een veertiende-eeuws handschrift," *Ons Geestelijk Erf* 31 (1964): 23–55.

19. On the use of this chant in the monasteries of the region, see Barbara Haggh, "Medieval Plainchant from Cambrai: A Preliminary list of Hymns, Alleluia Verses, and Sequences," *Revista de Musicologia* 16.4 (1993): 2326–34.

20. On this association, see Caroline Bynum, "Women Mystics and Eucharistic Devotion in the Thirteenth Century," *Women's Studies* 11 (1984): 115–28; and Miri Rubin, *Corpus Christi: The Eucharist in Late Medieval Culture* (Cambridge: Cambridge University Press, 1991), 302–15. On the attention of male religious to the Eucharist, see David Burr, *Eucharistic Presence and Conversion in Late Thirteenth-Century Franciscan Thought* (Philadelphia: American Philosophical Society, 1984); Marsha Dutton, "Eat, Drink, and Be Merry: The Eucharistic Spirituality of the Cistercian Fathers," in *Erudition at God's Service*, ed. John Sommerfeldt (Kalamazoo, MI: Cistercian Publications, 1987); Caroline

the consecrated host not through their devotional practices but through their similar salutary effects. For example, Guiard of Laon's sermon, *On the Twelve Fruits of the Sacrament*, is copied here (fols. 60r-73r). As we saw in the previous chapter, this sermon enjoyed widespread Latin and vernacular circulation in the thirteenth and fourteenth centuries.[21] Guiard was the bishop of Cambrai, the chancellor of the University of Paris in 1237, and a well-known supporter of the women's religious movement in the southern Low Countries.[22] Dubbed the *doctor eucharisticus* for his contributions to sacramental theology, Guiard appears in the *Life* of Lutgard of Aywières, where he engages Lutgard in a spiritual conversation.[23] He also makes an appearance in the *Life* of Margaret of Ypres, in which he voices his concern for her health during a period of fasting.[24] Guiard had traveled throughout the Diocese of Cambrai instructing locals on the role of the transubstantiated host in the confession of faith, and he was a vocal advocate for celebrating the eucharistic sacrament by adopting into the universal Christian calendar the feast of Corpus Christi as designed by Juliana of Mont-Cornillon.[25] By choosing to bind together a eucharistic sermon by one of the region's greatest supporters of the mulieres religiosae with examples of their *Lives*, the compiler of MS 8609–20 implicitly instructed users on how to make meaning of this manuscript. Guiard's sermon offered a theology of the Eucharist that focused closely on the sanctifying and salubrious effects of communion that were propelled by the physiology of mastication.[26] The twelve "fruits" of his treatise were twelve effects of grace made visible through ingestion of the consecrated host. He imagined the Host as a medication (*digestivum*; *aromata apothece*) that took effect on the communicant's soul, dispersing grace that animated and revivified the sinful body, conforming it to the body of Christ.[27] Guiard discussed the manner in which the Eucharist conformed the recipient to

---

Bynum, *Jesus as Mother: Studies in the Spirituality of the High Middle Ages* (Berkeley: University of California Press, 1982), 122–24.

21. Wybren Scheepsma, *The Limburg Sermons: Preaching in the Medieval Low Countries at the Turn of the Fourteenth Century* (Leuven: Brill, 2008), 165.

22. *La vie et les oeuvres de Guiard de Laon, 1170–env1248*, ed. Petrus Boeren (The Hague: Nijhoff, 1956); excerpts from Guiard's unedited treatises are included in the section "Textes inédits de Guiard de Laon," 310–47. Guiard's treatise on the twelve fruits also circulated in an abbreviated version, *On the Eight Fruits of the Venerable Sacrament*.

23. *VLA* II.40.

24. *VMY*, ch. 14.

25. Scheepsma, *Limburg Sermons*, 173; Charles Caspers, *De eucharistische vroomheid en het feest van Sacramentsdag in de Nederlanden tijdens de Late Middeleeuwen* (Louvain: Peeters, 1992), 192–96.

26. *La vie et les oeuvres de Guiard de Laon*, 279; "Textes inédits de Guiard de Laon," 332.

27. *La vie et les oeuvres de Guiard de Laon*, 252–53; "Textes inédits de Guiard de Laon," 329.

Christ through medical action. He was particularly interested in digestion, which dispersed comforting and conforming passions throughout the body. For Guiard, the medicine of the Eucharist worked in tandem with the generation of imitative passions within the communicant. He called attention to the grief experienced by Mary, requiring his audience to conjure similar affective states in order for the medicinal host to take effect. At the same time, Guiard conceived of the Eucharist as the *verbum dei*, the word that fused divinity with matter. This therapeutic word, for Guiard, had profound physical and psychological effects.[28] His conception of the Eucharist as the word of God emphasized the verbal mediation of the sacrament's efficacy, consecrated and thus transformed at the moment the priest uttered those efficacious words *Hoc est corpus meum*. Guiard's sermon is followed by a second sermon on the Eucharist.[29] Rubricated as *Sermo de sacramento altaris*, this sermon bears all the rhetorical trappings of a lively performance, so that its lessons were presented through the persuasive language and charismatic presence of a priestly authority, one who claimed the power to effect sacramental change. Together, these two sermons reflect performed speech.[30]

An anonymous treatise on the body and blood of Christ strengthens the association between eucharistic medicine and local female saints in MS 8609–20. Rubricated as *Incipit tractatus de corpore et sanguine Domini*, the treatise established a direct connection between the Eucharist and the mulieres religiosae. The treatise specifically cites the example of Marie of Oignies, asserting that she considered the Eucharist as medicine, and used it as her personal healing unguent that nurtured her through an illness lasting many days.[31] His exhortation on the transformational power of the Host praises the sacrament as the premier pharmaceutical, the "preferred remedy" for all wounds.[32] The manuscript's section on eucharistic texts concludes with a cascade of miscellaneous songs on the sacrament, including Hildebert of Lavardin's *De sumptione sacrae Eucharistiae* (On Taking the Holy Eucharist)

---

28. *La vie et les oeuvres de Guiard de Laon*, 250–51; "Textes inédits de Guiard de Laon," 325.

29. Incipit: *sanctorum virtus permaxima humilitas est*. Fols. 66v-73r.

30. I take factitive utterances from Roy Rappaport, who adopted it from a paper presented by Fehean O'Doherty. Rappaport dubbed these words, "performatives." According to Rappaport's formulation, in these words "the effect is completed in the gesture or utterance itself." In this particular case, the phrase "This is my body" actually accomplished the transubstantiating act. Roy Rappaport, *Ritual and Religion in the Making of Humanity* (Cambridge: Cambridge University Press, 1999), 114–15. On "efficacy phrases," see Claire Jones, "Formula and Formulations: 'Efficacy Phrases' in Medieval English Medical Manuscripts," *Neuphilologische Mitteilungen* 2 (1998): 199–210.

31. Fol. 79v.

32. Fol. 76r: "remedia potius"; fol. 96r: "medicalis virtus memorati sacramenti."

and others that serve as poetic homage to its effects as a "powerful medi-cine" and "sacred medicine."[33] The songs elicit communal participation, as the women of La Cambre would have gathered together, most likely in the presence of a clerical visitor, to perform this tribute to the Eucharist as a sacred medicine. As performed words, the songs elicited a therapeutic process that required the nuns to gesture, emote, and transform themselves in a manner that embodied the words on the page. The nuns synchronized their gestures and affects when they performed these songs as a community. The nuns were not seen as the sole beneficiaries of this practice, however; by offering their songs of praise as a communal therapeutic praxis, as I will show, the women of La Cambre could also aid the members of the laity who sought their prayers.

In its emphasis on the physical and hygienic transformation attendant upon reception of the Eucharist, the texts copied in this manuscript reflect long-standing Christian teaching. Ignatius of Antioch had described the Host as "the medicine of immortality," and Christ himself had long been depicted as healer or doctor, patterned on images of Aesclepius and Serapis.[34] But the healing power of the Eucharist had assumed a new theological urgency in the thirteenth century, when sacramental efficacy became canonically linked to bodily health at the Fourth Lateran Council in 1215. As we have seen, in the required confession that preceded Mass, according to Canon 21, the priest was likened to a doctor who healed the sick with the Host. The council's decrees clarified that the Eucharist was no mere metaphorical medi-cine, nor the priest a base analogue of the physician. Rather, their practices had real bodily effects. And thus Canon 22 ordered that physicians seek the accompaniment of priests when attending the sick so that the state of the soul, which conditioned the health or sickness of the body, might be properly cared for, "for when the cause ceases so does the effect."[35] The healing power of the transubstantiated host underwrote the power of the saints whose *Lives*

---

33. Fol. 99v.

34. Ignatius of Antioch, *Epistle to the Ephesians* 20.2, in *The Apostolic Fathers: Greek Texts and English Translations*, ed. Michael Holmes (Grand Rapids: Baker Academic, 2007), 199; Herman Kessler, "A Sanctifying Serpent: Crucifix as Cure," in *Studies on Medieval Empathies*, ed. Karl Morrison and Rudolph Bell (Turnhout: Brepols, 2013), 162.

35. *Constitutiones Concilii quarti Lateranensis una cum commentariis glossatorum*, ed. Antonius Gar-cía y García (Vatican City: Bibliotheca Apostolica Vaticana, 1981). Several scholars have remarked on the influence of these canons on medieval understandings of health. See Jessalyn Bird, "Medicine for Body and Soul: Jacques de Vitry's Sermons to Hospitallers and Their Charges," in *Religion and Medi-cine in the Middle Ages*, ed. Joseph Ziegler and Peter Biller (York: York Medieval Press, 2001), 91–134; Marcia Kupfer, *The Art of Healing: Painting for the Sick and the Sinner in a Medieval Town* (University Park: Pennsylvania State University Press, 2003), 133–35.

were collected in the manuscript.[36] This cluster of eucharistic texts rationalized the therapeutic efficacy of saints' *Lives*: Guiard's sermon and pastoral activity throughout the region linked theological discourse on the therapeutic efficacy of the sacrament with hagiographic literature and the performance of living sanctity. Both the Eucharist and living saints contained an overabundance of grace, with the potential to trigger physiological change.

It is from this therapeutic appreciation of sacramental theology in the region that we should understand the reading event established by the *Lives* that follow in succession, only disrupted by a brief paragraph of text, a fragment from a treatise on the grace of the Eucharist (137r):[37] five *Lives* of regional saints, four of whom were among the mulieres religiosae of Liège. They include the *Lives* of Lutgard of Aywières (100r-128v), Christina Mirabilis (128v-137r), Alice of Schaerbeek (138r-146v), and Ida of Nivelles (147r-178r). The fifth *Life* in this section is devoted to the *liégeois* priest Odo (178r-179v), who served the mulieres religiosae in his parish. The fragment on the grace of the Eucharist appears in the limited space remaining after the conclusion of the *Life* of Christina Mirabilis, and it features a curt enumeration of the sacrament's salubrious effects, including the remission of sin, the subjugation of demons, and defense against temptation, which enabled plentiful bodily goods such as the "cure for infirmity," provision of optimal health (*valetudinem*), and deterrence of death.[38] The inclusion of this excerpt suggests that the scribe(s) considered it relevant to address the benefits of the Eucharist while reading from this series of *Lives*, thus linking them once again to sacramental considerations.

How, exactly, the makers of MS 8609–20 understood the experience of the *Lives* of these saints to be therapeutically efficacious is suggested by a meditative *scriptum* on the passion of Christ and the mourning of the Virgin Mary.[39] This meditation, known as *Quis dabit*, was imagined as the words Mary uttered after the death of Christ. It was one of the most widely circulated devotional texts of the later Middle Ages.[40] The meditation provided rich visual images for the reader, taking her through every scene as she transitioned from the point of view of Christ to Mary to other onlookers. The

---

36. Kupfer, *The Art of Healing*, 135.

37. Fol. 137r. Incipit: *Mare non habundat tot guttis . . . quantum habundat sacramentum altaris karismatibus*.

38. Fol. 137r: "curat quondam infirmitate."

39. Incipit: *Quis dabit capiti meo aquam*, Jeremiah 9:1. This meditation on tears has a complex textual history with many borrowings; see Thomas Bestul, *Texts of the Passion: Latin Devotional Literature and Medieval Society* (Philadelphia: University of Pennsylvania Press, 1996), 136–40. According to Bestul, the meditation lacks a fixed text and is found in several recensions.

40. Bestul, *Texts of the Passion*, 136.

text, like the others copied throughout the manuscript, trained the user to conjure appropriate emotions—namely, grief and compassion; it engineered an effect, leading its reader to be transformed, physically in the form of posture and the production of tears, as well as emotionally by arousing certain affects. Like the songs on the medicinal sacrament, this meditation was likely designed for a group effort, producing a communal therapy. The Cistercian adviser to La Cambre would lead the nuns in the meditation so that, together, they conjured these feelings and gestures in a performed practice that promised affective and physiological transformation.

Mary Carruthers has shown that many monastic authors used textual meditations to cultivate tears as a physical preparation for scholastic thought. Medieval monastic meditative texts inherited the Galenic model of humoral theory in which the optimal balance of the body's natural qualities (hot, cold, wet, dry) determined the health and functioning of the rational capacity of the soul.[41] Scholastic authors such as Thomas Aquinas and Peter of Celle generated tears by physically prostrating themselves in certain strained positions while meditating on texts that aroused grief, fear, and anxiety; doing so, they believed, prepared the mind, clearing it for rational cogitation.[42] It is unlikely that *Quis dabit* was copied into MS 8609–20 for such purposes, as it was made for a women's community that was not trained to engage in scholastic disputation; however, we might still understand this text within the long monastic tradition that hailed the physiological effects of meditation. Even in nonclerical communities, passion meditation could take the form of medical regimen by fostering the affective disposition that made eucharistic reception more efficacious, more salubrious.[43] Bartholomaeus of Montagnana, for example, recommended meditation for a young patient roiled with strong emotion.[44]

That the *Quis dabit* meditation in MS 8609–20, like the other texts copied into this manuscript, was used as a technique for fostering physiological change

41. On the physiological preparation for meditation, see Mary Carruthers, "On Affliction and Reading, Weeping and Argument: Chaucer's Lachrymose Troilus in Context," *Representations* 93 (2006): 9.

42. Carruthers, "On Affliction," 11.

43. Daniel McCann discusses English passion texts and paraprofessional lay readers in his "Heaven and Health: Middle English Devotion to Christ in Its Therapeutic Contexts," in *Devotional Culture in Late Medieval England and Europe: Diverse Imaginations of Christ's Life* (Turnhout: Brepols, 2014), 350; on lay readers of medical texts, see also Michael Solomon, *Fictions of Well-Being: Sickly Readers and Vernacular Medical Writing in Late Medieval and Early Modern Spain* (Philadelphia: University of Pennsylvania Press, 2010).

44. Bartholomaeus de Montagnana, *Consilia CCCV* (Venice, 1564), fol. 19v; cited in Naama Cohen-Hanegbi, *Caring for the Living Soul: Emotions, Medicine, and Penance in the Late Medieval Mediterranean* (Leuven: Brill, 2017), 118.

is borne out by the scripta that surround it, creating a powerful textual inter-play that linked reading on the life and passion of Christ with verbal processes of healing, with efficacious words. Much of the detail for Mary's lament in *Quis dabit* was taken from the Gospel of Nicodemus. This adaptation is useful for further decoding the manuscript, as an excerpt from the Gospel of Nico-demus appears several folios later, in a series of fragmentary texts dedicated to the healing capacity of Christ and his cross.[45] The Gospel of Nicodemus was a fifth-century apocryphal passion narrative that became popular in the thirteenth century.[46] In the particular selection from the Gospel that is copied here, Pilate asks the company of Jesus's followers about his healing miracles. The crowd reports that Jesus healed a leper, repaired a paralyzed leg, and raised Lazarus from the dead.[47] The scribe followed this excerpt with copies of the legends of the finding of the cross and its exaltation, both appealing to the cross as an agent of physical healing: in the story of its finding, the true cross is distinguished from two other crosses by its capacity to revive a dead youth, and the exaltation narrative included two important miracle stories in which salubrious water and blood gushed from a wounded image of Christ that was painted by Nicodemus.[48] This cluster of scripta brings together Christ's pas-sion with the healing effects of the Eucharist—his bodily death on the cross is featured as the remedy for sin and sickness. The passion had therapeutic effects that were textually mediated in the process of reading the manuscript.[49] Just as ingesting the sacrificial body in the consecrated host carried hygienic effects within the communicant, so also did the process of digesting the words of the passion narrative compel therapeutic effects for the reader.[50] The therapeutic effects of reading meditations on the life of Christ were not unlike those prom-ised by the process of reading saints' *Lives*. As constructed by MS 8609–20, both served to arouse salutary passions.

Following the exaltation of the cross, the scribe copied a series of texts that can only be described as incantatory. First, he included a litany of worthies

---

45. Zbigniew Izydorczyk, *Manuscripts of the Evangelium Nicodemi: A Census* (Turnhout: Brepols, 1993).

46. Villers' library housed a copy of the Gospel of Nicodemus, bound with the Cure of Saint Tiberius, the Epistle of Pilate, and the *Life* of Saint Anselm of Canterbury. Izydorczyk, *Manuscripts of the Evangelium Nicodemi*, 30–31.

47. Fol. 199v.

48. Barbara Baert, *A Heritage of Holy Wood: Legend of the True Cross in Text and Image* (Leiden: Brill, 2004), 133.

49. McCann, "Heaven and Health," 346. McCann explains that the *Priking of Love* fashions Christ's body into a pharmacy while at the same time articulating the body as a book for study and meditation.

50. On reading as a digestive process, see Carruthers, "On Affliction," 8–10; Carruthers, *The Book of Memory: A Study of Memory in Medieval Culture* (Cambridge: Cambridge University Press, 2008), 165–73.

who suffered with Saint Ursula, essentially a cast of characters in the narrative of her life. The community at La Cambre possessed relics from Saint Ursula and her band of virgins, suggesting the possibility that this scriptum served as a mnemonic for recounting her legend as one meditated before the sacred materials.[51] The Ursuline names should be read in conjunction with another inscription, the Ursuline visions of Elizabeth of Schönau, which appears at fol. 185r. The account reports on Elizabeth's prophetic authentication of the relics of Ursula and her troupe of virgin martyrs, which had been discovered in Cologne in the early twelfth century.[52] The hagiographic material from Elizabeth's visions in MS 8609–20 thereby endorses the intercessory power of Ursula's relics housed at La Cambre. Thus, the manuscript provided its own certificate of authentication in the copy of Elizabeth's visions, which served to affirm the salvific work accomplished by the nuns' recitation of the litany in the presence of the relics. Another miracle-working object at La Cambre suggests that such a practice might be quite routine, and would envelop the local lay community. In the nuns' custody was a "certain image of the mother of God" at which many blind, deaf, and diseased individuals found cure.[53] The local sick could access these therapeutic objects through the abbey church, which may have been open to the parish, as is suggested by archaeological evidence revealing the presence of a chapel on the north side of the abbey church. The chapel was separated from the nuns' enclosure and open to the public through a walk along the north side of the nave.[54] Furthermore, we know that the nuns of La Cambre maintained a porteress who distributed

---

51. The Ursuline revelations from Elizabeth of Schönau, *Ordo revelationis de gloriosis sodalibus sanctae Ursulae,* fols. 185–192. Cistercians in the German Empire expressed a particular interest in the dissemination of Saint Ursula's relics; see Ernest McDonnell, *The Beguines and Beghards in Medieval Culture: With a Special Emphasis on the Belgian Scene* (New Brunswick: Rutgers University Press, 1954), 296–97.

52. *Die Visionen der hl. Elizabeth und die Schriften der Aebte Ekbert und Emecho von Schönau,* ed. F. W. F. Roth (Brünn: Verlag der Studien aus dem Benedictiner- und Cistercienser Orden, 1884); Elizabeth's visions have been translated by Anne Clark as *Elizabeth of Schönau: The Complete Works* (New York: Paulist, 2000). On Elizabeth's role in authenticating the relics, see Laurence Moulinier, "Élisabeth, Ursule et les Onze mille Vierges: Un cas d'invention de reliques à Cologne au XIIe siècle," *Médiévales* 22–23 (1992): 173–86.

53. Philippe Numan, *Miracles Lately Wrought by the Intercession of the Glorious Virgin Marie, at Mont-aigu,* trans. Robert Chambers (Antwerp: Arnold Coinings, 1606), 8. Although the collection was printed in 1606, it refers to a Jewish man attacking the image with a boar-spear in 1232, thus positing its presence at La Cambre at this time. That the author of the miracle collection could imagine the space of La Cambre as available to Jewish people, among others, suggests that the abbey maintained certain points of access, at which visitors could see their relics and images, here most likely in the church.

54. Thomas Coomans, "Cistercian Nunneries in the Low Countries: The Medieval Architectural Remains," in *Studies in Cistercian Art and Architecture,* ed. Meredith Parsons (Kalamazoo, MI: Cistercian Publications, 2005), 61–131.

alms to the poor, because in 1234 they received a donation for this very purpose from the castellan of Brussels, Lionnet I.[55] So it is possible that the relics
of the Ursuline virgins worked to attract sick pilgrims and generated cure
while hearing the story of their heroic travails. These components of the
manuscript place it clearly within the physical space of the cloister and reveal
the production of the codex as a response to the specific circumstances of
the women at La Cambre, whose prayers extended their service beyond the
cloister.

The nuns' service beyond the cloister is also made clear in a series of healing charms copied into the manuscript (figure 10).[56] The charms were not
marginal, but were rather included as part of the scribal planning, rubricated,
and marked with crosses. These charms are particularly helpful for understanding the relationship between the Cistercian nuns of La Cambre and
their social networks outside the cloister. The presence of a series of charms
copied centrally into this manuscript provides evidence that the women who
used MS 8609–20 wanted a textual source to support their healing prayers.
While we may have little evidence that women read formal medical treatises,
the charms here provide yet another glimpse into processes of oral transmission of therapeutic knowledge. Some of the charms have no known textual
exemplars, suggesting that they represent a moment of oral communication
in the creation of this manuscript.[57] Because so many of the charms were
obstetric, they also suggest that the nuns of La Cambre, many of whom
likely lived as beguines before taking permanent vows as Cistercians, maintained their healthcare ties to the community they previously served.[58]

The first charm copied into MS 8609–20, on fol. 199r, promised to assist
against *caducus morbus*, or epilepsy. The charm asked its user to create a

55. Aubertus Miraeus and Joannes Foppens, *Opera diplomatica et historica*, vol. 1, ch. 162, 745.
For a discussion of the development of the position of the porter as a charitable post, and its pos-
sible origins in Cistercian women's charitable practices, see Anne Lester, "The Porter of Clairvaux:
Space, Place, and Institution; An Example of the Evolution of the Spirituality of Charity during the
Thirteenth Century," in *Le temps long de Clairvaux: Nouvelles recherches, Nouvelles perspectives (XIIe–XXIe
siècle)*, ed. Arnaud Baudin and Alexis Grélois (Troyes: Conseil Départmental de l'Aube, 2017), 117–34.

56. Lea Olsan, "The Marginality of Charms in Medieval England," in Kapaló, Pòcs, and Ryan,
The Power of Words, 122–42.

57. What was the exemplar for these charms? The booklists of Villers include only one obvious
medical work, *textus phisicorum et methafisice in uno volumine*, but this codex likely arrived at Villers
after the production of MS 8609–20. See Albert Derolez, ed., *Medieval Booklists of the Southern Low
Countries* (Brussels: Paleis der Academiën, 2001), 4:227. Derolez notes that this book would have
arrived about 1328, when Gislenus of Binche transferred to Villers from Aulne, bringing with him
a number of books.

58. Yvette of Huy, for example, dressed as a Cistercian nun and maintained ties with her family
members at Villers, Orval, and Trois-Fontaines. Although she never took vows as a Cistercian, Yvette
served the leperous while living as a recluse.

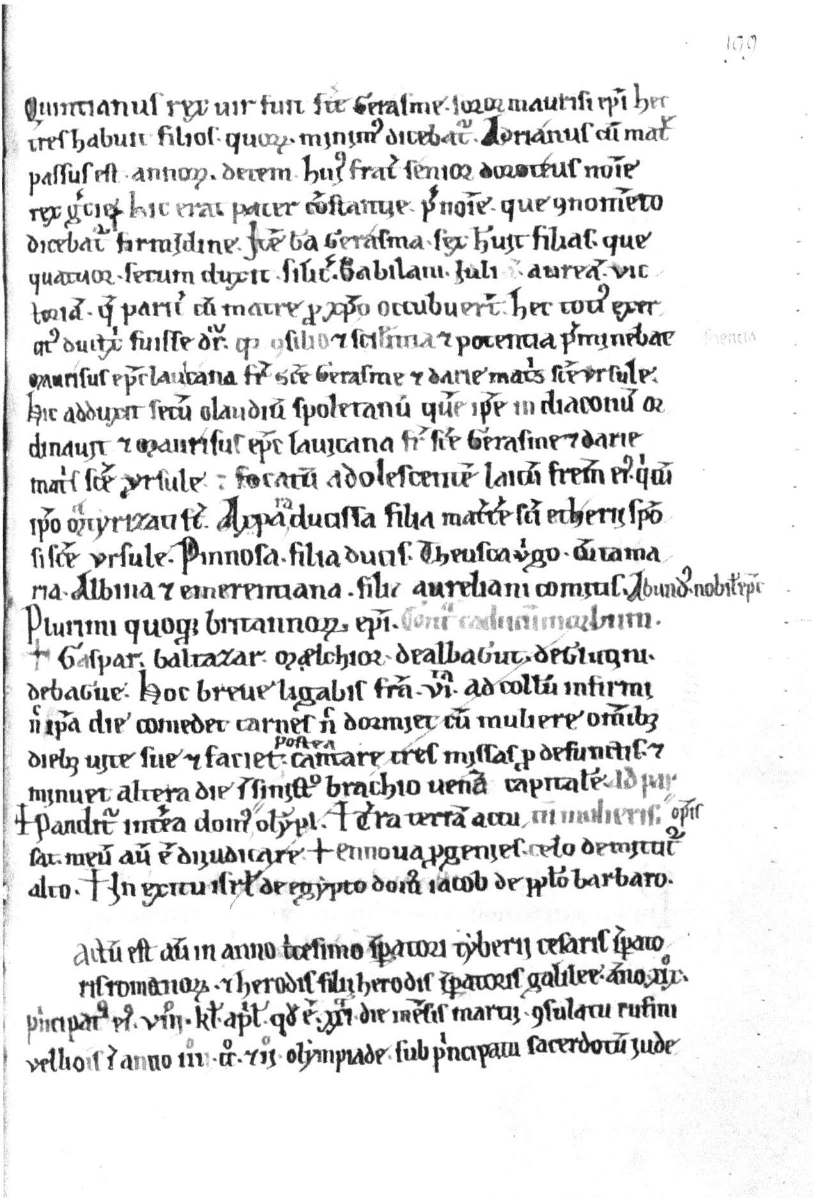

Quinciannuſ rex uir fuit ſce ſeraſme · ioɔz maurisi epi hec
treſ habuit filioſ quoꝝ minimū dicebat · Ioriánuſ cū mat
paſſuſ eſt annoꝝ · decem · huⁱ frat ſenioꝛ dɔꝛdeuſ noīe
rex ꝗ uɩɡ hic erat pater cōſtancie · p̄noīe · que gnometo
dicebat firmldine · fue̅ ba ſeraſma ſex huⁱc filiaſ que
quatuoꝛ ſecum dux̄it · ſiliē̅ · Babilani · ſulı · z aurea · vic
toʃid · ꝗ partī cū matre p̄ xp̄o occubuerit · hec toū ex̄it
at̄ duux̄ı fuiſſe d̄r · ꝗ z uſilio z ſciſſima z pocencia p̄minebat
omaurisuſ epī clautana · fr̄ ſce ſeraſme z darie maūs ſce vr̄ſule
hic adduxit ſecū claudiū ſpoletanū qᵘe ipe in diaconū oꝛ
dinaūt z omaurisuſ epī lauicana · fr̄ ſce ſeraſme z darie
maūs ſce vr̄ſule · z ſocratū adoleſcenciē laicū fr̄em eⁱ qᵘi
ip̄o oꝛiyrizau te · Appa ducaſſa filia matⁱe ſcī echerni ſp̄o
ſiſce vr̄ſule · Pinnoſa · filia duuſ · Theuſca v̄go · ɢtama
ria · Albina z emerenciana · filie aurelianī comſul · Abundᵒ nobilı p̄r
Plurimi quoꝗ britannoꝛ epī · · · · · · · · ·
✝ Gaſpar · baltazar · melchior · dealbabut · deciuqnu ·
debacue · Hoc breue ligabiſ frā · vi · ad coltū inf̄irmi
ñ ipa die comedet carnet ñ doꝛmiet cū muliere omīb3
die3 uɩte ſue · z fariet catmare treſ myſſaſ p̄ deſunctiſ z
minuet altera die · ſi inſtº brachio uenā capitalē · lɔ par
✝ Pandrū intⁱa dom̄ olypi · ✝ eⁱra uⁱa accu m mulieriſ opⁱ
ſat meū aū e̅ diiudicare · ✝ ennoua pꝛgeniet cⁱ to demiſcuſ
alto · ✝ In exⁱcu iſr̄l de egypto dorū iacob de pⁱ to barbaro ·

Actū eſt aū in anno tⁱceſimo ſp̄acⁱoꝛ tyberii ceſariſ ip̄aio
riſ romanoꝛ · z herodiſ filii herodiſ ip̄acⁱoſ galilee · ano xix
p̄ncⁱpat · eⁱ · vⁱij · kⁱ aplⁱ · qd e̅ xxⁱi die meſiſ marciſ · gſulacu rufini
velhoſ z anno iij · ū · vⁱij · olympiade · ſub p̄ncⁱpatu ſacerdociū iude

FIGURE 10. A series of charms, with markings of later censure. Brussels, KBR, MS 8609–20, fol. 199r.

ligature, tying it around the neck of the infirm and calling on the magi Gaspar, Balthazar, and Melchior. It was a well-known charm, commonly called the "Three Kings Charm," and was included in Bernard of Gordon's *Lily of Medicine* as well as Roger Bacon's *Opus majus*.[59] The remedy for epilepsy is followed by a series of four charms for assistance in childbirth, clearly rubricated with the words *ad partum mulieris*. These include a commonly used charm, *Panditur interea domus olympi*, which was based on the opening to the tenth book of Vergil's *Aeneid*.[60] This charm is followed by a less familiar one, *Terra terram accusat meum autem est judicium*. The line is related to a story from the Gospel of John (8:1–11) in which a crowd asked Jesus how to punish a woman who was accused of adultery; he responded by writing in the dirt of the earth. Though the content of what, exactly, he wrote is not indicated, theologians beginning with Ambrose of Milan were undeterred from speculation, with one of the most favored responses being *Terra terram accusat* (Earth accuses earth).[61] Offered without commentary as a charm in this manuscript it evoked the power of words. The content or significance of Jesus's words was unimportant; it was their effect that mattered.[62] The third birthing charm echoes another line from Vergil, *[En]nova progenies cello demittitus alto* (A new generation is let down from heaven above). This phrase was part of the well-known "peperit charm" in which, after the invocation of a series of "holy mothers," these words were to be copied on a slip of parchment and attached to the leg of a parturient woman.[63] And the final charm, *In exitu Israel de egypto domus Jacob de populo barbaro* (When Israel went out of Egypt, the house of Jacob from a barbarous people) derives from psalm 113, which was commonly used as a funerary song. While I have found no

---

59. Skemer, *Binding Words*, 181.

60. Thomas Fayreford attested to its efficacy in his commonplace book; see Peter Murray Jones and Lea T. Olsan, "Performative Rituals for Conception and Childbirth in England, 900–1500," *Bulletin of the History of Medicine* 89 (2015): 14.

61. Jennifer Knust and Tommy Wasserman, "Earth Accuses Earth: Tracing Jesus's Writing on the Ground," *Harvard Theological Review* 103 (2010): 407–46. George Aichele connects the passage to the logocentrism of John's Gospel; see his "Reading Jesus Writing," *Biblical Interpretation* 12 (2004): 353–68.

62. The phrase is also connected to the Carolingian "Lothair Crystal," an amulet given as a kind of apotropaic talisman to Queen Theutberga by King Lohair II upon the reconciliation of their marriage. On this interpretation of the Lothair Crystal, see Valerie Flint, "Susanna and the Lothair Crystal: A Liturgical Perspective," *Early Medieval Europe* 4 (1995): 61–86.

63. This charm is copied in the famous late fourteenth-century Anglo-French medical miscellany, London, British Library, MS Sloane 3564, where it instructed users to write these words on a "foille"; see Tony Hunt, *Popular Medicine in Thirteenth-Century England: Introduction and Texts* (Woodbridge: Boydell & Brewer, 1990), 92. For an extended discussion of the "peperit" charm, see Jones and Olsan, "Performative Rituals," 8–9.

other textual analogues for this birthing charm, as we saw in chapter 4, psalm texts played a significant role in religious women's caritative practices.[64]

The charms in MS 8609–20 are highly condensed. In those charms with a known textual tradition, such as the "peperit charm," the Vergilian phrases appear as one component of a more elaborate, multistep charm that included instructions for gesture, invocation of holy figures, and specific prayers.[65] Here, however, only the Latin words, apparently meant for inscription, were provided. This condensed version of the charms points to an oral tradition that would have communicated the totality of the procedure. The text of all four charms derives from literary or biblical traditions that would have been well known within the cloister. Appearing as charm texts, then, they represent appropriations of culturally significant texts for the purpose of healing. That they were in fact appropriated as *charms* indicates that these traditional texts were reinscribed with meaning through the act of performing them. If performed properly, they were understood to bring about physiological transformation, from illness to health, from struggle to ease in labor.

Bearing in mind the oral and performative expositions that stood behind the text of these charms, we can imagine how they would have interacted with other texts in MS 8609–20 and with other material objects at La Cambre. The charms in MS 8609–20 are embedded among prayers, meditations, and saints' *Lives*, suggesting the possibility that the manuscript as a whole was consulted during the birthing process. The nuns of La Cambre may have read from its *Lives* and sung its chants, perhaps also making use of the Ursuline relics, while attending to laboring women or to other caregiving needs. That ecclesiastical authorities sought to terminate and erase the memory of their caritative outreach to pregnant women is indicated by the later marks of censure that scratched through the charms' text.[66]

---

64. Other amuletic charms that included psalm texts can be found in Hebrew tradition; see Carmen Caballero-Navas, *The Book of Women's Love and Jewish Medieval Medical Literature on Women: Sefer ahavat nashim* (London: Kegan Paul, 2004), 174–76. I thank Carmen Caballero-Navas for assisting me with this scriptum. Another ritual for speeding up birth directs the practitioner to write a verse from Psalm 115 on parchment and then to read it over the head of a woman, tying it with a seal and binding it to her finger with a red silk thread. Jones and Olsan, "Performative Rituals," 14.

65. In other cases of the "peperit" charm, for example, there is a brief historiale, the invocation of a series of holy mothers, instructions to write the Latin phrase on parchment and affix it to the laboring woman, and an adjuration for the child to come out, as well as, in some cases, an exorcism of demons. See Marianne Elsakkers, "In Pain You Shall Bear Children: Medieval Prayers for a Safe Delivery," in *Women and Miracle Stories: A Multi-Disciplinary Exploration* ed. Anne-Marie Korte (Leiden: Brill, 2004), 179–210.

66. The same black line appears earlier in the manuscript, in the *Life* of Lutgard next to marginal comments that read: "vacat . . . vacat." The section corresponds to chapters 25 and 26 in the *AASS*

Similar in form to the five charms in MS 8609–20 are a string of incantatory verbal utterances with a medical Latin patterning, but no clear significance: *lacrimae balneum, mors vita, lingua doctor, oculus ductor, facies speculum, cor hospicium.* The words express illocutionary force, but contain no obvious meaning.[67] Thirteenth-century grammatical theory conceived of such interjections as emerging from the passions of the soul. Considered in this light, these words of interjection were "vessels of affect."[68] Their very incompleteness managed the expression of inexpressible feelings.[69] These gestural interjections provide another example of the performed communal utterances that the manuscript structured for its readers. Here, they strike the reader as pleas for immediate therapeutic action.

By embodying the saint's life textually, the manuscript copy of the *Life* became a verbal relic.[70] The manuscript copy of the *Life* was part of the

---

version of her *Life*. The first tells of how a young nun of the Cistercian order who was very ill and could not properly fast or follow the Rule languished in the infirmary until Lutgard assisted her with prayers. This healing, declared a miracle by Thomas, provides an important temporal dimension to the layers of mediation of Lutgard's textual *Life*. Thomas reports that the woman who was assisted by Lutgard was now a *vetula* and had affirmed the veracity of this anecdote. In this way, Lutgard's past actions were brought closer to the present by recording the *vetula's* memory of her interaction with and bodily transformation at the hands of Lutgard. The second rescinded miracle relates that another young nun, Hespelendis, suffered from a pathological depression. She requested that Lutgard pray for her, and, assenting, Lutgard gave very specific directions as to when her cure would be delivered—on Good Friday, during the adoration of the cross, at the moment when the priest lifted the cross, saying, "Behold." Thomas reports that, indeed, at this exact moment in the liturgy, Hespelendis experienced an infusion of grace comforting her body.

67. John Searle and Daniel Vanderveken, *Foundations of Illocutionary Logic* (Cambridge: Cambridge University Press, 1985), 46–48.

68. This is Daniel McCann's phrase; McCann explores nonverbal prayer in the *Cloud of Unknowing*, viewing its interjections through the grammatical theory of Hugh of St. Victor, John of Garland, Roger Bacon, and Thomas Aquinas. These authors insist that interjections express affections of the soul. McCann, "Words of Fire and Fruit: The Psychology of Prayerwords in the *Cloud of Unknowing*," *Medium Aevum* 84 (2015): 223.

69. John of Garland asserted that emotions are "expressed better in an incomplete sentence (*per oratione inperfectam*)," in a chapter on word order, suggesting that interjections be placed at the beginning of sentences. *The Parisiana Poetria of John of Garland*, ed. and trans. Traugott Lawler (New Haven: Yale University Press, 1974). On John of Garland's observations about affective interjections, see McCann, "Words of Fire and Fruit," 214. McCann notes also that many liturgical expressions, such as *amen, alleluia, deo gratias*, were seen as interjections that express pure affect, no reason. Aquinas compared human interjections to the bark of a dog or the roar of lion—sounds that signified internal pleasure and pain with immediacy. Thomas Aquinas, *Commentary on the Politics*, I.1.1/b, in McCann, "Words of Fire and Fruit," 217.

70. Skemer, *Binding Words*, 236 and 50. Skemer borrows the term "verbal relics" from Raymond Van Dam, who used it to describe the exchange of hagiographic stories about Gregory of Tours. Van Dam noted that healing miracles took place during public recitations of the stories from Gregory's *Life*, so that the reading of the *Life* was an occasion in which audience/hearers expected Gregory to reenact miracles. Raymond Van Dam, *Saints and Their Miracles in Late Antique Gaul* (Princeton: Princeton University Press, 1993), 138.

saint's material identity, just like her relics and tomb.[71] In its presence, and through its utterance, the power of the saint revivified and was made present to a fresh audience. Listening to the narratives of cure, auditors imagined the process of miraculous healing, the "transformational patterns" made visible in them.[72] These narratives were culturally understood as therapeutic texts. For example, the Italian physician Gentile of Foligno recommended to a woman suffering from the pain of an ulcerous bladder that she engage the memory of astonishing stories as a means of transforming sorrow to delight.[73] And the English theologian Thomas Chobham praised the beneficial effects made possible by musicians who performed narrative songs recounting the lives of saints.[74] The scripta within MS 8609–20 linked the reading and hearing of *Lives* of mulieres religioisae with the infusion of grace that was believed to fuel sacramental change, to effect physical transformation. The process of reading, or actively hearing these *Lives* read, prepared audiences for similar transformation. When audiences heard the dramatic performance of reading, they learned to expect the kind of conversion and physiological transformation the original eyewitnesses to the living saint had experienced.

Efficacious Performances at Vrouwenpark

A second book produced at Villers further demonstrates that the Cistercian community in the thirteenth- and early fourteenth-century Low Countries experienced this corpus of *Lives* as efficacious texts. Brussels, KBR, MS 4459–70 was copied in 1320 for the Cistercian women's community of Vrouwenpark.[75] A colophon inscribed on a half sheet after the front flyleaf

---

71. Jocelyn Wogan-Browne, "The Apple's Message: Some Post-Conquest Hagiographic Accounts of Textual Transmission," in *Late Medieval Religious Texts and Their Transmission*, ed. Alistair Minnis (Cambridge: D.S. Brewer, 1993), 45. Alice of Schaerbeek presents a special case because she was a resident of La Cambre, her bones were buried there, and a copy of her *Life* in MS 8609–20 resided there. On her burial, see *The Life of Alice of Schaerbeek*, trans. Martinus Cawley (Lafayette, OR: Our Lady of Guadalupe Abbey, 2000), 31. Cawley notes that, by the time the Bollandists were investigating her, there was no longer a record of Alice's grave.

72. Giselle de Nie, "*Mutatio Sensus*: Poetics of Holiness and Healing in Paulinus of Périgueux's *Life of Saint Martin*," in *Studies on Medieval Empathies* (Turnhout: Brepols, 2013), 85.

73. Gentile of Foligno, *Consilia* (Pavia, 1488), in Cohen-Hanegbi, *Caring for the Living Soul*, 115: "remoratio rerum mirabilium."

74. Christopher Page, "Music and Medicine in the Thirteenth Century," in *Music as Medicine: The History of Music Therapy since Antiquity*, ed. Peregrine Horden (Aldershot: Ashgate, 2000), 118.

75. Suzan Folkerts has undertaken a thorough codicological analysis of this manuscript; see *Vorbeeld op schrift: De overlevering en toe-eigening van de vita van Christina Mirabilis in de late middeleeuwen* (Hilversum: Verloren, 2010), 266–70. Other scholars have examined the manuscript and provided in-depth bibliographic descriptions; see Willem Lourdaux, *Bibliotheca Vallis Sancti Martini in Lovanio*

indicates that the manuscript was created by a brother John of St. Trond from Villers, who was appointed as the confessor to the nuns of Vrouwenpark. It conveys that, for brother John, the use of this manuscript could wield intercessory power. In his message, John of St. Trond prays that those who read this book might assist his soul's journey to heaven by performing the texts within it. That is, he expected that the encounter with this book might effect the transmission of divine grace, that his sins might be purged and his soul ferried to heaven.[76] The creation and use of this codex were a means of facilitating access to grace, to salvation.

Manuscript 4459–70 is an omnibus text, but one with internal coherence. The manuscript includes seventeen different fourteenth-century hands and eleven codicological units.[77] The codicological units were produced at roughly the same time and in the same scriptorium.[78] A table of contents on the recto of the half sheet was written c. 1330, and the texts within the book reflect the order described in the table, so that it has remained in its current composite form since that time.[79] The contents are not foliated, which suggests that they acted as more of an inventory than a navigational aid. The codex was likely used by John or other Villers advisers as they communed with the nuns of Vrouwenpark. There are signs that the nuns may have had some role in selecting its contents. For example, the book includes a birth indulgence that would seem appropriate only for a women's community with explicit ties to the healthcare of people outside their walls. Further evidence of collaboration between John and the religious women of Vrouwenpark are two scripta said to be transcriptions directly from religious women. These include fifteen brief notes on visionary experiences reported by a Cistercian nun and a short text describing a mystical conversation reported by a beguine from Tongres between herself and Christ.[80] Although the book was a miscellany produced by numerous hands, in its reception and use among

(Leuven: Universitaire Pers, 1978), 480–87; and Albert Ampe, *Jan van Ruusbroec 1293–1381: Tentoonstellingscatalogus; Catalogi vantentoonstellingen georganiseerd in de koninklijke Bibliotheek Albert I* (Brussels: Koninklijke Bibliotheek, 1981), 22–24.

76. On a half-sheet, after the flyleaf: "Quamobrem precatur lecturos in eo quod dicere velint anima eius cum animabus omnium fidelium defunctorum per Dei misericordiam et per Ihesu Christi sanguinis aspersionem et per intercessionem beate Marie ac omnium sanctorum sanctarumque requiescant in pace. Amen, amen."

77. Folkerts, *Vorbeeld op schrift*, 126.

78. Distinct black and red decorative elements are scattered throughout the manuscript. Folkerts, *Vorbeeld op schrift*, 126.

79. Folkerts, *Vorbeeld op schrift*, 126. Some fragmentary texts and insertions are not included in the contents.

80. At fols. 148v-50r; 252r-v. M. Nuyttens has suggested that the author of the conversation was William, abbot of Affligem, and that the beguine was Beatrice of Dendermonde; see his "Abbaye de

the nuns of Vrouwenpark and their Cistercian advisers we can see it as one with internal logic and coherence.[81] That logic, I argue, hinges on the reading event as a performance of grace, a technology for transmitting divine grace through prayer to humans and other material objects in Vrouwenpark and its surroundings.

Manuscript 4459–70 contains the *Lives* of four local Cistercian saints from the *liégeois* corpus: Alice of Schaerbeek, Beatrice of Nazareth, Walter of Bierbeek, and Prior Werric of Aulne.[82] It also includes the *Lives* of four, non-Cistercian saints from the region, two of whom were in the *liégeois* corpus: Margaret of Ypres, Christina Mirabilis, Elizabeth of Hungary, and Anthony of Padua. In addition to the *Lives* of saints, the manuscript presents descriptions of mystical experiences, collations, prayers, charms, benedictions, spiritual letters, and a papal bull. Nearly all of the texts are what we might consider "efficacious"—they either provide ritual words to effect change, offer theological explanations for physical and spiritual transformation, or demonstrate through narrative the power of words. In the century prior to the creation of MS 4459–70, theologians had fiercely argued the distinction between official church sacraments and the broader realm of sacramental activity.[83] While Peter Lombard reduced the sacraments to seven (from as many as twelve, according to Peter Damian) based on the certainty of their efficacy, a whole array of sacramental blessings, rites, and incantations continued to proliferate and remained in use by both priests and laypeople.[84] Theologians beginning with Alexander of Hales made room

---

Zwijveke à Termonde," in *Monasticon Belge* VII: *Province de Flandre Orientale*, ed. U. Berlière (Liège: Revue Belge de Philologie et d'Histoire, 1980), 473–75.

81. The miscellaneous nature of MS 4459–70 has elicited the attention of scholars. For example, D. A. Stracke deemed it a "collective codex" produced by the cooperation of numerous scribes. D. A. Stracke, "Arnulf van Leuven, O. Cist. versus gelukz. Hermann Jozef, O. Praem," *Ons Geestelijk Erf* 24 (1950): 27–50. Jacques Foret also examined it, commenting on the compound nature of the book. Wybren Scheepsma called attention to its sundry yet still coherent nature, asserting that it "gathers together a wide variety of disparate texts, whereby a common thread seems to be that they are connected in one way or another with the mystical movement of which Villers formed the center." Scheepsma, *Limburg Sermons*, 90.

82. Whether Walter of Bierbeek's entry in MS 4459–70 merits categorization as a *Life* is debatable. It has otherwise been classified as *collationes* or even as an anecdote; this story of a converted knight who entered Himmerod Abbey also appears in Caesarius of Heisterbach's book on Mary in the *Dialogus miraculorum*.

83. Derek Rivard, *Blessing the World: Ritual and Lay Piety in Medieval Religion* (Washington, DC: Catholic University of America Press, 2008), 41; Jaroslav Pelikan, *The Growth of Medieval Theology, 600–1300* (Chicago: University of Chicago Press, 1978); Gary Macy, *Theologies of the Eucharist in the Early Scholastic Period: A Study of the Salvific Function of the Sacrament According to Theologians, 1080–1220* (New York: Oxford University Press, 1984).

84. Rivard, *Blessing the World*, 41–43. Thirteenth-century theologians argued vehemently over the issue of linguistic efficacy and its relation to the sacraments. Some theologians argued that

for sacramentals, that is, objects that might be lifted through the power of formulaic verbal blessings into a state of physical efficacy. The texts copied into MS 4459–70 provided not only the scripts for efficacious reading performances, but also numerous guarantors of their efficacy. The manuscript appears to promise readers that, through performance, their words could be made to move, persuade, or transform the material world.[85]

The character of the texts copied in MS 4459–70, their concern for transforming action, becomes apparent in a series of benedictions that follow the manuscript copy of the *Lives* of Elizabeth of Hungary and Alice of Schaerbeek. They were common benedictions, found in various monastic missals in use through the fourteenth century.[86] The first blessing in the series of four is for water (*benedictio aque*), which would have been confected by the visiting priest. One would suspect that a priest would know the formula for blessing water and that he would carry his own more complete missal. The presence of the blessing in this manuscript thus raises the possibility that it was inscribed for use by the women of Vrouwenpark. The blessing requests the water's hallowing because only through "celestial benediction" can it be rendered "effective" in warding off diabolic temptation and providing health to the whole community who made use of it.[87] A second benediction involves bread and salt and expresses a wish for grace to enter these materials for the benefit of human and animal health, stating that the person or animal ingesting the foodstuff, once endowed with grace through this ritual blessing, would encourage healing in heart or eyes, nostrils, hands or feet.[88] The third benediction (*benedictio domus vel loci*) was a standard in the Roman rite, requesting the endowment of grace among the inhabitants of the monastery.[89] The blessing identifies the monastic house with the health of

---

virtus inhered in the material of the sacraments that caused them to be vehicles of grace; others insisted that the efficacy of the sacrament stemmed from a pact with God whereby certain conditions (proper words, ordained minister, faithful audience) satisfied the occasion of an effect. On this debate, see Irène Rosier-Catach, *La parole efficace: Signe, rituel, sacré* (Paris: Éditions du Seuil, 2004).

85. On the intentional quality of words in charms, see Matthew Milner, "The Physics of Holy Oats: Vernacular Knowledge, Qualities, and Remedy in Fifteenth-Century England," *Journal of Medieval and Early Modern Studies* 43.2 (2013): 219–45. Milner argues for the "specific rationality" of charms whereby laypeople used their vernacular understanding of sacramental theology, specifically the intentionality of grace, to explain the efficacy of verbal remedies.

86. Three of the benedictions were part of the Germano-Roman pontifical. They were copied throughout the twelfth and thirteenth centuries in monastic settings. Examples can be found in the Chester-le-Street additions to Durham Cathedral Library A.IV.19; Leofric Missal, Bamberg Lit. 53; and in the missal of Robert of Jumièges, MS Rouen Y6.

87. Fol. 57v: "Facias efficatem"; "sanitatis dulcedine."

88. Fol. 57v: "medicinam celestem" ; "ut sanitas fiat eis in ore in ventre in corde in oculis in auribus in naribus. In manibus in pedibus." Cyrille Vogel and Reinhard Elze, eds., *Le pontifical romano-germanique du dixième siècle* (Vatican City: Bibliotheca Apostolica Vaticana, 1963), Ordo 184.

89. Fol. 57.

its collective inhabitants, in this way also including the conversae in the health-securing plea of the benediction.[90] The final blessing in the series, *benedictio aque contra vermes segetum* (blessing for water against grain worms) seeks to expel vermin from crops.[91] All four blessings are listed in the table of contents, suggesting their importance among the collected scripta in MS 4459–70. The benedictions are one of many examples in this codex demonstrating that the inhabitants of Vrouwenpark were interested in gathering together efficacious texts—readings that promised physical transformation and changed status, that assisted in channeling divine grace into the elements of their environment.

We can understand these benedictions as "factitive utterances," statements that were meant to infuse the materials of the environment with grace. As such, the benedictions cast significance on the scripta that follow, so many of which combine gesture, word, and objects to effect transformation in the physical environment or in members of the community at Vrouwenpark. For example, the liturgy for a *commune sanctorum* (a "common of the saints," used for a whole category of saints such as martyrs or apostles) commences with a line from Proverbs, *Mulierem fortem quis inveniet?* (31:10) and resembles the commune sanctorum for virgin martyrs in the primitive Cistercian breviary. It is noteworthy that this liturgical cursus differs slightly in its readings and responsories from the standard Cistercian breviary.[92] The rubricator indicates to readers that the Mass formulary is for use with multiple female saints, including the "feast of Saint Elizabeth, Marie of Egypt, and the other chosen ones."[93] This variation indicates that the makers and users of this manuscript were interested in celebrating Mass for a wider range of female saints, in making their liturgical performances meaningful to the local community by addressing their preferred saints.[94]

A prayer for Saint Audoenus, Frankish miracle worker and bishop of Rouen, suggests additional dimensions for the use of efficacious words at La Cambre. Audoenus's reputation for effecting miracles was enhanced in

---

90. Rivard, *Blessing the World*, 80.

91. Vogel and Elze, *Le pontifical romano-germanique du dixième siècle*, Ordo 214b.

92. Chrysogonus Waddell, ed., *The Primitive Cistercian Breviary* (Fribourg: Academic Press Fribourg, 2007), 630–36.

93. Fol. 64r: "Iste cursus potest dici in festo btē elyzabus, marie egypciache, et aliorum electarum. Missa Gaudeamus."

94. On the use of Mass liturgies among cloistered women, see Felice Lifshitz, *Religious Women in Early Carolingian Francia: A Study of Manuscript Transmission and Monastic Culture* (New York: Fordham University Press, 2014), 185–92, which provides manuscript evidence showing that early Carolingian nuns engaged in a variety of clerical activities in exchange for donations. Jean Leclercq, "Eucharistic Celebrations without Priests in the Middle Ages," *Workshop* 55 (1980): 160–68; Ian Christopher Levy, "The Eucharist and Canon Law in the High Middle Ages," in *A Companion to the Eucharist in the Middle Ages*, ed. Ian Levy, Gary Macy, and Kristen Van Ausdall (Leiden: Brill, 2012), 399–446.

the eleventh century when two separate miracle collections dedicated to his work began circulating.[95] The prayer included here is nonnarrative, requesting blessings and grace. The words of the prayer are highly incantatory, falling like staccato exhortations: "Jesus of Nazareth"; "King of the Jews"; "Kyrie Elysion"; "Christi Elysion."[96] As we glimpsed in MS 8609–20, there is also here a penchant for affective exclamation. Liturgical patterns such as these, Augustine held, were verbal interjections that expressed healthful joy.[97] The words of the oratio provided the community with a medium for modulating their affective states, for stimulating internal joy. The oratio also includes gestic instructions to the user to make the sign of the cross with her hands while chanting the antiphon, "Adesto Deus unus omnipotens." The user would perform these gestures while uttering a new series of injunctions, such as "Sanctificas" and "Benedicas." The string of utterances and gestures in this prayer worked together as "spoken actions" that begged for transformation, rendering the supplicant into a likely candidate for grace, commanding benediction that promised to transform the self through sanctification and grace.[98] It is in this context of the manuscript's multiform performative texts that the *Lives* within it take on the tenor of performances or "presentations" of the saint. Just as the blessings, oratio, and Mass formulary required communal participation in paraliturgical performance wherein biblical time (here, the crucifixion) is made present, so too did the *Lives* gain this present performative meaning from the texts with which they were embedded.[99] Within this manuscript, the reading event is performative in that it reanimates, or makes present, the saint. Only by viewing the *Lives* from their reception within the context of the complete manuscript can we understand them as having operated this way. Embedded with liturgical and sacramental scripts, the *Lives* promised to effect parallel transformations in their participants.

---

95. On the spread of his cult, see Felice Lifshitz, "Eight Men In: Rouennais Traditions of Archepiscopal Sanctity," *Haskins Society Journal*, 1990, 63–74.

96. Fols. 64v-65r.

97. McCann, "Words of Fire and Fruit," 218–19.

98. "Spoken actions" refers to theatrical speech in which uttered language, rather than descriptive language, propels the action in a story; Manfred Pfister, *Theory and Analysis of Drama* (Cambridge: Cambridge University Press, 1988). J. L. Austin referred to the phenomenon as a "performative utterance," in which the uttering of a statement is tantamount to the doing of an action; J. L. Austin, *How to Do Things with Words*, ed. J. O. Urmson and Marina Sbisá (Cambridge, MA: Harvard University Press, 1962), 5–8.

99. Mary Suydam, "Visionaries in the Public Eye: Beguine Literature as Performance," in *The Texture of Society: Medieval Women in the Southern Low Countries*, ed. Ellen Kittell and Mary Suydam (New York: Palgrave, 2004), 131–152, 136.

Scripted word and gesture are brought together again in a series of verses attributed to Arnulf, abbot of Villers.[100] The verses are rife with references to the salubrious work of prayer. Playing on the verbal resonance of *salve*, meaning both "Be well" and "Hail," the opening line of each song entreats the healing power of Christ: *salve meum salutare / salve, salve, Ihesu chare*. Like the prayerful meditation in the coda to the Lambert-le-Bègue Psalter (British Library, MS Additional 21114), this one leads the user from the feet of Christ on the cross, up to his knees, then his hands, side wound, breast, heart, and finally, his face. At the start of each canto the song directs its performer to utter "Salve," as simultaneously a greeting to Christ's limb, an exhortation for salvation, and a plea for cure. "Sweet Jesus, heal everything, restore, make full like pious medicine," it demands. "Cure me and I will be saved."[101]

Arnulf's songs are disrupted on fol. 150v by an indulgence, two additional prayers (or hymns), and a drawing of Christ's side wound, bordered above and below by illustrations of the *arma Christi* (see figure 8 in chapter 4). The indulgence is placed inelegantly at the top of the page, as an introduction to or explanation of the illustrations and words under it. The indulgence, authorized by Pope Leo, granted forty days to those who contemplated the arms of Christ.[102] Below the indulgence is a horizontal row of instruments of the passion, under which is the wound and the inscription of two prayers dedicated to the wound, *Salve plaga lateris* and *O fons aque paradisi*. Like Arnulf's song, the prayers call specifically for the therapeutic intervention of the blood that flowed from Christ's side wound, the "true medicine" (*vera medicina*) and "medicine of people" (*medicina populi*). The wound is situated directly in the center of the manuscript page; around its periphery, the scribe has written a verbal claim that it represented the actual size of Christ's side wound.[103] This claim strengthened the link between the manuscript page, the words that it supported, and the salvific sacrifice of body and blood that was celebrated

---

100. Although this codicological unit of the manuscript (fols. 145–52) contains Richard of Saint Victor's discussion of nature and grace, an account of the visionary experiences of a virgin, an oratio, and two indulgences, only Arnulf's oratio is listed in the contents.

101. Fol. 150r: "Salve meum salutare salve meum Jhesu care . . . dulcis Ihesu totum sana tu restaura tu complana tam pio medicamine . . . me sanibis hic spero. Sana me et salvus ero."

102. Fol. 150v: "Quicumque hoc cotidie inspexerit in commemoratione passionis et armorum Iesu Christi XL dies indulgentiarum datas a Leone papa et ab eodem confirmatas."

103. On the image, see Flora Lewis, "The Wound in Christ's Side and the Instruments of the Passion: Gendered Experience and Response," in *Women and the Book: Assessing the Visual Evidence*, ed. Lesley Smith and Jane Taylor (London: British Library, 1997), 204–29. Lewis insists on the polyvalence of wound images in manuscripts, pointing to royal uses, childbirth talismans, and male appropriation of feminine imagery.

in the sacrament.[104] The exactitude of measurement asserted the power of the image, rendering it a sort of contact relic.[105] The practice of measuring the length of a tomb, a person's body or limb for a candle, the distance to a shrine, or the size of Christ's wound was thought to materialize and thus re-present the thing measured, so that the measurement absorbed the power and personhood of the template.[106] The wound image in MS 4459–70, in its authentication through measurement, rendered the crimson parchment into a real, bloody wound. The image made present its exemplar, just as the scriptum of the *Life* made present the saint. In the presence of this relic of Christ, the manuscript provided the words of prayer for users to petition for health, thereby enhancing the power of those words to take effect.

Arnulf's *carmina*, the two prayers, the side wound and arma Christi illustrations, and the written indulgence provided a brilliant multimediality by which the user was transformed into one freed from sin, one received of grace, one healed. The songs, then, may have acted as a vehicle for contemplating the pictured arms, moving the reader to each of Christ's broken limbs, imagining the force of injury, and beseeching personal healing through the wounded body before them. The indulgence provided to those who completed the round of prayers acted as proof of efficacy. Through the specular, gestic, and verbal performance of this text, time in purgatory was reduced, the punishment from sin was diminished, and thus humans were recuperated. The "medicine of Christ" referred to in Arnulf's song was the avenue for redemption of sin and thus for bodily health.[107] The chanting of these *carmina* was the medicine that generated physiological change.

---

104. Surrounding the wound are the words "Hec est mensura vulneris lateris domini nostri Christi. Nemo dubitet quia ipse apparuit cuidam et ostendit ei vulnera sua." On the illustration, see Rudolf Berliner, "Arma Christi," in *"The Freedom of Medieval Art" und andere Studien zum christlichen Bild* (Berlin: Lukas Verlag, 2003). Berliner has argued that MS 4459–70 was the oldest literary indulgence for viewing the arma Christi.

105. Caroline Bynum, *Christian Materiality: An Essay on Religion in Late Medieval Europe* (Brooklyn: Zone Books, 2001), 97–99. Bynum's discussion of "the measure of Christ" centers on the medieval presumption that the measure of a person is in some sense their replicated self; such an approach to measurement is seen in the practice of donating a unit of wax equal to a body's measure in exchange for a saint's favor. According to Bynum, "To measure is to absorb the power of the measured self by contact with it." See also David S. Areford, "The Passion Measured: A Late Medieval Diagram of the Body of Christ," in *The Broken Body: Passion Devotion in Late-Medieval Culture*, ed. A. A. MacDonald, H. N. B. Ridderbos, and R. M. Schlusemann (Groningen: Egbert Forsten, 1998), 211–38.

106. On "metric relics," see Kathryn Rudy, *Virtual Pilgrimages in the Convent: Imagining Jerusalem in the Late Middle Ages* (Turnhout: Brepols, 2011), 97–107.

107. Jessica Barr has commented on the healing function of the prayer/wound/text nexus; see her "Reading Wounds: Embodied Mysticism in a Fourteenth-Century Codex," *Magistra* 19.1 (2013): 27–29, 37. See also Ann Eljenholm Nichols, "The Footprints of Christ as Arma Christi: The Evidence

Notes at the bottom of fol. 150v alert the reader to flip two pages, where they will discover another series of drawings and another indulgence (figure 11). The second indulgence established a list of popes who authorized it and specified the number of days for which it was effective—three years' remission from purgatory from Saint Peter, one hundred days from thirty popes, forty days from twenty-eight bishops, and forty days from Pope Leo. This list thereby assured the practitioner of the efficacy of performing the contemplative process. This second indulgence makes more explicit the function of bodily health in the practice of this prayer, indicating that "whoever daily considers these with a devout mind will find no evil death."[108] Furthermore, it specifically addressed women, recommending contemplation of the arms as a healing practice for parturient women because "this practice will provide the best remedy for women in labor."[109] The song and indulgences suggest something of the urgency underlying the making of this manuscript to assure its users of the efficacy of the texts it supports. The indulgences—authorized by a string of powerful clerics—acted as proof that words the nuns uttered could indeed establish *salus*.

The childbirth indulgence harkens back to the wound, resignifying the wound as an obstetric amulet. Flora Lewis has shown that the arma Christi and wound images were often associated with talismans against fatal or difficult childbirth.[110] The blood of Christ here was analogous to the blood of childbirth, both providing salvation and renewed life.[111] In fact, the arma Christi indulgence had a long history of therapeutic uses, where it had been employed as a textual amulet for healing, often worn around the neck. As discussed in the previous chapter, fifteenth-century English arma Christi illustrations were designed especially for women, who used them for apotropaic purposes and for protection in childbirth, and, in an earlier period, devotional images of Christ's passion and side wound were sources of semantic motifs for healing bodily wounds.[112] Like the obstetric

---

of Morgan B.54," in *The Arma Christi in Medieval and Early Modern Material Culture*, ed. Lisa Cooper and Andrea Denny-Brown (Aldershot: Ashgate, 2014), 113–42.

108. Fol. 152v: "Item qui cotidie devota mente inspexerit nonquam mala morte peribit."

109. Fol. 152v: "Item mulieribus in partu laborantibus prestat optimum remedium."

110. Lewis, "The Wound in Christ's Side," 217; on the wound and birthing, see also Mary Morse, "Seeing and Hearing: Margery Kempe and the Mis-en-Page," *Studia Mystica* 20 (1999): 15–42.

111. Bynum, *Christian Materiality*, 197.

112. Skemer, *Binding Words*, 259–68; Olsan, "Latin Charms of Medieval England," 130. Elsewhere Olsan lists medical practitioners who invoked the wound of Christ in their healing charms, calling on the "virtue" of Christ's wounds to eject infections; see her "Charms and Prayers in Medieval Medical Theory and Practice," *Social History of Medicine* 16 (2003): 360. Miri Rubin discusses wound imagery and Host salutations, as well as indulgences provided to those who gazed at, wore,

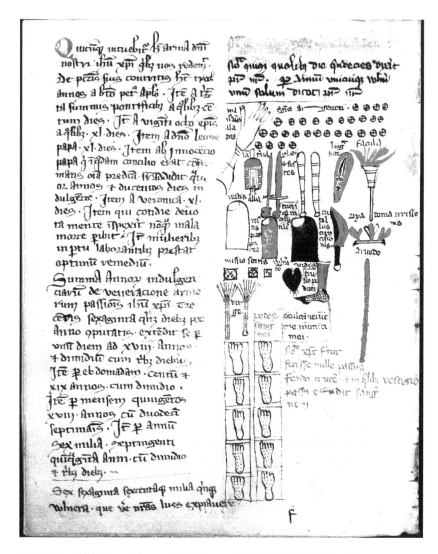

FIGURE 11. Indulgences with arma Christi. Brussels, KBR, MS 4459–70, fol. 152v.

charms in KBR MS 8609–20, this series of images, songs, and indulgences offers another example of a prayerful remedy for safe labor in a manuscript used in Cistercian women's communities. It provides a further indication that Cistercian nuns in the thirteenth- and early fourteenth-century Low

---

or kissed a representation of the wound, the *mensura vulneris*. She finds none of this activity prior to 1300. Rubin, *Corpus Christi*, 303–6.

Countries were possibly administering healthcare, in the form of both physical and spiritual caregiving, to petitioners from outside of their cloister walls. We know, for example, that the nuns of Vrouwenpark were permitted to receive family and friends, so it is possible that they provided care to outsiders.[113] In fact, so passionately did they guard this approval that, when the 1242 General Chapter sought to enforce greater restrictions on enclosure, the nuns of Vrouwenpark rebelled by threatening visitor abbots and departing from the chapter house.[114]

Religious women's verbal efficacy is further established in this manuscript by a cluster of texts dedicated to elucidating the beneficial effects of participation in the feast of Corpus Christi. A transcription of papal records related to the foundation of the feast, these texts carried regional significance, as the feast was conceived, designed, and promoted in the Diocese of Liège by two mulieres religiosae, Juliana of Mont-Cornillon and Eve of St. Martin. They include a bull of canonization for the Franciscan "living saint," Louis of Toulouse, approved by Pope John XXII, who was responsible for elevating the feast of Corpus Christi to universal observance in the Christian calendar.[115] Also copied here is a list of reasons given by Pope Urban IV for his initial confirmation of the feast and for his support of its regional promotion. Clear marginal numeration made the treatise manageable for readers unfamiliar with the scholastic style. The *rationes* emphasized the logic behind the promotion of the feast, which, he claimed, assisted in the fight against heretics, conferred grace, and elevated the status of the Host as a cure for human infirmity. The treatise, in fact, suggested that the Host itself was experiencing its own infirmity, being wounded and degraded by the lack of reverence Christians paid it. The author likened the feast to a cure that would heal (*salubriter*) the Host as well as the Christian community. The treatise therefore imagined the feast, a liturgical procession, as an efficacious practice, one with the capacity to heal through participation.

Notes made hastily under this text by a later reader provide additional context that tells us about the interests of the book's readers. The notes indicate that a bull of approval was given to the "monialibus" of Liège, and that the feast was to be celebrated after Pentecost. The nuns referenced here are Juliana of Mont-Cornillon and her helpmate, Eve, the recluse of the Church of St.

---

113. Sara Moens, "Beatrice's World: The Rise of Cistercian Nunneries in the Bishoprics of Liège and Cambrai," *Ons Geestelijk Erf* 89.3–4 (2020): 256.

114. Moens, 259.

115. His *Life* is copied at fols. 239v-244v. That both his *Life* and his canonization bull are included in the manuscript emphasizes the intertextuality of the scripta. The *Lives* in this manuscript gain meaning in relationship to other scripta copied within.

Martin of Liège.[116] While living, Juliana experienced what she believed were divine revelations urging her to develop an annual liturgical celebration for the institution of the sacrament of the Eucharist.[117] Acting upon these visions, she recruited an assistant, John, from Mont-Cornillon and began to elaborate a liturgical office, what would eventually become *Animarum cibum.*[118] After scrutiny of her office by clerics, including Hugh of St. Cher, Jacques Pantaleon (who later became Pope Urban IV), and Guiard of Laon, Juliana's feast was eventually adopted before undergoing significant revisions by Thomas Aquinas.[119] The notes, then, indicate that readers were actively connecting the mulieres religiosae to sacramental and liturgical performances.

The treatise on Urban IV's rationale for adopting the feast is followed by a letter from his papal successor, Clement V, which paid tribute to the memory of Urban, honoring him for his interest in and promotion of the feast of Corpus Christi regionally. A copy of Pope Urban IV's 1264 bull, *Transiturus de hoc mundo,* is also featured here. This bull provided authorization for the feast of Corpus Christi to be celebrated on the Thursday after Pentecost, praising in particular the renewal of Christ's body and blood in the Host, in which "wonderful things are transformed," an idea he explains using scholastic language that aligned the transformation of bread and wine into body and blood with the transformation of sinful humanity into the body Christ.[120] Drawing a direct connection between salvation from sin and the salvific effects of the Host, Urban praised

---

116. The Cistercian compiler of this manuscript refers to Juliana as a nun, though it is not certain what vows she would have taken.

117. The *Life* of Juliana is bound in a small volume of eighty folios alongside Fulbert of Chartres's sermon on the Nativity of the Virgin and Jerome's address to Paula and Eustochium, the subject of which is the Assumption of the Virgin. Paris, Bibliothèque de l'Arsenal, MS 945 was likely made at Villers in the late thirteenth century. The textual association with the Virgin Mary seems appropriate given that the *Life* of Juliana records that "she had a most tender devotion to the Holy mother of God. In the midst of her labors she would frequently cast herself upon her knees and with great fervor and devotion recite the Ave Maria," and when meditating on the virtues of the Virgin, "she endeavored to put into practice the particular virtue on which she was meditating." But the association of Juliana and the Virgin makes sense therapeutically as well. As prioress at Mont-Cornillon, Juliana recommended that her sisters perform the Aves and the Magnificat as a means of "exciting in others" a kind of joy.

118. Catherine Saucier, "Sacrament and Sacrifice: Conflating Corpus Christi and Martyrdom in Medieval Liège," *Speculum* 87 (2012): 682–723. Saucier shows that the liturgy for the feast reflected the precise terms of twelfth-century eucharistic debates among Liège clerics.

119. On the process of revision, see J. Cottiaux, "L'office liégeois de la Fête-Dieu, sa valeur et son destin," *Revue d'Histoire Ecclésiastique* 58 (1963): 5–81, 8; Anneke Mulder-Bakker, *Lives of the Anchoresses: The Rise of the Urban Recluse* (Philadelphia: University of Pennsylvania Press, 2005), 106; Rubin, *Corpus Christi,* 164–75.

120. The bull is edited in Jean Guiraud, ed., *Les Registres d'Urbain IV (1261–1264)* (Paris: Fontemoing, 1901), 423–25: "si digne recipitur, sibi recipiens conformatur."

the Host as a universal cure for all wounds, which was necessary because all humans were made sick at the fall. Analogizing the infectious apple of Eden to the health-giving Eucharist, he insisted that "because food ruined man in death, food cured him in life."[121]

Urban IV's bull was sent directly to Eve of St. Martin, a measure of the affection he held for the mulieres religiosae of Liège. Before becoming pope, Urban had been a canon of St. Lambert beginning in 1232 and had involved himself in Juliana's struggle for control of her leprosarium.[122] In 1245 he wrote the *Libellus de Regula et Vita Beginarum* to assist with the governance of beguines in Liège, urging their regularity and adherence to customs.[123] After instituting the feast of Corpus Christi in Laon and Verdun, he acceded to the papal throne in 1261 and, out of affection, brought with him Juliana's prayer book.[124] From his papal seat, Urban IV addressed to Eve his bull officially approving the feast of Corpus Christi. After her death, in 1264, her tomb in a chapel at the Church of St. Martin became a central focus of the feast, at which the canons would stop to pay her tribute after the Mass.[125]

These texts supporting the feast of Corpus Christi are copied along with a *third* indulgence, this one for participation in the feast. The indulgence is included as part of a letter from Hugh of St. Cher, regent master of theology at Paris, Dominican provincial in Paris, and later cardinal-legate to Germany. Hugh was a supporter of the eucharistic feast in Liège, promoting it in sermons delivered along his legatine route.[126] He had served as the evaluator of Juliana's feast, probably about 1235–36, and became an advocate for it, as well as for the mulieres religiosae who enlivened the region he visited as cardinal.[127] He ensured that the feast was celebrated annually by the canons of St. Martin, and he instituted it in the Diocese of Liège. The letter from Hugh copied into MS 4459–70 was originally written in April of 1252 and guaranteed to the Church of St. Mary in the abbey of Villers a forty-day indulgence for anyone who attended the Corpus Christi Mass.[128] Like the

---

121. "quia per mortem homo corruerat, et per cibum relevaretur ad vitam."

122. Mulder-Bakker, *Lives of the Anchoresses*, 130.

123. The work is no longer extant. But an edited version attempts to reconstruct it from notes found in a charter of Henry of Guelders. Jean Paquay, "L'archidiaconat liégeois d'Urbain IV," *Leodium* 2 (1903): 60–63. See the discussion in chapter 2.

124. Mulder-Bakker, *Lives of the Anchoresses*, 133.

125. Mulder-Bakker, 80.

126. Rubin, *Corpus Christi*, 174–75.

127. Mulder-Bakker, *Lives of the Anchoresses*, 89.

128. Barbara Walters, Vincent Corrigan, and Peter Ricketts, eds., *The Feast of Corpus Christi* (University Park: Pennsylvania State University Press, 2006), 12.

indulgences that preceded it in the manuscript, this one served to convince readers of the efficacious capacity of the Host, and of its celebratory feast. The indulgence promoted the path to salvation for participants in this ritual, who memorialized the crucifixion and ingested the body of Christ.

Let me conclude where the manuscript concludes, with attention to a series of texts about religious women and the men of Villers who ministered to them. The final inscriptions include a Tongres beguine's mystical dialogue, letters from Thomas, a Villers monk, to his sister Alice, a nun of Vrouwen-park, and excerpts from the Chronicle of Villers. These scripta allow us to capture a sense of the salutary significance attributed to religious women's performed words in this region. The Tongres beguine's words demonstrate a real interest in seeking out, recording, and sharing the inner visionary experiences of women, thereby endorsing their value. The beguine's spiritual experience was considered valuable enough by the monks of Villers to be translated into Latin and transmitted, along with a series of women's *Lives*, in this codex.[129] Her visionary experience, just like those of all "holy virgins," as Caesarius of Heisterbach asserted, might generate delight and promote health.[130] Meanwhile, the letters from Thomas demonstrate an interest in training and cultivating women's performed words. Thomas, his brothers, Godfrey and Renier, and his father, Renier, had all entered Villers in the first quarter of the thirteenth century, and their sister Alice took vows at Vrou-wenpark.[131] Only two letters survive from a more extensive correspondence that Thomas maintained with his sister. These two letters express an interest in Alice and her sisters' performance of prayer and in the role of the Divine Office as a means of transforming the self from sin to salvation. For example, Thomas instructed Alice that participating in the psalmody "magnifies the soul, purifies the mouth, gladdens the heart," and catalyzes a host of other personal transformations, including, "mak[ing] a person illustrious, open[ing] the senses, vanquish[ing] sins, mak[ing] peace between body and soul."[132] The psalm prayers of Alice and her sisters effected real change.

---

129. On the translation, possibly from Dutch, of this account, see Walter Simons, "Staining the Speech of Things Divine: The Uses of Literacy in Medieval Beguine Communities," in *The Voice of Silence: Women's Literacy in a Men's Church*, ed. Thérèse de Hemptinne and María Eugenia Góngora (Turnhout: Brepols, 2004), 97–98.

130. Caesarius of Heisterbach, bk. VIII, ch. lxxix: "quam sint iocundae, quam salutiferae visiones sanctarum virginum."

131. On Godfrey, see chapter 2; his *Life* is considered part of the *liégeois* corpus.

132. Thomas of Villers, "Deux lettres inédites," ed. Edmund Mikkers, *Collectanea Ordinis Cisterciensium Reformatorum* 10 (1948): 172: "animam magnificat, os purificat, cor laetificat"; "hominem clarificat, sensus aperit, omne malum occidit . . . pacem inter corpus et animam facit." On the letters, see Anthony Ray, "Brothers and Sisters in Christ, Brothers and Sisters Indeed: Two Thirteenth-Century

Their performed words of the psalter eliminated sin, sharpened the affects, and brought wellness to the body and soul.

The manuscript witness of the first collections of *Lives* of the thirteenth-century mulieres religiosae from this region suggests that the performance of those *Lives* wrought therapeutic effects. The audition of their *Lives*, and quite possibly even the physical presence of their *Lives* within the codex, had achieved among beguine and Cistercian women's communities in the region a status not unlike that of Margaret of Antioch, though on a strictly local level. Their healing grace did not dissipate after their deaths, but remained in their bones and in their *Lives*, an embodiment of the saintly self in parchment and performance. The association, in KBR MSS 8609–20 and 4459–70, between the *Lives* of religious women in the region and salutary texts reveals a concern to establish the efficacy of daily words and practices, of blessings, prayers, liturgical celebrations, and other rituals. Reading the *Lives* recreated the therapeutic experience of their grace-filled presence when alive in a manner that transformed those who experienced it, providing healing *gaudium*. Nearly all of the scripta copied into both manuscripts provide some kind of platform for arousing hygienic passions, and in doing so, they position Cistercian nuns as skilled purveyors of this practice of prayer. As a form of therapeutic practice, their prayers extended beyond the cloister walls. Even in a censored birthing charm, we can detect traces of lives that labored for the health of their communities. In prayers, the guardianship of relics and images, the recitation of charms, the performance of psalms, and the reading of *Lives*, Cistercian nuns found ways to build salutary communities and to practice forms of care that heretofore have remained invisible.

Letters of Thomas, Cantor of Villers, to His Sister Alice, Nun of Parc-les-Dames," in *Partners in Spirit: Women, Men, and Religious Life in Germany, 1100–1500*, ed. Fiona Griffiths and Julie Hotchin (Turnhout: Brepols, 2014), 213–36. Ray argues, contrary to current scholarly emphasis on women's capacity to spiritually inspire clerical men, that Thomas was the spiritual leader in his relationship with Alice and, potentially, with the other women of her community.

Afterword

On 29 December 1840 on a city street in Ghent, Marie-Anne Piesens, a beguine of Ter Hooie, took a terrible fall. After witnesses carried her home, her sisters called a surgeon to repair Marie-Anne's wounded left leg. The surgeon employed a number of remedies, but to no effect. He then summoned a second surgeon, who also failed to make any progress. The two physicians deemed the beguine incurable and declared her leg permanently paralyzed. Unsatisfied by this outcome, however, Marie-Anne took matters into her own hands. She devised a means of perambulating with the aid of crutches, so that her wounded leg crept across the ground, lagging behind her. Her device was admittedly imperfect. At the slightest movement, the foot would tremble uncontrollably, and sharp pain surged beyond her knee. In time, the foot would atrophy, and her entire left leg seemed to desiccate. After two years of suffering in this manner, Marie-Anne called for additional doctors to treat her affliction, but after much intervention they, too, agreed that the leg remained quite incurable. At this point she turned to spiritual interventions. In April of 1843, Marie-Anne commenced a novena to Saint Philomena, the virgin martyr who had five years previously earned an official liturgical celebration. She also employed a material remedy, massaging her leg nightly with oil from a lantern that burned before the saint's image at the church of the Dominicans in Ghent. On the last day of this procedure, while praying, the beguine experienced for the first time since her fall a sense of relief. Shocked and encouraged, she continued this therapeutic practice, and soon reported that she could walk with only one crutch and with little pain. She eventually gave up crutches and cane entirely, hopping up and down the stairs with no resulting pain whatsoever. Several of her sisters, including Jeanne D'Hoedt, Pélagie Donche, and Hélène Hessels, witnessed the transformation. The therapeutic treatment that Marie-Anne devised had really worked, and was reported as the successful intervention of Saint Philomena.[1]

Across an ocean, another cure. In the francophone prairie of Grand Coteau, Louisiana, Mary Wilson, a recent convert and postulant of the convent of the Sacred Heart, found herself quite unwell. It was December of 1866, and the young woman was suffering from a severe gastric disease that left her arms and feet contracted, her fingernails blue, and the whole of her mouth wounded and clotted with blood.[2] A physician treated her with chloroform for her headaches, cupped her wasted limbs with hot glass, and prescribed mustard and turpentine for her wounds. He considered these interventions merely palliative, however, and professed Mary incurable.[3] Meanwhile, throughout her illness, Mary's sisters "lavished upon the patient all possible care, natural and professional," including "spiritual and supernatural remedies."[4] Mary Wilson's material needs were also accommodated by the labor of the Eaglin and Hawkins families, previously enslaved Black domestic servants who were counted in the 1870 federal census among residents of the Sacred Heart estate. David and Julie Anne Eaglin and three younger members of the Hawkins family, Marceline, Elmire, and John, served the community alongside a white Frenchman, Stanislas Billand.[5] These servants

---

1. "Nouvelles: Ecclésiastiques et Politiques," *Journal Historique et Littéraire* 10 (1843–44): 461–73, at 465–66.

2. Francis Benausse, SJ, *Account of the Cure of Miss Mary Wilson, Novice in the Community of the Sacred Heart, Grand Coteau, Louisiana* (Baltimore: John Murphy, 1873), 4–5.

3. Letter to Mary A. Perry from F. M. Nachon, SJ, 18 December 1866, Archives of the New Orleans Province, Society of Jesus, New Orleans.

4. *Morning Star and Catholic Messenger*, New Orleans, Sunday, 1 March 1868.

5. Julie and David Eaglin were born in Maryland, and possibly came to southern Louisiana as part of the Maryland Jesuits' sale of over 250 enslaved peoples. It is not clear that they were part of the sale. Dave was from Maryland, and sold to Mother Xavier Murphy in 1833. He joined his sister Jenny Eaglin Hawkins, who had been living at Grand Coteau since her sale in 1824. The surnames Eaglin and Hawkins are recorded among the 1838 sale and ship manifest of enslaved people transported from Maryland to Louisiana. "Articles of Agreement between Thomas F. Mulledy, of Georgetown, District of Columbia, of one part, and Jesse Beatty and Henry Johnson, of the State of Louisiana, of the other part, 19th June 1838," box 40, file 10, item 3a-h, Maryland Province

provided the cooking, cleaning, daily maintenance, and body knowledge that also enhanced the therapeutic environment from which Mary Wilson benefited during her convalescence. The subprioress, Victoria Pizarro Martinez, also assisted in Mary's care. She began to call upon a remote resource by commencing a novena for a blessed Jesuit from Diest, John Berchmans (b. 1599). When Mary cried out in anguish, Mother Martinez applied a small, portable picture of John Berchmans to Mary's aching limbs and prayed for his intercession. On the morning of 14 December 1866, after touching a picture of the Jesuit to her blistered lips, Mary Wilson sat up for the first time in many weeks and proclaimed, "I am well. Blessed Berchmans has cured me."[6]

These miracle stories lay bare the patterns of health and care that are braided throughout this book. Their temporal distance from the subjects of this book reinforces a lingering mode of recording healthcare interactions, the long endurance of a health maintenance system that conceals certain forms of care and valorizes others. The social organization of care labor has meant that status obligations as wife, mother, sister, daughter, and servant presume informal and naturalized obligations to meet dependency needs.[7] Those needs are often accommodated in intimate settings, in homes and small communities, at bedsides, in kitchens and baths. Stories of miracle cure lift up and expose those otherwise sequestered moments, providing a window into past experiences of health and infirmity. But in doing so they also shift therapeutic efficacy to a supernatural realm, all the while maintaining the gendered and raced allocation of daily responsibility for the care of vulnerable bodies. Obligations to perform the unremunerated tasks of cleaning, feeding, comforting, and restoring wellness are cast in miracle cures as filial, self-sacrificing, and charitable labors; caregiving is naturalized as compassionate, maternal, or servile while cure is anchored in a supernatural origin, a complex mystery decipherable by an elite few. These miracle tales

---

Archives, Booth Family Center for Special Collections, Georgetown University, Washington, DC; "Manifest of the Katherine Jackson," National Archives, Fort Worth, TX, Georgetown Slavery Archive. The agreement includes a "Julie Anne," aged twenty-two, and "David," aged fourteen, which would match the roughly approximated ages of fifty and forty-five recorded in the census, but the Julie Anne and Dave at Grand Coteau were already present in Louisiana by 1833. The Jesuits founded a school in Grand Coteau in 1838, less than a mile from Sacred Heart, and the enslaved people from both communities traveled back and forth. Maureen Chicoine, RSCJ has outlined the history of human trafficking at Grand Coteau in an unpublished pamphlet, "We Speak Your Names" (https://rscj.org/system/files/news/attachments/we_speak_your_names_final_program_web.pdf). I am grateful to Maureen Chicoine for helping me to navigate these records, and to Cathy Mooney for the encouragement and introduction.

  6. Benausse, *Account of the Cure of Miss Mary Wilson*, 8.
  7. Evelyn Nakano Glenn, *Forced to Care: Coercion and Caregiving in America* (Cambridge, MA: Harvard University Press, 2010), 1–11.

make transcendent the skill and body knowledge that caregivers produced and shared, a textual process that has only further exasperated the masking of that very skill and knowledge and alienated it from our historical trajectories of medicine and healthcare. Care of the soul, the affects, the embodied self, are excised from their foundational role in establishing therapeutic relationships. We are left with the awe of cure, forgetting the profound skill of care.

These fragments of the past—hints of possible traditions of care knowledge and their erasure—continue to materialize even as I grasp toward closure. There are many avenues for bringing this history of care to a close. Each one, however, opens additional doors that replicate patterns of marginalization, erasures of care providers and their body knowledge. Take, for example, the 1320 expulsion of "dishonorable" beguines from St. Christopher's in Liège, following the publication of the decrees of the Council of Vienne, in particular *Cum de quibusdam mulieribus*, which called for greater examination of the orthodoxy of beguines and enforcement of "discipline" in beguine communal life.[8] Investigations of beguines in Thérouanne, Arras, Cambrai, Tournai, and Liège proceeded in the following years, causing some women to shirk use of the term "beguine" as a self-identifier. Nevertheless, women who lived according to pious ideals and engaged in active charity continued to gather in various communal formations. Their need for access to *cura animalium* meant that, in this tentative environment, clerics sometimes imposed on them forms of enclosure and identifying clothing, rendering their work scarcely distinguishable from that of traditional female monastics, and thus scarcely detectable in the sources.[9]

Or perhaps we complete this tale with the 1322 trial of the noble woman Jacoba Felicie, brought by the Faculty of Medicine at the University of Paris. Jacoba stood accused of inspecting urine, "touching, palpating, and holding" (*tangendo, palpando, et tenendo*) her patients, prescribing them syrups and potions, and telling them, "I shall make you well, god willing, if you have faith in me (*credideritis*)." She visited patients in homes and hospital, many of whom had searched in vain for cure from the hands of other trained physicians. She did these things, as the record of the trial attests, with marvelous outcomes for the benefit of prestigious clients. But Jacoba had not

---

8. *Decrees of the Ecumenical Councils*, ed. and trans. Norman Tanner (London: Sheed and Ward, 1999), 1:374; on the expulsion and the effects of the Council of Vienne on beguine communities in the southern Low Countries, see Walter Simons, *Cities of Ladies: Beguine Communities in the Medieval Low Countries, 1200–1565* (Philadelphia: University of Pennsylvania Press, 2001), 133–34.

9. Alison More, "Dynamics of Regulation, Innovation, and Invention," in *Observant Reform in the Late Middle Ages and Beyond*, ed. James D. Mixon and Bert Roest (Leiden: Brill, 2015), 85–110.

been approved by an official *studium*, nor would she, as a woman, ever be admitted to one, and hence her practices and those of women like her were forbidden.[10]

Another possible terminus is the 1326 papal bull, *Super illius specula*, issued by John XXII, which levied immediate excommunication on practitioners of sorcery.[11] The bull framed magical rites as heretical in practice, meaning that intention or ignorance was no cover for dabbling in rites, crafting images, or uttering words that smacked of superstition. Concern about nebulously defined "superstitious" practices took hold throughout European courts, perhaps nowhere more so than in the kingdom of France, where women who were said to possess supernatural powers, manufacture potions, or use incantations became particularly suspect in the eyes of clerics and inquisitors.[12] By 1398, the Faculty of Theology in Paris would issue twenty-eight articles condemning as superstitious certain practices that might appear as falling within the parameters of Christian devotion, but subject to certain discerning clerical eyes, actually concealed demonic forces. These practices included nefarious invocations, impious rituals, baptizing gold or silver images, even saying prayers, fasting and performing ablutions (*jejunia et balneationes*), and participating in Masses that involved demons.[13] In this climate, devout and unenclosed single women dabbling in herbs and soothing words were especially suspicious.

But all these possible points of exit suppress an enduring pattern that keeps replicating itself in systems of caregiving throughout history. These decrees silence traces that continue to murmur scarcely audibly below the surface of their vocalizations of order, like the silent screams of a recurring

---

10. The text of her trial can be found in *Chartularium universitatis Parisiensis*, ed. Henri Denifle (Paris: Delalain, 1889), II.255–67; a translated excerpt was produced by Mary Martin McLaughlin for *The Portable Medieval Reader* (New York: Viking, 1959), 635–40. On the trial in feminist historiography, see Monica Green, "Getting to the Source: The Case of Jacoba Felicie and the Impact of the *Portable Medieval Reader* on the Canon of Medieval Women's History," *Medieval Feminist Forum* 42 (2006): 49–62.

11. As Michael Bailey states, it is "generally held" to have been issued in 1326; 1327 is also a possibility. Bailey, *Fearful Spirits, Reasoned Follies: The Boundaries of Superstition in Late Medieval Europe* (Ithaca: Cornell University Press, 2013), 79–80.

12. This suspicion had only increased apace since the trial and execution of Marguerite Porete. In June of 1315, three women were burned in Paris, accused of manufacturing the potion that killed Jean of Châteuvillain, bishop of Chalons-sur-Marne and testator in Marguerite's inquisition. The following year, Isabelle de Feriennes was implicated in a plot to label the Countess Mahaut of Artois as a devotee of magic and sorcery who sought to use potions to kill Louis X. In defending herself, Mahaut exposed Isabelle for having been repeatedly imprisoned for using incantations and sorceries, along with other damnable deeds and crimes. On these events, see Sean Field, *Courting Sanctity: Holy Women and the Capetians* (Ithaca: Cornell University Press, 2019), 221–22.

13. *Chartularium*, IV.32–36.

nightmare. Many of the traces I encountered when writing this book simply alluded me, their voices too faint to reassemble into a coherent chorus
of any kind; for example, the list of recipes in cipher nuzzled into a Villers
lectionary or the attribution of the label *sage femme*, a common term for midwife, to the visionary Elizabeth of Spalbeek.[14] These fragments have resisted
meaning-making. And now they resist closure. I can offer no periodizing ter-
minations here, only reconfigurations and replications, alternate projections,
and recovery methods. I close with one final ripple, then; not an ending, but
an opening.

Antwerp, 1603: Margaret vaden Perre, a lay sister in the cloister of the
third order of Saint Francis, has been living with a cancer so virulent that her
breasts had become purplish, rock-hard, and unsightly.[15] Her right breast is
so swollen that it occludes her armpit, sending shocks of pain up and down
her back; meanwhile, the left breast leaks a bloody matter from its nipple,
though sometimes the fluid escapes from another passageway, her ears. The
lay sister consults a series of clinicians, including a "skillfull woman" named
Magdalen, who applies herbal plasters that only worsen the condition.
A famous surgeon from Harentals, M. Peter, then substitutes a new plaster,
but his remedy also fails. An old Portuguese surgeon by the name of Vento
Rodriguez counsels Margaret to make an issue in her arm to draw out the
humor of the cancer. When this intervention also proves unsuccessful, Margaret tries "diverse remedies" taught to her by several friends and neighbors.
She is visited by an elderly maid named Anne Cammarts who practices surgery under the alias Abacucx.[16] After a series of prescribed purgations neglect
to provide relief, Margaret seeks help from yet another cunning woman,
Gertrude Munsters, who discovers that the cancer has metastasized, and thus
rubs Margaret's back with ointment and applies plates of lead and linen to
her breasts. Gertrude finally advises Margaret that physic can offer her no
lasting remedy. It is only at this point in the story that a care practitioner
who has been with Margaret for the duration of her malady comes into view,
her conventual sister Marie Clemens. Marie is the guardian of the infirmary
and, with the permission of Mother Superior, takes to escorting Margaret

---

14. Vienna, Österreichische Nationalbibliothek, Codex 1134; reference to Elizabeth of Spalbeek
as "sage femme" is discussed in Field, *Courting Sanctity*, 141.

15. *Historie vande miraculen die onlancx in grooten getale ghebeurt zyn door de intercessie ende voorbid-
den van die Heylighe Maget Maria op een plaetse genoemt Scherpenheuvel bij die stadt Sichen in Brabant* was
first published in Dutch in 1604, and then rapidly translated into Spanish, French, English, and Latin;
Philippe Numan, *Miracles Lately Wrought by the Intercession of the Glorious Virgin Marie, at Mont-aigu
in Brabant* (Antwerp: Arnold Coinings, 1606), 163–70.

16. This name both baffles and delights. Could it derive from the prophet Habbukuk (Abacus)
who appears in some iterations of the Tree of Jesse?

on a weeklong pilgrimage to the site of a small Marian statue lodged in an oak tree on a hill (Montaigu) near Diest. They have sat for three Masses in the shrine chapel when Margaret reports experiencing a sense of wholeness. Home from their journey, Marie inspects Margaret's breasts and finds them "perfectly cured and in good order." Margaret's recovery is declared a miracle. Marie Clemens's craft and care are suppressed by the narrative, which traces Margaret's path to cure across interactions with a hierarchy of official practitioners. Marie's role in Margaret's recovery of health is absorbed into the unfathomable mystery and supernatural power of divine cure. To recognize Marie's labor is not to deny the mystery or to reject the gods. It is to place equal value on the means of Margaret's daily sustenance, the skill it involved, and the continuum it shares with other practitioners who offer cure; her care labor made possible all other generative acts.

Bibliography

Manuscripts and Archival Sources

Archives de l'État, Liège
    Dominicains, chartes, no. 22 July 1266
    Béguinage de Saint-Christophe
Archives of the New Orleans Province, Society of Jesus, New Orleans
Biblioteca Apostolica, Rome
    MS Pal. Lat. 1990
Bibliothèque de l'Arsenal, Paris
    MS 945
Bibliothèque municipale, Valenciennes
    MS 329
Bibliothèque nationale de France, Paris
    MS Latin 1077
    Nouvelles acquisitions françaises, MS 6539
Bibliothèque de l'Université de Liège, Liège
    MS 431
Bodleian Library, Oxford
    MS Douce 381
British Library, London
    MS Additional 21114
    MS Additional 60629
    MS Harley 2558
    MS Harley 2930
    MS Harley 3717
    MS Sloane 1611
    MS Sloane 2435
Fitzwilliam Museum, Cambridge
    MS 288
Harvey Cushing/John Hay Whitney Medical Library, Yale University
    Library, New Haven
    MS 19
KBR, Brussels

MS 4459–70

MS 8609–20

MS 8895–96

MS 11130–32

MS II–1047

MS II–1658

MS IV–1013

MS IV–1066

Maryland Province Archives, Booth Family Center for Special
    Collections, Georgetown University. Washington, DC, box 40, file 10

The Morgan Library, New York

MS 155

MS 183

MS 440

National Archives, Georgetown Slavery Archive, Fort Worth, TX
    Records of the U.S. Customs Service, Record Group 36

Österreichische Nationalbibliothek, Vienna

Codex 1134

Series Nova, MSS 12706–12707

Princeton University Library, Princeton

MS 138.44

Rijksarchief Leuven, Leuven

Kierkarchiv Vlaams

Klein Begijnhof

Staatsbibliothek Preussischer Kulturbesitz, Berlin

Theol. Lat. Qu. 195

MS 50

Stadsarchief Tongeren, Tongeren

Begijnhof

Sint-Jacobsgasthuis

Ushaw College, Durham

MS 29

Walters Art Gallery, Baltimore

MS 68

Wellcome Library, London

MS 632

Printed Primary Sources

Aesopus. *Anonymus Neveleti*. Edited by Wendelin Foerester. Heilbronn: Henninger, 1882.

Alan of Lille. *The Art of Preaching.* Translated by Gillian Rosemary Evans. Piscataway, NJ: Gorgias Press, 2010.

Albertus Magnus. *The Book of Minerals.* Translated by Dorothy Wyckoff. Oxford: Clarendon Press, 1967.

——. *On Animals: A Medieval Summa Zoologica.* Translated by Kenneth Kitchell and Irven Resnick. Columbus: Ohio State University Press, 2018.

——. *On the Body of the Lord.* Translated by Sr. Albert Marie Surmanski. Washington, DC: Catholic University of America Press, 2017.

Anonymous. "The History of the Foundation of the Venerable Church of Blessed Nicholas of Oignies and the Handmaid of Christ Mary of Oignies." Translated by Hugh Feiss. In *Mary of Oignies: Mother of Salvation,* edited by Anneke Mulder-Bakker, 167–75. Turnhout: Brepols, 2006.

Arnald of Villanova. *Aphorismi de gradibus.* In *Opera medica omnia,* vol. 2, edited by Michael McVaugh, 137–228. Grenada-Barcelona: Seminarium Historiae Medicae Granatensis, 1975.

——. *De cautelis medicorum.* Translated by Henry Sigerist. In *Henry Sigerist on the History of Medicine,* edited by Felix Marti-Ibañez, 132–40. New York: MD Publications, 1960.

——. *Regimen sanitatis ad regem Aragonum.* In *Opera medica omnia,* vol. 10.1, edited by Michael McVaugh, Luis García-Ballester, and Juan Paniagua. Barcelona: Editions Universitat Barcelona, 1996.

Augustine. *The City of God against the Pagans.* Translated by R. W. Dyson. Cambridge: Cambridge University Press, 1998.

Bacon, Roger. *De secretis operibus artis et naturae et de nullitate magicae.* In *Fratris Rogeri Bacon Opera quaedam hactenus inedita,* vol. 1, edited by John Brewer, 523–51. London: Longman, 1859. Translated by Tenney Davis as *On the Nullity of Magic* (New York: AMS Press, 1982).

——. *Fratris Rogeri Bacon De retardatione accidentium senectutis.* Edited by Andrew G. Little and Edward Withington. Oxford: Clarendon Press, 1928.

——. *The Opus Maius of Roger Bacon.* Edited by Henry Bridges. London: Williams and Norgate, 1900.

Bartholomaeus de Montagnana. *Consilia CCCV.* Venice, 1564.

Benausse, Francis, SJ. *Account of the Cure of Miss Mary Wilson, Novice in the Community of the Sacred Heart, Grand Coteau, Louisiana.* Baltimore: John Murphy, 1873.

Bonaventure. "The Tree of Life." In *The Soul's Journey into God, the Tree of Life, and the Life of St. Francis,* translated by Ewert Cousins, 117–76. New York: Paulist Press, 1978.

Boniface VIII. "Periculoso." In *Corpus iuris canonici,* edited by Aemilius Richter and Emil Friedberg, vol. 1, c. 119. Leipzig: Bernhard Tauchnitz, 1829.

Brouette, Émile. *Recueil des chartes et documents de l'abbaye du Val-Saint-Georges à Salzinnes (1196–1300).* Cîteaux: Commentarii Cistercienses. Achel: Abbaye cistercienne, 1971.

Caesarius of Heisterbach. *Dialogus miraculorum.* Edited by Nikolaus Nösges. Turnhout: Brepols, 2009. Translated by Henry von Essen Scott and Swinton Bland as *Dialogue on Miracles* (London: Routledge, 1929).

Cartulaire de l'abbaye de Marquette. Edited by Maurice Vanhaeck. Lille: Secretariat de la Société, 1937.

Cartulaire de l'abbaye de Zwyveke-lez-Termonde. Edited by Alphons De Vlaminck. Ghent: Annoot-Braeckman, 1869.

Cartulaire de l'abbaye du Val-Benoit. Edited by Joseph Cuvelier. Brussels: Kiessling, Ibreghts, 1906.

Cartulaire de l'hôpital Saint-Jean de Bruxelles. In *Actes des XIIe et XIIIe siècles,* edited by Paul Bonenfant. Brussels: Publications de la Commission Royale d'Histoire, 1953.

Cartulaire du béguinage du Cantipret à Mons. Edited by Léopold Devillers. Brussels: Archives Générale du royaume, 1865 (repr. 2001).

Cartulaire du béguinage de Saint Elisabeth à Gand. Edited by Jean Bethune. Bruges: Zuttere, 1883.

Cassian, John. *Collationes patrum in scetica eremo.* PL 49:477–1328.

Chartularium universitatis Parisiensis. Edited by Henri Denifle. Paris: Delalain, 1889.

Chroniques liégeoises. Edited by Sylvain Balau. Brussels: P. Imbreghts, 1915.

Les codifications cisterciennes de 1237 et de 1257. Edited by Bernard Lucet. Paris: Centre National de la Recherche Scientifique, 1977.

Constitutiones Concilii quarti Lateranensis una cum commentariis glossatorum. Edited by Antonius García y García. Vatican City: Bibliotheca Apostolica Vaticana, 1981.

De B. Nicolao et Sociis Narratio. AASS Nov. IV, 277–79.

De B. Waltero de Birbeke. AASS January II, 447–50.

Decrees of the Ecumenical Councils. Edited and translated by Norman Tanner. 2 vols. London: Sheed and Ward, 1999.

De Ryckel, J., ed. *Vita S. Beggae, Ducissae Brabantiae Andetennensium, Begginarum et Beggardorum.* Leuven: Oorbeeck, 1631.

Despy, Georges, and André Uyttebrouck. *Inventaire des archives de l'abbaye de La Ramée à Jauchelette.* Brussels: Archives générales du Royaume, 1970.

De venerabili viro Godefrido Pachomio. Edited by R. Poncelet. *Analecta Bollandiana* 14 (1895): 263–68.

Elizabeth of Schönau. *Die Visionen der hl. Elizabeth und die Schriften der Aebte Ekbert und Emecho von Schönau.* Edited by F. W. F. Roth. Brünn: Verlag der Studien aus dem Benedictiner- und Cistercienser Orden, 1884. Translated by Anne Clark as *Elizabeth of Schönau: The Complete Works* (New York: Paulist, 2000).

Galen. *On Unnatural Tumors.* Translated by D. G. Lytton and L. M. Resuhr. *Journal of the History of Medicine and the Allied Sciences* 33.4 (1978): 531–49.

———. *Opera omnia.* Edited by C. G. Kühn. Hildesheim: Reprographischer Nachdruck der Ausgabe Leipzig, 1964–65.

Gentile of Foligno. *Consilia.* Pavia, 1488.

Gertrude of Helfta. *Oeuvres Spirituelles.* Edited and translated by Jacques Hourlier, Pierre Doyere, and Jean-Marie Clement. Paris: Éditions du Cerf, 1967–86.

Gilbertus Anglicus. *Compendium medicinae.* Lyon: Iacobum Saccon, 1510.

Giovanni Matteo Ferrari da Grado. *Consilia.* Lyon, 1535.

Goswin of Bossut. *Vita Arnulfi conversi Villariensis.* AASS June VII, 556–79. Translated by Martinus Cawley as "The Life of Arnulf, Laybrother of Villers," in *Send Me God: The Lives of Ida the Compassionate of Nivelles, Nun of la Ramée, Arnulf, Lay Brother of Villers, and Abundus, Monk of Villers, by Goswin of Bossut* (University Park: Pennsylvania State University Press, 2005), 125–98.

——. *Vita beatae Idae de Nivella sanctimonialis in Monasterio de Rameya*. In *Quinque prudentes virgines*, edited by Chrysostomo Henriquez, 199–297. Antwerp: Cnobbaert, 1630. Translated by Martinus Cawley as "The Life of Ida the Compassionate of Nivelles," in *Send Me God: The Lives of Ida the Compassionate of Nivelles, Nun of la Ramée, Arnulf, Lay Brother of Villers, and Abundus, Monk of Villers, by Goswin of Bossut* (University Park: Pennsylvania State University Press, 2005), 29–124.

Guiard of Laon. *La vie et les oeuvres de Guiard de Laon, 1170–env1248*. Edited by Petrus Boeren. The Hague: Nijhoff, 1956.

Guibert of Tournai. "Collectio de scandalis ecclesiae." *Archivum Franciscanum Historicum* 24 (1931): 33–62.

Guiraud, Jean, ed. *Les Registres d'Urbain IV (1261–1264)*. Paris: Fontemoing, 1901.

Henri of Mondeville. *Die Chirurgie des Heinrich von Mondeville (1306–1320)*. Edited by Julius Pagel. Berlin: Hirschwald, 1892.

Hildegard of Bingen. *Causae et curae*. Edited by Paulus Kaiser. Leipzig: B.G. Teubneri, 1903.

Hillinus. *Miraculi sancti Foillani*. AASS Oct. XIII, 417–26.

Historia monasterii Villariensis in Brabantia. Edited by Edmundus Martène and Ursinus Durand. In *Thesaurus novus anecdotorum*, 1267–1374. Paris: Delaulne, 1717.

Honorius III. *Honorii Romanorum pontificis opera omnia*. Edited by C. A. Horoy. 5 vols. Paris, 1879–83.

Hoornaert, Rodolphe. "La plus ancienne règle de béguinage de Bruges." *Annales de la Société d'Émulation de Bruges* 72 (1930): 1–79.

Hunayn ibn Ishaq (Johannicius). "Johannicius: Isagoge ad Techni Galieni." Edited by Gregor Maurach. *Sudhoffs Archiv* 62 (1978): 148–74.

Iacopo da Varazze. *Legenda aurea: Edizione critica*. Edited by Giovanni Paolo Maggioni. Florence: SISMEL, 2001. Translated by William Granger Ryan as *The Golden Legend: Readings on the Saints* (Princeton: Princeton University Press, 1993).

Ibn Sīnā (Avicenna). *Liber canonis*. Venice: Bonetum Locatellum Bergomensem, 1507. Translated by Cameron Gruner as *The Canon of Medicine* (New York: AMS Press, 1973).

Ignatius of Antioch. *Epistle to the Ephesians*. In *The Apostolic Fathers: Greek Texts and English Translations*, edited by Michael Holmes, 182–201. Grand Rapids: Baker Academic, 2007.

Innocent III. *Encomium charitatis*. PL 217:761–64.

——. *Libellus de eleemosyna*. PL 217:745–62.

Inventaire des Archives de l'abbaye du Val-Benoit. Edited by Joseph Cuvelier. Liège: Léon de Thier, 1902.

Iuliana virgo. AASS April I, 443–77. Translated by Barbara Newman as "The Life of Juliana of Mont Cornillon," in *Living Saints of the Thirteenth Century*, edited by Anneke Mulder-Bakker (Turnhout: Brepols, 2011), 143–302.

Jacques de Vitry. *The Exempla or Illustrative Stories from the Sermones vulgares of Jacques de Vitry*. Edited by Thomas Crane. London: The Folklore Society, 1890.

——. *Lettres de Jacques de Vitry, 1160/70–1240 évêque de Saint-Jean d'Acre*. Edited by R. B. C. Huygens. Leiden: Brill, 1960.

——. *Vita Mariae Oigniacensis*. Edited by R. B. C. Huygens. Turnhout: Brepols, 2012. Translated by Margot King as "The Life of Mary of Oignies," in *Mary of Oignies: Mother of Salvation*, edited by Anneke Mulder-Bakker (Turnhout: Brepols, 2006), 22–127.

John of Gaddesden. *Johannis Anglici Rosa Anglica seu Rosa Medicinae*. Edited by Winifrid Wulff. London: Simkin Marshall, 1929.

John of Garland. *The Parisiana Poetria of John of Garland*. Edited and translated by Traugott Lawler. New Haven: Yale University Press, 1974.

Lambert of Liège. "L'Antigraphum Petri et les lettres concernant Lambert le Bègue, conservés dans le manuscript de Glasgow." Edited by Arnold Fayen. *Compte-Rendu des Séances de la Commission Royale d'Histoire* 68 (1899): 255–356.

Luykx, Theo. *Johanna van Constantinopel, gravin van Vlaanderen en Henegouwen: Haar leven (1199/1200–1244), haar regeering (1205–1244) vooral in Vlaanderen*.: Verhandelingen van de koninklijke Vlaamsche Academie voor Wetenschappen, Letteren en schoone Kunsten van België, Klasse der Letteren, 5. Antwerp, 1946.

Miraeus, Aubertus, and Joannes Foppens, eds. *Opera diplomatica et historica*. 4 vols. Louvain: Diplomatum belgicorum nova collectio, 1723–48.

Nicholas of Poland. "Antipocras, Streitschrift für mystische Heilkunde in Versen des Magisters Nikolaus von Polen." Edited by Karl Sudhoff. *Sudhoffs Archiv für Geschichte der Medizin* 9 H ½ (1915): 31–52. Translated by William Eamon as *Antipocras: Composed and So Named by Brother Nicholas of the Preaching Friars; Also Called by Another Name, The Book of Empirical Things* (PDF file, history. nmsu.edu/people/faculty/eamon, 2014).

Numan, Philippe. *Miracles Lately Wrought by the Intercession of the Glorious Virgin Marie, at Mont-aigu*. Translated by Robert Chambers. Antwerp: Arnold Coinings, 1606.

Paquay, Jean. "L'archidiaconat liégeois d'Urbain IV." *Leodium* 2 (1903): 60–63.

Peter of Blois. *De duodecim utilitatibus tribulationis*. PL 207:992–93.

A Philosophy Reader from the Circle of Miskawayh. Edited and translated by Elvira Wakelnig. Cambridge: Cambridge University Press, 2014.

Pietro d'Abano. *Conciliator differentiarum philosophorum*. Venice: Luca Giunta, 1520.

Qūsta ibn Lūqā. *De animae et spiritus discrimine*. In Constantine the African, *Constantini Africani opera*, translated by Joannes Hispalensis, 308–17. Basel: Henricum Petrum, 1536.

Raepsaet, Henry, ed. *Archives de l'hôpital Notre Dame, à Audenarde*. In *Messager des Sciences historiques de Belgique*, 332–61. Ghent: Hebbelynck, 1832.

Regimen sanitatis salerni. London: Alsop, 1649.

Schoolmeesters, Èmile, ed. *Les regestes de Robert de Thourotte*. Liège: D. Cormaux, 1906.

Stephen of Lexington. "Registrum epistolarum Stephani de Lexinton abbatis de Stanlegia et de Savigniaco." *Analecta Sacri Ordinis Cisterciensis* 2 (1946): 1–118; 8 (1952): 181–378.

Teodorico Borgognoni. *Chirurgia*. In *Ars chirurgia Guidonis Cauliaci*. Venice, 1546. Translated by Eldridge Campbell and James Colton as *The Surgery of Theodoric* (New York: Appleton, 1955).

Thomas Aquinas. *Sententia super libros De generatione et coruptione expositione*. Salamanca: Leonardo Hutz, 1496.

——. *Summa contra Gentiles*. Translated by Vernon J. Bourke. South Bend: University of Notre Dame Press, 1975.

Thomas of Cantimpré. *De S. Christina Mirabili virgine*. AASS July V, 637–60. Translated by Margot King and Barbara Newman as "The Life of Christina the Astonishing," in *Thomas of Cantimpré: The Collected Saints' Lives; Abbot John of Cantimpré, Christina the Astonishing, Margaret of Ypres, and Lutgard of Aywières* (Turnhout: Brepols, 2008), 127–60.

——. *De vita S. Lutgardis*. AASS June III, 237–63. Translated by Margot King and Barbara Newman as "Life of Lutgard of Aywières," in *Thomas of Cantimpré: The Collected Saints' Lives; Abbot John of Cantimpré, Christina the Astonishing, Margaret of Ypres, and Lutgard of Aywières* (Turnhout: Brepols, 2008), 211–96.

——. *Liber de natura rerum*. Berlin: De Gruyter, 1973.

——. *Vita Ioannis Cantipratensis*. In "Une oeuvre inédite de Thomas de Cantimpré, la 'Vita Ioannis Cantipratensis,'" edited by Robert Godding, *Revue d'Histoire Ecclésiastique* 76 (1981): 241–316. Translated by Barbara Newman as "The Life of Abbot John of Cantimpré," in *Thomas of Cantimpré: The Collected Saints' Lives; Abbot John of Cantimpré, Christina the Astonishing, Margaret of Ypres, and Lutgard of Aywières* (Turnhout: Brepols, 2008), 57–124.

——. *Vita Margarite de Ypris*. In "Frères Prêcheurs et movement dévot en Flandre au XIIIe siècle," edited by Gilles G. Meersseman, *Archivum Fratrum Praedicatorum* 18 (1948): 106–30. Translated by Margot King and Barbara Newman as "The Life of Margaret of Ypres," in *Thomas of Cantimpré: The Collected Saints' Lives; Abbot John of Cantimpré, Christina the Astonishing, Margaret of Ypres, and Lutgard of Aywières* (Turnhout: Brepols, 2008), 163–208.

Thomas of Villers. "Deux lettres inédites." Edited by Edmund Mikkers. *Collectanea Ordinis Cisterciensium Reformatorum* 10 (1948): 161–73.

Vita Beatricis. Edited and translated by Roger de Ganck as *The Life of Beatrice of Nazareth* (Kalamazoo, MI: Cistercian Publications, 1991).

Vita beatae Aleyde Scharembekana. AASS June II, 471–77. Translated by Martinus Cawley as *The Life of Alice of Schaerbeek* (Lafayette, OR: Guadalupe Translations, 2000).

Vita Beatae Juettae reclusae. AASS January XIII, 863–89. Translated by Jo Ann McNamara as "The Life of Yvette, Anchoress of Huy," in *Living Saints of the Thirteenth Century: The Lives of Yvette, Anchoress of Huy; Juliana of Cornillon, Author of the Corpus Christi Feast; and Margaret the Lame, Anchoress of Magdeburg*, edited by Anneke Mulder-Bakker (Turnhout: Brepols, 2011), 49–141.

Vita beati Simonis: La vie du bienheureux frère Simon, convers à l'abbaye d'Aulne. Edited by Franciscus Moschus. Tournai: Desclée, 1968.

Vita B. Goberti. AASS August IV, 370–95.

Vita B. Ida Lewensi. AASS October XIII, 107–24. Translated by Martinus Cawley as *Ida the Gentle of Léau* (Lafayette, OR: Guadelupe Translations, 1998).

Vita B. Odiliae Viduae Leodiensis. Edited by C. De Smedt. *Analecta Bollandiana* 13 (1894): 190–287.

Vita domni werrici. In *Catalogus codicum hagiographicorum bibliothecae Regiae Bruxellensis*, 1:445–63. Brussels: Typis Polleunis, Ceuterick et Lefébure, 1886.

Vita Idae de Lovanio. AASS April II, 157–189. Translated by Martinus Cawley as *Ida the Eager of Louvain* (Lafayette, OR: Gaudelupe Translations, 2000).

Vogel, Cyrille, and Reinhard Elze, eds. *Le pontifical romano-germanique du dixième siècle.* Vatican City: Bibliotheca Apostolica Vaticana, 1963.

Wace. *La vie de St. Marguerite, poème.* Edited by Aristide Joly. Paris: Vieweg, 1879.

Waddell, Chrysogonus, ed. *The Primitive Cistercian Breviary.* Fribourg: Academic Press Fribourg, 2007.

William of St. Thierry. *De natura corporis et animae.* PL 180:695–726. Translated by Benjamin Clark in *Three Treatises on Man: A Cistercian Anthropology,* edited by Bernard McGinn (Kalamazoo, MI: Cistercian Publications, 1977), 101–52.

Secondary Sources

Agrimi, Jole, and Chiara Crisciani. "Savoir médical et anthropologie religieuse: Les représentations et fonctions de la *vetula* (XIIIe–XVe siècle)." *Annales: Économies, Société, Civilisations* 48.5 (1993): 1281–1308.

Aichele, George. "Reading Jesus Writing." *Biblical Interpretation* 12 (2004): 353–68.

Albert, Jean-Pierre. "La légende de sainte Marguerite un mythe maïeutique?" *Razo* 8 (1988): 19–33.

Allen, Judson. *The Ethical Poetic of the Later Middle Ages.* Toronto: University of Toronto Press, 1982.

Ampe, Albert. "Een oud *Florilegium eucharisticum* in een veertiende-eeuws handschrift." *Oons Geestelijk Erf* 31 (1964): 23–55.

——. *Jan van Ruusbroec 1293–1381: Tentoonstellingscatalogus; Catalogi vantentoonstellingen georganiseerd in de koninklijke Bibliotheek Albert I.* Brussels: Koninklijke Bibliotheek, 1981.

Amundsen, Darrel W., and Gary B. Ferngren. "Medicine and Religion: Pre-Christian Antiquity." In *Health/Medicine and the Faith Traditions,* edited by Martin Marty and Kenneth Vaux, 53–92. Philadelphia: Fortress, 1982.

Archambeau, Nicole. "Healing Options during the Plague: Survivor Stories from a Fourteenth-Century Canonization Inquest." *Bulletin of the History of Medicine* 85.4 (2011): 531–59.

——. "Miracle Mediators as Healing Practitioners: The Knowledge and Practice of Healing with Relics." *Social History of Medicine* 31.2 (2017): 209–30.

Areford, David S. "The Passion Measured: A Late Medieval Diagram of the Body of Christ." In *The Broken Body: Passion Devotion in Late-Medieval Culture,* edited by A. A. MacDonald, H. N. B. Ridderbos, and R. M. Schlusemann, 211–38. Groningen: Egbert Forsten, 1998.

Austin, J. L. *How to Do Things with Words.* Edited by J. O. Urmson and Marina Sbisá. Cambridge, MA: Harvard University Press, 1962.

Aymar, Alphonse. "Le sachet accoucheur et ses mystères." *Annales du Midi* 38 (1926): 273–347.

Baert, Barbara. *A Heritage of Holy Wood: Legend of the True Cross in Text and Image.* Leiden: Brill, 2004.

Bailey, Michael. "The Disenchantment of Magic: Spells, Charms, and Superstition in Early European Witchcraft Literature." *American Historical Review* 111.2 (2006): 383–404.

——. *Fearful Spirits, Reasoned Follies: The Boundaries of Superstition in Late Medieval Europe.* Ithaca: Cornell University Press, 2013.

Balty-Guedson, Marie G. "Bayt al-Hikmah et politique culturelle du calife al-Mamun." *Medicinia nei Secoli* 6 (1994): 275–91.

Barboud, Jean, and Pierre Gillon. "Cinq calendriers diététiques provenant de manuscrits de la Bibliothèque nationale de Paris: Réflexions sur l'origine et la destination de ces calendriers." In *XXX Congrès international d'histoire de la médecine (Düsseldorf 31 sept.–5 oct. 1986)*, edited by Hans Schadewaldt and K. H. Leven, 179–87. Düsseldorf: Organisationskommittee des XXX. Int. Kongresses, 1988.

Barnhouse, Lucy. "Disordered Women? The Hospital Sisters of Mainz and Their Late Medieval Identities." *Medieval Feminist Forum* 3 (2020): 60–97.

Barr, Jessica. "Reading Wounds: Embodied Mysticism in a Fourteenth-Century Codex." *Magistra* 19.1 (2013): 27–39.

Barrat, Alexandra. "Language and the Body in Thomas of Cantimpré's *Life of Lutgard of Aywières*." *Cistercian Studies Quarterly* 30.3 (1995): 339–47.

Barre, M. Louis Carolus. "Un nouveau parchemin amulette et la légende de Sainte Margarite patronne des femmes en couche." *Académie des Inscriptions et Belles-Lettres Comptes Rendus* 123.2 (1979): 256–75.

Bartlett, Robert. *Why Can the Dead Do Such Great Things? Saints and Worshippers from the Martyrs to the Reformation*. Princeton: Princeton University Press, 2015.

Bashir, Shahzad. "On Islamic Time: Rethinking Chronology in the Historiography of Muslim Societies." *History & Theory* 53.4 (2014): 519–44.

Baumgarten, Elisheva. *Mothers and Children: Jewish Family Life in Medieval Europe*. Philadelphia: University of Pennsylvania Press, 2007.

——. "A Separate People: Some Directions for Comparative Research on Medieval Women." *Journal of Medieval History* 34.2 (2008): 212–28.

Berliner, Rudolf. "Arma Christi." In *"The Freedom of Medieval Art" und andere Studien zum christlichen Bild*, edited by Robert Suckale, 97–191. Berlin: Lukas Verlag, 2003.

Berman, Constance. *The White Nuns: Cistercian Abbeys for Women in Medieval France*. Philadelphia: University of Pennsylvania Press, 2018.

Bestul, Thomas. *Texts of the Passion: Latin Devotional Literature and Medieval Society*. Philadelphia: University of Pennsylvania Press, 1996.

Biehl, João. *Will to Live: AIDS Policies and the Politics of Survival*. Princeton: Princeton University Press, 2007.

Biller, Peter. "Words and the Medieval Notion of Religion." *Journal of Ecclesiastical History* 36.3 (1985): 351–69.

Bird, Jessalyn. "Medicine for Body and Soul: Jacques de Vitry's Sermons to Hospitallers and Their Charges." In *Religion and Medicine in the Middle Ages*, edited by Joseph Ziegler and Peter Biller, 91–108. York: York Medieval Press, 2001.

Black, Winston. "William of Auvergne and the Rhetoric of Penance." In *Learning to Love: Schools, Law, and Pastoral Care in the Middle Ages*, edited by Tristan Sharp, 419–42. Toronto: PIMS, 2017.

Blumenfeld-Kosinski, Renate. *The Strange Case of Ermine of Rheims: A Medieval Woman between Demons and Saints*. Philadelphia: University of Pennsylvania Press, 2015.

Bolton, Brenda. "Some Thirteenth-Century Women in the Low Countries: A Special Case?" *Nederlands Archief voor Kerkgeschiedenis/Dutch Review of Church History* 61.1 (1981): 7–29.

Bonenfant, Paul. *Hôpitaux et bienfaisance publique dans les anciens Pays-Bas, des origines à la fin du XVIIIe siècle.* Brussels: Société belge d'histoire des hôpitaux, 1965.

Bono, James. "Medical Spirits and the Medieval Language of Life." *Traditio* 40 (1984): 91–130.

Boquet, Damien, and Piroska Nagy. "Medieval Sciences of Emotions in the 11th–13th Centuries: An Intellectual History." *Osiris* 31 (2016): 21–45.

Borgnet, A., and S. Bormans. *Ly myreur des histors ou chronique et geste de Jean des Preis dit d'Outremeuse.* 7 vols. Brussels: Publications de la Commission Royale d'Histoire, 1864–87.

Borland, Jennifer. "Female Networks and the Circulation of a Late Medieval Health Guide." In *Moving Women Moving Objects*, edited by Tracy Hamilton and Mariah Proctor-Tiffany, 108–36. Leiden: Brill, 2019.

Botana, Federico. *The Works of Mercy in Italian Medieval Art.* Turnhout: Brepols, 2011.

Bott, Nicholas T., Clifford Sheckter, and Arnold Milstein. "Dementia Care, Women's Health, and Gender Equity: The Value of Well-Timed Caregiver Support." *JAMA Neurology* 74.7 (2017): 757–58.

Boudot, Jean-Patrice, Franck Collard, and Nicolas Weill-Parot, eds. *Médecine, astrologie et magie entre Moyen Âge et Renaissance: Autour de Pietro d'Abano.* Florence: Sismel, 2013.

Boudreaux, Anna. "Les remèdes du vieux temps: Remedies and Cures of the Kaplan Area in Southwest Louisiana." *Southern Folklore Quarterly* 35.2 (1971): 121–40.

Bowers, Barbara, ed. *The Medieval Hospital and Medical Practice.* Aldershot: Ashgate, 2007.

Bowker, Geoffrey, and Susan Leigh Star, eds. *Sorting Things Out: Classification and Its Consequences.* Boston: MIT Press, 1999.

Boynton, Susan. "Prayer as Liturgical Performance in 11th- and 12th-Century Monastic Psalters." *Speculum* 82 (2007): 892–931.

Bozóky, Edina. *Charmes et prières apotropaïque.* Typologie des Sources du Moyen Âge Occidental, fasc. 86. Turnhout: Brepols, 2003.

——. "Medieval Narrative Charms." In *The Power of Words: Studies on Charms and Charming in Europe*, edited by James Kapaló, Èva Pòcs, and William Frances Ryan, 101–16. Budapest: Central European Press, 2013.

Brantley, Jessica. *Reading in the Wilderness: Private Devotion and Public Performance in Late Medieval England.* Chicago: University of Chicago Press, 2007.

Brassart, Modeste. *Notes historiques sur les hôpitaux et établissements de charité de la ville de Douai.* Douai: Adam d'Aubers, 1842.

Brenner, Elma. *Leprosy and Charity in Medieval Rouen.* Woodbridge: Boydell, 2015.

Brodman, James. *Charity and Religion in Medieval Europe.* Baltimore: Johns Hopkins University Press, 2009.

——. "Religion and Discipline in the Hospitals of Thirteenth-Century France." In *The Medieval Hospital and Medical Practice*, edited by Barbara Bowers, 123–32. New York: Routledge, 2007.

Brooks, Lisa. *Our Beloved Kin: A New History of King Philip's War.* New Haven: Yale University Press, 2018.

Broomhall, Susan. *Women's Medical Work in Early Modern France.* Manchester: Manchester University Press, 2004.

Brouette, Émile. "Abbaye de Villers à Tilly." In *Monasticon Belge* IV-2, 341–405. Liège: Revue Belge de Philologie et d'Histoire, 1968.

Brown, Jennifer N. *Three Women of Liège: A Critical Edition and Commentary on the Middle English Lives of Elizabeth of Spalbeek, Christina Mirabilis, and Marie d'Oignies.* Turnhout: Brepols, 2008.

Brown, Miranda. "'Medicine' in Early China." In *Routledge Handbook of Early Chinese History*, edited by Paul Goldin, 465–78. New York: Routledge, 2018.

Brown, Peter. *The Cult of Saints: Its Rise and Function in Latin Christianity.* Chicago: University of Chicago Press, 1981.

——. *Through the Eye of the Needle: Wealth, the Fall of Rome, and the Making of Christianity in the West, 350–550.* Princeton: Princeton University Press, 2012.

Brundage, James. *Medieval Canon Law.* New York: Longman, 1995.

Bull, Marcus. *The Miracles of Our Lady Rocamadour: Analysis and Translation.* Suffolk: Boydell & Brewer, 1999.

Bullough, Vern. *The Development of Medicine as a Profession: The Contribution of the Medieval University to Modern Medicine.* New York: Karger, 1966.

Burnett, Charles. "European Knowledge of Arabic Texts Referring to Music: Some New Material." *Early Music History* 12 (1993): 1–17.

——, ed. Marie-Thérèse d'Alverny, *Transmission des textes philosophiques et scientifiques au Moyen Âge.* Aldershot: Variorum, 1994.

Burr, David. *Eucharistic Presence and Conversion in Late Thirteenth-Century Franciscan Thought.* Philadelphia: American Philosophical Society, 1984.

Bylebyl, Jerome. "The Medical Meaning of *Physica.*" *Osiris* 6 (1990): 16–41.

Bynum, Caroline Walker. *Christian Materiality: An Essay on Religion in Late Medieval Europe.* Boston: MIT Press, 2011.

——. *Holy Feast and Holy Fast: The Religious Significance of Food to Medieval Women.* Los Angeles: University of California Press, 1987.

——. *Jesus as Mother: Studies in the Spirituality of the High Middle Ages.* Berkeley: University of California Press, 1982.

Caballero-Navas, Carmen. *The Book of Women's Love and Jewish Medieval Medical Literature on Women: Sefer ahavat nashim.* London: Kegan Paul, 2004.

——. "She Will Give Birth Immediately: Pregnancy and Childbirth in Medieval Hebrew Medical Texts Produced in the Mediterranean West." *Dynamis* 2 (2014): 377–401.

Cabré, Montserrat. "Women or Healers? Household Practices and the Categories of Healthcare in Late Medieval Iberia." *Bulletin of the History of Medicine* 82.1 (2008): 18–51.

Carolus-Barré, Louis. "L'abbaye de la Joie-Notre-Dame á Berneuil-sur-Aisne (1234–1430)." In *Mélanges à la mémoire du père Anselme Dimier*, edited by Benoît Chauvin, 487–504. Arbois: Chauvin, 1984.

Carruthers, Mary. *The Book of Memory: A Study of Memory in Medieval Culture.* Cambridge: Cambridge University Press, 2008.

——. *The Craft of Thought: Meditation, Rhetoric, and the Making of Images, 400–1200*. Cambridge: Cambridge University Press, 2000.

——. "On Affliction and Reading, Weeping, and Argument: Chaucer's Lachrymose Troilus in Context." *Representations* 93 (2006): 1–21.

Caspers, Charles. *De eucharistische vroomheid en het feest van Sacramentsdag in de Nederlanden tijdens de Late Middeleeuwen*. Louvain: Peeters, 1992.

——. "Indulgences in the Low Countries c. 1300–1520." In *Promissory Notes on the Treasury of Merits*, edited by R. N. Swanson, 65–99. Leiden: Brill, 2006.

Ceccaroni, Sandro. *La storia millenaria degli ospedali della città e della diocesi di Spoleto*. Spoleto: Ente Rocca di Spoleto, 1978.

Chenu, M. D. "Spiritus: Vocabulaire de l'âme au XIIe siècle." *Revue des Sciences Philosophiques et Théologiques* 41 (1957): 209–32.

Cifuentes, Lluís. "Teodorico Borgognoni." In *Medieval Science, Technology, and Medicine: An Encyclopedia*, edited by Thomas Glick, Steven Livesey, and Faith Wallis, 95–96. New York: Routledge, 2005.

Cipriani, Mattea. "*Questio satis iocunda est*: Analisi delle fonti di *questiones* et *responsiones* del *Liber de natura rerum* di Tommaso di Cantimpré." *Rursus Spicae* 11 (2017): 1–58.

Coakley, John. *Women, Men, and Spiritual Power: Female Saints and Their Male Collaborators*. New York: Columbia University Press, 2006.

Coens, Maurice. "Les saints vénérés à Huy d'après un psautier récemment rapatrié et le martyrologe de la collégiale." *Analecta Bollandiana* 76 (1958): 316–35.

Cohen-Hanegbi, Naama. *Caring for the Living Soul: Emotions, Medicine, and Penance in the Late Medieval Mediterranean*. Leuven: Brill, 2017.

Collet, Alain. "Traité d'hygiène de Thomas le Bourguignon (1286)." *Romania*, 1991, 450–87.

Collins, Patricia Hill. *Black Feminist Thought: Knowledge, Consciousness, and the Politics of Empowerment*. New York: Routledge, 2002.

Coomans, Thomas. "Cistercian Nunneries in the Low Countries: The Medieval Architectural Remains." In *Studies in Cistercian Art and Architecture*, edited by Meredith Parsons, 61–131. Kalamazoo, MI: Cistercian Publications, 2005.

——. *L'abbaye de Villers-en-Brabant: Construction, configuration et signification d'une abbaye cistercienne gothique*. Brussels: Commentarii cistercienses, 2000.

——. "Moniales cistercienne et mémoire dynastique: Églises funéraires princières et abbayes cisterciennes dans les anciens pays-bas médiévaux." *Cîteaux* 56 (2005): 87–146.

——. "Saint-Christophe à Liège: La plus ancienne église médiévale du movement Béguinal." *Bulletin Monumental* 164 (2006): 359–76.

Copeland, Rita. *Rhetoric, Hermeneutics, and Interpretation in the Middle Ages*. Cambridge: Cambridge University Press, 1995.

Cottiaux, J. "L'office liégeois de la Fête-Dieu, sa valeur et son destin." *Revue d'Histoire Ecclésiastique* 58 (1963): 5–81.

Courtoy, Ferdinand. "Les reliques de la passion dans le comte de Namur au XIII siècle." *Anciens Pays* 14 (1957): 85–98.

Csordas, Thomas. *Body/Meaning/Healing*. New York: Palgrave, 2002.

Dagenais, John. *The Ethics of Reading in Manuscript Culture: Glossing the Libro de Buen Amor*. Princeton: Princeton University Press, 1994.

Dangler, Jean. *Mediating Fictions: Literature, Women Healers, and the Go-Between in Medieval and Early Modern Iberia*. Lewisburg: Bucknell University Press, 2001.

Daniell, Christopher. *Death and Burial in Medieval England, 1066–1550*. New York: Routledge, 1998.

Daris, Joseph. "Notes historiques sue Huy." *Analects pour Server à l'Histoire Ecclésiastique de la Belgique* 14 (1877): 36–77.

Das, Shinjini. *Vernacular Medicine in Colonial India: Family, Market, and Homeopathy.* Cambridge: Cambridge University Press, 2019.

Daston, Lorraine, and Katherine Park. *Wonders and the Order of Nature, 1150–1750*. Boston: Zone Books, 1998.

Davis, Adam. "Hospitals, Charity, and the Culture of Compassion." In *Approaches to Poverty in Medieval Europe: Complexities, Contradictions, Transformations, 1100–1500*, edited by Sharon Farmer, 23–45. Turnhout: Brepols, 2016.

——. *The Medieval Economy of Salvation: Charity, Commerce, and the Rise of the Medieval Hospital*. Ithaca: Cornell University Press, 2019.

Davis, Natalie Zemon. "Hosts, Kin, and Progeny: Some Features of Family Life in Early Modern France." In *The Family*, edited by Alice Rossi, Jerome Kagan, and Tamara Hareven, 87–114. New York: Norton, 1978.

Deane, Jennifer Kolpacoff. "Beguines Reconsidered: Historiographical Problems and New Directions." *Commentaria* 34.61 (2008): n.p.

Delattre, Jean-Luc. "La foundation des hôpitaux de Saint-Nicolas et du Saint-Sépulchre à Nivelles au XIIe siècle." In *Hommage au Professeur Paul Bonenfant (1899–1965)*, edited by Georges Despy, 595–99. Brussels: Université Libre de Bruxelles, 1965.

Delaurenti, Béatrice. *La puissance des mots: Virtus verborum; Débats doctrinaux sur le pouvoir des incantations au Moyen Âge*. Paris: Éditions du Cerf, 2007.

——. "Pietro d'Abano et les incantations: Présentations, édition et traduction de la *differentia* 156 du *Conciliator*." In *Médecine, astrologie et magie entre Moyen Âge et Renaissance: Autour Pietro d'Abano*, edited by Jean-Patrice Boudet, Franck Collard, and Nicolas Weill-Parot, 39–105. Florence: Sismel, 2013.

Delmaire, Bernard. "Les béguines dans le nord de la France au premier siècle de leur histoire (vers 1230–1350)." In *Les religieuses en France au XIIIe siècle*, edited by Michel Parisse, 121–62. Nancy: Presses Universitaires de Nancy, 1985.

Demaitre, Luke. *Leprosy in Premodern Medicine: A Malady of the Whole Body*. Baltimore: Johns Hopkins University Press, 2007.

——. *Medieval Medicine: The Art of Healing from Head to Toe*. Santa Barbara: ABC Clio, 2013.

Deploige, Jeroen. "How Gendered Was Clairvoyance in the Thirteenth Century? The Case of Simon of Aulne." In *Speaking to the Eye: Sight and Insight in Text and Image, 1150–1650*, edited by Thérèse de Hemptinne, Veerle Fraeters, and Mariá Eugenia Góngora, 95–126. Turnhout: Brepols, 2013.

Derolez, Albert, ed. *Medieval Booklists of the Southern Low Countries*. Brussels: Paleis der Academiën, 2001.

Des Marez, Guillaume. "Le droit privé à Ypres au XIIIe siècle." *Bulletin de la Commission Royale pour la Publication des Anciennes Lois et Ordonnances de Belgique* 12 (1927): 210–460.

Dillon, Emma. *The Sense of Sound: Musical Meaning in France, 1260–1330*. Oxford: Oxford University Press, 2012.

Dimier, Marie-Anselme. "Un découverte concernante le bienheureux Simon d'Aulne." *Cîteaux* 21 (1970): 302–5.

Domingo, Carmel Ferrargud. *Medicina i promoció social a la baixa edat mitjana: Corona d'Aragó 1350–1410*. Madrid: Consejo Superior de Investigaciones Científicas, 2005.

Doyno, Mary Harvey. *The Lay Saint: Charity and Charismatic Authority in Medieval Italy, 1150–1350*. Ithaca: Cornell University Press, 2019.

Draelants, Isabelle. "The Notion of Properties: Tensions between *Scientia* and *Ars* in Medieval Natural Philosophy and Magic." In *The Routledge History of Medieval Magic*, edited by Sophie Page and Catherine Rider, 169–86. New York: Routledge, 2019.

Duffy, Eamon. *Marking the Hours: The English People and Their Prayers, 1240–1570*. New Haven: Yale University Press, 2010.

——. "Two Healing Prayers." In *Medieval Christianity in Practice*, edited by Miri Rubin, 164–72. Princeton: Princeton Univeristy Press, 2009.

Dutton, Marsha. "Eat, Drink, and Be Merry: The Eucharistic Spirituality of the Cistercian Fathers." In *Erudition at God's Service*, edited by John Sommerfeldt, 1–31. Kalamazoo, MI: Cistercian Publications, 1987.

Eamon, William, and Gundolf Keil. "Plebs amat empirica: Nicholas of Poland and His Critique of the Medical Establishment." *Sudhoffs Archiv* 50.1 (1987): 180–96.

Edwards, Suzanne. *The Afterlives of Rape in Medieval English Literature*. New York: Palgrave, 2016.

Effros, Bonnie. "Symbolic Expressions of Sanctity: Gertrude of Nivelles in the Context of Merovingian Mortuary Custom." *Viator* 27 (1996): 1–10.

El Cheikh, Nadia Maria. *Women, Islam, and Abbasid Identity*. Cambridge, MA: Harvard University Press, 2015.

Elliott, Dyan. *Proving Woman: Female Spirituality and Inquisitional Culture in the Later Middle Ages*. Princeton: Princeton University Press, 2004.

Elsakkers, Marianne. "In Pain You Shall Bear Children: Medieval Prayers for a Safe Delivery." In *Women and Miracle Stories: A Multi-Disciplinary Exploration*, edited by Anne-Marie Korte, 179–210. Leiden: Brill, 2004.

Espinas, Georges, ed. *La vie urbaine de Douai au Moyen Âge*. Paris: August Picard, 1913.

Falmagne, Thomas. *Un text en contexte: Les "Flores Paradisi" et le milieu culturel de Villers-en-Brabant dans la première du 13e siècle*. Turnhout: Brepols 2001.

Fancy, Nahyan. *Science and Religion in Mamluk Egypt: Ibn al-Nafis, Pulmonary Transit, and Bodily Resurrection*. New York: Routledge, 2013.

Farmer, Sharon. "The Leper in the Master Bedroom: Thinking through a Thirteenth-Century Exemplum." In *Framing the Family: Narrative and Representation in the Medieval and Early Modern Families*, edited by Diane Wolfthal and Rosalynn Voaden, 79–100. Tempe: Arizona Center for Medieval and Renaissance Studies, 2005.

Fassler, Margot, and Rebecca Baltzer. *The Divine Office in the Latin Middle Ages: Methodology and Source Studies, Regional Developments, Hagiography*. Oxford: Oxford University Press, 2000.

Feierman, Steve. "Explanation and Uncertainty in the Medical World of Ghamboo." *Bulletin of the History of Medicine* 74.2 (2000): 317–44.

Feiss, Hugh. "Introduction to the Texts for the Mass and Divine Office in Honour of Mary of Oignies." In *Mary of Oignies: Mother of Salvation*, edited by Anneke Mulder-Bakker, 177–83. Turnhout: Brepols, 2006.

Féry-Hue, Françoise. "Le régime du corps d'Aldebrandin de Sienne: Tradition manuscrite et diffusion." In *Santé, médecine et assistance au Moyen Âge*, 113–34. Paris: Actes du Congrès national des Sociétés Savantes, 1987.

Field, Sean. *Courting Sanctity: Holy Women and the Capetians*. Ithaca: Cornell University Press, 2019.

——. "On Being Beguine in France, c. 1300." In *Labels and Libels: Naming Beguines in Northern Medieval Europe*, edited by Letha Böhringer, Jennifer Kolpacoff Deane, and Hildo van Engen, 117–33. Turnhout: Brepols, 2014.

Finucane, Ronald. *Miracles and Pilgrims: Popular Beliefs in Medieval England*. New York: St. Martin's, 1977.

——. "Sacred Corpse, Profane Carrion: Social Ideals and Death Rituals in the Later Middle Ages." In *Mirrors of Mortality: Studies in the Social History of Death*, edited by Joachim Whaley, 40–60. New York: Routledge, 1981.

Fissell, Mary. "Introduction: Women, Health, and Healing in Early Modern Europe." *Bulletin of the History of Medicine* 82.1 (2008): 1–17.

Flint, Valerie. "Susanna and the Lothair Crystal: A Liturgical Perspective." *Early Medieval Europe* 4 (1995): 61–86.

Folkerts, Suzan. *Vorbeeld op schrift: De overlevering en toe-eigening van de vita van Christina Mirabilis in de late middeleeuwen*. Hilversum: Verloren, 2010.

Freed, John. "Urban Development and the 'Cura monialium' in Thirteenth-Century Germany." *Viator* 3 (1972): 311–28.

Fuentes, Marissa J. *Dispossessed Lives: Enslaved Women, Violence, and the Archive*. Philadelphia: University of Pennsylvania Press, 2016.

Furth, Charlotte. *A Flourishing Yin: Gender in China's Medical History, 960–1665*. Los Angeles: University of California Press, 1999.

Galarneau, Charlene. *Communities of Health Care Justice*. Newark: Rutgers University Press, 2016.

García-Ballester, Luis. "Artifex factivus sanitatus: Health and Medical Care in Medieval Latin Galenism." In *Knowledge and the Scholarly Medical Traditions*, edited by Donald Bates, 127–50. Cambridge: Cambridge University Press, 1995.

——. "Construction of a New Form of Learning and Practicing Medicine in Medieval Latin Europe." *Science in Context* 8.1 (1995): 75–102.

——. *Galen and Galenism: Theory and Medical Practice from Antiquity to the European Renaissance*. Aldershot: Ashgate, 2002.

García-Ballester, Luis, Michael McVaugh, and Augustín Rubio-Vela. *Medical Licensing and Learning in Fourteenth-Century Valencia*. Philadelphia: Transactions of the American Philosophical Society, 1989.

Geary, Patrick. *Living with the Dead in the Middle Age*. Ithaca: Cornell University Press, 1994.

Gentilcore, David. *Medical Charlatanism in Early Modern Italy*. Oxford: Oxford University Press, 2006.

George, Philippe. "À Saint-Trond, un import-export de reliques des Onze Mille Vierges au XIIIe siècle." *Bulletin de la Société Royale Le Vieux-Liège* 12 (1991): 209–28.

Getz, Faye. "Charity, Translation, and the Language of Medical Learning in Medieval England." *Bulletin of the History of Medicine* 64 (1990): 1–17.

——, ed. *Healing and Society in Medieval England: A Middle English Translation of the Pharmaceutical Writings of Gilbertus Anglicus.* Madison: University of Wisconsin Press, 1991.

Glenn, Evelyn Nakano. *Forced to Care: Coercion and Caregiving in America.* Cambridge, MA: Harvard University Press, 2010.

Glymph, Thavolia. *Out of the House of Bondage: The Transformation of the Plantation Household.* Cambridge: Cambridge University Press, 2008.

Gómez, Pablo. "The Circumstances of Body Knowledge in the Seventeenth-Century Black Spanish Caribbean." *Social History of Medicine* 26.3 (2013): 383–402.

——. *The Experiential Caribbean: Creating Knowledge and Healing in the Early Modern Atlantic.* Chapel Hill: University of North Carolina Press, 2017.

——. "Incommensurable Epistemologies? The Atlantic Geography of Healing in the Early Modern Caribbean." *Small Axe*, 2014, 95–107.

Good, Byron. *Medicine, Rationality, and Experience: An Anthropological Perspective.* Cambridge: Cambridge University Press, 1993.

Goodich, Michael. *Miracles and Wonders: The Development of the Concept of Miracle, 1150–1350.* New York: Routledge, 2007.

Gravdal, Kathryn. *Ravishing Maidens: Writing Rape in Medieval French Literature and Law.* Philadelphia: University of Pennsylvania Press, 1991.

Green, Monica. "Books as a Source of Medical Education for Women in the Middle Ages." *Dynamis* 20 (2000): 331–69.

——. "Documenting Medieval Women's Medical Practice." In *Practical Medicine from Salerno to the Black Death*, edited by Luis García-Ballester, Jon French, Jon Arrizabalaga, and Andrew Cunningham, 322–52. Cambridge: Cambridge University Press, 1994.

——. "Gender, Health, Disease: Recent Work on Medieval Women's Medicine." *Studies in Medieval and Renaissance History*, ser. 3, 5 (2005): 1–46.

——. "Gendering the History of Women's Healthcare." *Gender & History* 20.3 (2008): 487–518.

——. "Getting to the Source: The Case of Jacoba Felicie and the Impact of the *Portable Medieval Reader* on the Canon of Medieval Women's History." *Medieval Feminist Forum* 42 (2006): 49–62.

——. *Making Women's Medicine Masculine: The Rise of Male Authority in Pre-modern Gynaecology.* Oxford: Oxford University Press, 2008.

——. "The Possibilities of Literacy and the Limits of Reading: Women and the Gendering of Medical Literacy." In *Women's Healthcare in the Medieval West: Texts and Contexts*, edited by Monica Green, 1–76. Aldershot: Ashgate, 2000.

——. "Richard de Fournival and the Reconfiguration of Learned Medicine in the Mid-Thirteenth Century." In *Richard de Fournival et les sciences au XIIIe siècle*, edited by Joelle Ducos and Christopher Luclean, 179–206. Florence: SISMEL, 2018.

——. "Salerno." In *Medieval Science, Technology, and Medicine: An Encyclopedia*, edited by Thomas Glick, Steven Livesey, and Faith Wallis, 452–53. New York: Routledge, 2005.

——, ed. and trans. *The Trotula: A Medieval Compendium of Women's Medicine*. Philadelphia: University of Pennsylvania Press, 2001.

——. "Women's Medical Practice and Healthcare in Medieval Europe." *Signs* 14 (1989): 434–73.

Greilsammer, Myriam. "The Midwife, the Priest, and the Physician: The Subjugation of Midwives in the Low Countries at the End of the Middle Ages." *Journal of Medieval and Renaissance Studies* 21.2 (1991): 285–325.

Griffiths, Fiona. "Brides and Dominae: Abelard's *Cura monialium* at the Augustinian Monastery of Marbach." *Viator* 34 (2003): 57–88.

Grundmann, Herbert. *Religious Movements in the Middle Ages*. South Bend: University of Notre Dame Press, 1999.

Guerts, Kathryn Linn. *Culture and the Senses: Bodily Ways of Knowing in an African Community*. Berkeley: University of California Press, 2002.

Guidera, Christine. "The Role of Beguines in Caring for the Ill, Dying, and the Dead." In *Death and Dying in the Middle Ages*, edited by Edelgard DuBruck and Barbara Gusick, 51–72. New York: Peter Lang.

Haggh, Barbara. "Medieval Plainchant from Cambrai: A Preliminary List of Hymns, Alleluia Verses, and Sequences." *Revista de Musicologia* 16.4 (1993): 2326–34.

Halevi, Leor. "Wailing for the Dead: The Role of Women in Early Islamic Funerals." *Past & Present* 183 (2004): 3–39.

Hankart, Robert. "L'Hospice de Cornillon à Liège." *Vie Wallonne* 40 (1966): 5–49.

Harkness, Deborah. "A View from the Streets: Women and Medical Work in Elizabethan London." *Bulletin of the History of Medicine* 82.1 (2008): 52–85.

Harpham, Geoffrey Galt. "The Fertile Word: Augustine's Ascetics of Interpretation." *Criticism* 28.3 (1986): 237–54.

Harrington, Anne. *The Cure Within: A History of Mind-Body Medicine*. New York: Norton, 2008.

Harris, Carissa. *Obscene Pedagogies: Transgressive Talk and Sexual Education in Late Medieval Britain*. Ithaca: Cornell University Press, 2018.

Hartman, Saidiya. *Scenes of Subjection: Terror, Slavery, and Self-Making in Nineteenth-Century America*. Oxford: Oxford University Press, 1997.

Hasse, Dag Nikolaus. *Avicenna's "De anima" in the Latin West: The Formation of a Peripatetic Philosophy of the Soul, 1160–1300*. London: Warburg, 2000.

Haug, Andreas. "Performing Latin Verse: Text and Music in Early Medieval Versified Offices." In *The Divine Office in the Latin Middle Ages*, edited by Margot Fassler and Rebecca Baltzer, 278–99. Oxford: Oxford University Press, 2000.

Hayum, Andrée. *The Isenheim Altarpiece: God's Medicine and the Painter's Vision*. Princeton: Princeton University Press, 1993.

Henderson, John. *The Renaissance Hospital: Healing the Body and Healing the Soul*. New Haven: Yale University Press, 2006.

Heng, Geraldine. *The Invention of Race in the European Middle Ages*. Cambridge: Cambridge University Press, 2018.

Henneau, Marie-Élisabeth. "Entre terres et cieux . . . le temps des fondations (XIIIe–XIVe siècles)." In *La Ramée: Abbaye cistercienne en Brabant Wallon*, edited by Thomas Coomans, 7–31. Brussels: Éditions Racine, 2002.

Herckenrode, Léon de. "Une amulette: Légende en vers de Sainte Marguerite, tirée d'un ancien manuscrit." *Bulletin de Bibliophile Belge* 4 (1847): 2–23.

Hill, Boyd. "The Brain and the Spirit in Medieval Anatomy." *Speculum* 40 (1965): 63–73.

Hill, Carol. *Women and Religion in Late Medieval Norwich*. Woodbridge: Boydell and Brewer, 2010.

Hochschild, Arlie Russell. *The Commercialization of Intimate Life: Notes from Home and Work*. Berkeley: University of California Press, 2003.

Hohenberg, Paul, and Lynn Hollen Lees. *The Making of Urban Europe, 1000–1950*. Cambridge, MA: Harvard University Press, 1985.

Holsinger, Bruce. *Music, Body, and Desire in Medieval Culture: Hildegard of Bingen to Chaucer*. Palo Alto: Stanford University Press, 2001.

hooks, bell. *Feminist Theory: From Margins to Center*. Boston: South End Press, 2007.

Horden, Peregrine. "Disease, Dragons, and Saints: The Management of Epidemics in the Dark Ages." In *Epidemics and Ideas: Essays on the Historical Perception of Pestilence*, edited by T. Ranger and P. Slack, 45–76. Cambridge: Cambridge University Press, 1992.

——. *Hospitals and Healing from Late Antiquity to the Later Middle Ages*. Aldershot: Ashgate, 2008.

——. "A Non-natural Environment: Medicine without Doctors and the Medieval European Hospital." In *The Medieval Hospital and Medical Practice*, edited by Barbara Bowers, 133–46. London: Routledge, 2007.

——. "Religion as Medicine: Music in Medieval Hospitals." In *Religion and Medicine in the Middle Ages*, edited by Peter Biller and Joseph Ziegler, 135–54. York: York University Press, 2001.

——. "What's Wrong with Early Medieval Medicine?" *Social History of Medicine* 24.1 (2011): 5–25.

Horden, Peregrine, and Richard Smith, eds. *Locus of Care: Families, Communities, Institutions, and the Provision of Welfare since Antiquity*. London: Routledge, 1997.

Howell, Martha. *Women, Production, and Patriarchy in Late Medieval Cities*. Chicago: University of Chicago Press, 1986.

Hughes, Andrew. *Medieval Manuscripts for Mass and Office: A Guide to Their Organization and Terminology*. Toronto: University of Toronto Press, 1982.

Hunt, Nancy Rose. "An Acoustic Register, Tenacious Images, and Congolese Scenes of Rape and Repetition." *Cultural Anthropology* 23.2 (2008): 220–53.

——. *A Nervous State: Violence, Remedies, and Reverie in Colonial Congo*. Durham: Duke University Press, 2016.

Hunt, Tony. *Popular Medicine in Thirteenth-Century England: Introduction and Texts*. Woodbridge: Boydell & Brewer, 1990.

Imbert, Jean, and Michel Mollat. *Histoire des hôpitaux en France*. Paris: Privat, 1982.

Izbicki, Thomas. *The Eucharist in Medieval Canon Law*. Cambridge: Cambridge University Press, 2013.

Izydorczyk, Zbigniew. *Manuscripts of the Evangelium Nicodemi: A Census.* Turnhout: Brepols, 1994.

Jacquart, Danielle, ed. *La scuola medica salernitana: Gli autori e i testi.* Florence: SISMEL, 2007.

———. *Le milieu médical en France du XIIe au XVe siècle.* Geneva: Droz, 1981.

Jacquart, Danielle, and Françoise Micheau. *La médecine arabe et l'Occident médiévale.* Paris: Maisonneuve et Larose, 1990.

Jenks, Stuart. "Medizinische Fachkräfte in England zur Zeit Heinrichs VI (1428/ 9–1460/61)." *Sudhoffs Archiv* 69.2 (1985): 214–27.

Johnson, Sherri Franks. *Monastic Women and Religious Orders in Late Medieval Bologna.* Cambridge: Cambridge University Press, 2014.

Johnston, Michael, and Michael Van Dussen, eds. *The Medieval Manuscript Book: Cultural Approaches.* Cambridge: Cambridge University Press, 2015.

Jones, Claire. "Formula and Formulations: 'Efficacy Phrases' in Medieval English Medical Manuscripts." *Neuphilologische Mitteilungen* 2 (1998): 199–210.

Jones, Peter Murray. "Music Therapy in the Later Middle Ages: The Case of Hugo van der Goes." In *Music as Medicine: The History of Music Therapy since Late Antiquity,* edited by Peregrine Horden, 120–44. Aldershot: Ashgate, 2000.

———. "Thomas Fayreford: An English Fifteenth-Century Medical Practitioner." In *Medicine from the Black Death to the French Disease,* edited by Roger French, John Arrizabalaga, Andrew Cunnigham, and Luis García-Ballester, 156–83. Aldershot: Ashgate, 1998.

Jones, Peter Murray, and Lea T. Olsan, "Performative Rituals for Conception and Childbirth in England, 900–1500." *Bulletin of the History of Medicine* 89 (2015): 1–42.

Jordan, Erin. "Roving Nuns and Cistercian Realities: The Cloistering of Religious Women in the Thirteenth Century." *Journal of Medieval and Early Modern Studies* 42.3 (2012): 597–614.

———. *Women, Power, and Religious Patronage in the Middle Ages.* New York: Palgrave, 2006.

Jordan, Mark. "The Disappearance of Galen in Thirteenth-Century Philosophy and Theology." In *Mensch und Natur im Mittelalter,* edited by Albert Zimmermann and Andreas Speer, 703–13. Berlin: Walter de Gruyter, 1992.

———. "Medicine and Natural Philosophy in Aquinas." In *Thomas von Aquin: Werk und Wirkung im Licht neuerer Forschungen,* edited by Albert Zimmermann, 233–46. Berlin: Walter de Gruyter, 1988.

Kauanui, J. Kēhualani. *Hawaiian Blood: Colonialism and the Politics of Sovereignty and Indigeneity.* Durham: Duke University Press, 2008.

Kaye, Joel. *A History of Balance: The Emergence of a New Model of Equilibrium and Its Impact on Thought.* Cambridge: Cambridge University Press, 2014.

Keen, Elizabeth. *The Journey of a Book: Bartholomew the Englishman and the Properties of Things.* Canberra: Australian National University Press, 2007.

Kessler, Herman. "A Sanctifying Serpent: Crucifix as Cure." In *Studies on Medieval Empathies,* edited by Karl Morrison and Rudolph Bell, 161–85. Turnhout: Brepols, 2013.

Kieckhefer, Richard. *Magic in the Middle Ages.* Cambridge: Cambridge University Press, 1989.

——. "Rethinking How to Define Magic." In *The Routledge History of Medieval Magic*, edited by Catherine Rider and Sophie Page, 15–25. New York: Routledge, 2019.

——. "The Specific Rationality of Medieval Magic." *American Historical Review* 99.3 (1994): 813–36.

——. *Unquiet Souls: Fourteenth-Century Saints and Their Religious Milieu*. Chicago: University of Chicago Press, 1984.

Killam, G. D., ed. *Critical Perspectives on Ngugi Wa Thiong'o*. Washington, DC: Three Continents, 1984.

Klaniczay, Gabor. "Dreams and Visions in Medieval Miracle Accounts." In *Ritual Healing: Magic, Ritual, and Medical Therapy from Antiquity to the Early Modern Period*, edited by Ildikó Csperegi and Charles Burnett, 147–70. Florence: SISMEL, 2012.

——. "The Power of Words in Miracles, Visions, Incantations, and Bewitchments." In *The Power of Words: Studies of Charms and Charming*, edited by James Kapaló, Éva Pócs, and William Ryan, 281–304. Budapest: Central European Press, 2013.

——. "Using Saints: Intercession, Healing, Sanctity." In *The Oxford Handbook of Medieval Christianity*, edited by John Arnold, 227–28. Oxford: Oxford University Press, 2014.

Klassen, Pamela. "The Politics of Protestant Healing: Theoretical Tools for the Study of Spiritual Bodies and the Body Politic." *Spiritus: A Journal of Christian Spirituality* 14 (2014): 68–75.

Kleinberg, Aviad. *Prophets in Their Own Country: Living Saints and the Making of Sainthood in the Late Middle Ages*. Chicago: University of Chicago Press, 1992.

Kleinman, Arthur. *Patients and Healers in the Context of Culture: An Exploration of the Borderland between Anthropology, Medicine, and Psychology*. Berkeley: University of California Press, 1980.

Klemm, Matthew. "Les complexions vertueuses: La physiologie des vertus dans l'anthropologie médicale de Pietro d'Abano." *Médiévales* 63 (2012): 59–74.

——. "A Medieval Perspective on the Soul as Substantial Form of the Body: Peter of Abano on the Reconciliation of Aristotle and Galen." In *Psychology and the Other Disciplines: A Case of Cross-Disciplinary Interaction*, edited by Paul Bakker, Sander de Boer, and Cees Leijenhorst, 275–95. Leiden: Brill, 2012.

Knowles, David. *Great Historical Enterprises: Problems in Monastic History*. Edinburgh: Nelson and Sons, 1963.

Knuttila, Simo. *Emotions in Ancient and Medieval Philosophy*. Oxford: Clarendon Press, 2006.

Koopmans, Rachel. *Wonderful to Relate: Miracle Stories and Miracle Collecting in High Medieval England*. Philadelphia: University of Pennsylvania Press, 2011.

Krause, Kathy. "Guérisseuses et sorcières: La médecine feminine dans les romans des XIIe et XIIIe siècles." *Equinoxe* 8 (1992): 161–73.

Kuczynski, Michael. "The Psalms and Social Action in Late Medieval England." In *The Place of the Psalms in the Intellectual Culture of the Middle Ages*, edited by Nancy Van Deusen, 191–214. New York: SUNY Press, 1999.

Kunst, Jennifer, and Tommy Wasserman. "Earth Accuses Earth: Tracing Jesus's Writing on the Ground." *Harvard Theological Review* 103 (2010): 407–46.

Kupfer, Marcia. *The Art of Healing: Painting for the Sick and the Sinner in a Medieval Town.* University Park: Pennsylvania State University Press, 2003.

Kupper, Jean-Louis. "La cité de Liège." In *Fête-Dieu (1246–1996): Actes du Colloque de Liège, 12–14 septembre 1996,* edited by André Haquin, 19–26. Louvain-la-Neuve: Institut d'Études Médiévales de l'Université Catholique de Louvain, 1999.

Lahtinen, Anu, and Mia Korpiola, eds. *Dying Prepared in Medieval and Early Modern Europe.* Turnhout: Brill, 2017.

Langwick, Stacey. *Bodies, Politics, and African Healing: A Matter of Maladies in Tanzania.* Bloomington: Indiana University Press, 2011.

Larson, Wendy. "Who Is the Master of This Narrative? Maternal Patronage of the Cult of Saint Margaret." In *Gendering the Master Narrative: Women and Power in the Middle Ages,* edited by Mary Erler and Maryanne Kowalewski, 94–104. Ithaca: Cornell University Press, 2003.

Lässig, Simone. "The History of Knowledge and the Expansion of the Historical Research Agenda." *German Historical Institute Bulletin* 59 (Fall 2016): 29–58.

Latour, Bruno. *Science in Action: How to Follow Scientists and Engineers through Society.* Cambridge, MA: Harvard University Press, 1988.

Lauwers, Michel. "L'expérience béguinale et récit hagiographique à propos de la *Vita Mariae Oigniacensis* de Jacques de Vitry." *Journal des Savants* 11 (1989): 61–103.

Le Blévec, Daniel. "Le rôle des femmes dans l'assistance et la charité." *Cahiers de Fanjeaux* 23: *La femme dans la vie religieuse du Languedoc (XIIIe–XIVe s)* (1998): 171–90.

Leclercq, Jean. "Eucharistic Celebrations without Priests in the Middle Ages." *Workshop* 55 (1980): 160–68.

Leroquais, Chanoine. *Les psautiers manuscrits latins des bibliothèques publiques de France.* Mâcon: Protat, 1940.

Lester, Anne. *Creating Cistercian Nuns: The Women's Religious Movement and Its Reform in Thirteenth-Century Champagne.* Ithaca: Cornell University Press, 2011.

——. "The Porter of Clairvaux: Space, Place, and Institution; An Example of the Evolution of the Spirituality of Charity during the Thirteenth Century." In *Le temps long de Clairvaux: Nouvelles recherches, Nouvelles perspectives (XIIe–XXIe siècle),* edited by Arnaud Baudin and Alexis Grélois, 117–34. Troyes: Conseil Départmental de l'Aube, 2017.

Levy, Ian Christopher. "The Eucharist and Canon Law in the High Middle Ages." In *A Companion to the Eucharist in the Middle Ages,* edited by Ian Levy, Gary Macy, and Kristen Van Ausdall, 399–446. Leiden: Brill, 2012.

Lewis, Flora. "The Wound in Christ's Side and the Instruments of the Passion: Gendered Experience and Response." In *Women and the Book: Assessing the Visual Evidence,* edited by Lesley Smith and Jane Taylor, 204–29. London: British Library, 1997.

Lienhardt, Godfrey. *Divinity and Experience: The Religion of the Dinka.* Oxford: Clarendon Paperbacks, 1988.

Lifshitz, Felice. "Eight Men In: Rouennais Traditions of Archepiscopal Sanctity." *Haskins Society Journal,* 1990, 63–74.

——. *Religious Women in Early Carolingian Francia: A Study of Manuscript Transmission and Monastic Culture.* New York: Fordham University Press, 2014.

Little, Lester. *Religious Poverty and the Profit Economy in Medieval Europe.* Ithaca: Cornell University Press, 1978.

Long, Pamela. *Artisan Practitioners and the Rise of the New Sciences.* Corvalis: Portland State University Press, 2011.

——. *Openness, Secrecy, Authorship: Technical Arts and the Culture of Knowledge from Antiquity to the Renaissance.* Baltimore: Johns Hopkins University Press, 2001.

Lourdaux, Willem. *Bibliotheca Vallis Sancti Martini in Lovanio.* Leuven: Universitaire Pers, 1978.

Machielson, Jan. "Heretical Saints and Textual Discernment: The Polemical Origins of the Acta sanctorum (1643–1940)." In *Angels of Light? Sanctity and the Discernment of Spirits in the Early Modern Period,* edited by Clare Copeland and Jan Machielsen, 103–41. Leiden: Brill, 2012.

Macy, Gary. *Theologies of the Eucharist in the Early Scholastic Period: A Study of the Salvific Function of the Sacrament According to Theologians, 1080–1220.* New York: Oxford University Press, 1984.

Makowski, Elizabeth. "Mulieres Religiosae, Strictly Speaking: Some Fourteenth-Century Canonical Opinions." *Catholic Historical Review* 85 (1999): 1–14.

Mallardo, Domenico. "L'incubazione nella cristianità medieval napoletana." *Analecta Bollandiana* 67 (1949): 465–98.

Mannaerts, Pieter. "An Exception to the Rule? The Thirteenth-Century Historia for Mary of Oignies." *Journal for the Alamire Foundation* 2 (2010): 233–69.

Marcos, Natalio Fernández. *Los Thaumata de Sofronio: Contribución al estudio de la incubatio Cristiana.* Madrid: Instituto Antonio de Nebrija, 1975.

Marrone, Steven P. "Thomas Aquinas, Roger Bacon, and the Magicians on the Power of Words." In *Contemplation and Philosophy: Scholastic and Metaphysical Modes of Medieval Philosophical Thought: A Tribute to Kent Emery,* edited by Andreas Speer, 218–31. Leiden: Brill, 2018.

Matus, Zachary. "Resurrected Bodies and Roger Bacon's Elixir." *Ambix* 60.4 (2013): 323–40.

Maus, Marcell. *The Gift: The Form and Reason for Exchange in Archaic Societies.* Translated by W. D. Halls. New York: Norton, 1990.

McCann, Daniel. "Heaven and Health: Middle English Devotion to Christ in Its Therapeutic Contexts." In *Devotional Culture in Late Medieval England and Europe: Diverse Imaginations of Christ's Life,* edited by Stephen Kelly and Ryan Perry, 335–62. Turnhout: Brepols, 2014.

——. "Medicine of Words: Purgative Reading in Richard Rolle's Meditations on the Passion." *Medieval Journal* 5.2 (2015): 53–83.

——. *Soul Health: Therapeutic Reading in Late Medieval England.* Cardiff: University of Wales Press, 2019.

——. "Words of Fire and Fruit: The Psychology of Prayerwords in the *Cloud of Unknowing.*" *Medium Aevum* 84 (2015): 213–30.

McCleery, Iona. "Christ More Powerful than Galen: The Relationship between Medicine and Miracles." In *Contextualizing Miracles in the Medieval West,* edited by M. M. Mesley and Louise Wilson, 127–54. Leeds: Medium Aevum, 2014.

McCracken, Peggy. "Women and Medicine in Medieval French Narrative." *Exemplaria* 5.2 (1993): 239–62.

McDonnell, Ernest. *The Beguines and Beghards in Medieval Culture: With a Special Emphasis on the Belgian Scene.* New Brunswick: Rutgers University Press, 1954.

McNamer, Sarah. *Affective Meditation and the Invention of Medieval Compassion.* Philadelphia: University of Pennsylvania Press, 2009.

McVaugh, Michael. "Bedside Manners in the Middle Ages." *Bulletin of the History of Medicine* 71 (1997): 201–23.

——. "The Experience-Based Medicine of the Thirteenth Century." *Early Science and Medicine* 14 (2009): 105–30.

——. "*Incantationes* in Late Medieval Surgery." In *Ratio et superstitio: Essays in Honor of Graziella Federici Vescovini*, edited by G. Marchetti and Valeria Sorge, 319–45. Turnhout: Brepols, 2003.

——. *Medicine before the Plague: Practitioners and Their Patients in the Crown of Aragon, 1285–1345.* Cambridge: Cambridge University Press, 2002.

McVaugh, Michael, and Luis García-Ballester. "Therapeutic Method in the Later Middle Ages: Arnau de Vilanova on Medical Contingency." *Caduceus* 11 (1995): 73–86.

Meersseman, Gerard. *Der Hymnos Akathistos im Abendland.* Freiburg: Universitätsverlag, 1958.

Metcalf, Peter. *Where Are You/Spirits: Style and Theme in Berawan Prayer.* Washington, DC: Smithsonian Press, 1989.

Meyer, Paul. "Le psautier Lambert le Bègue." *Romania* 29 (1900): 536–40.

——. "Notice du MS Sloane 1611." *Romania* 40.160 (1911): 532–58.

——. "Rapport sur d'anciennes poésies religieuses en dialecte liégois." *Revue des Sociétés Savants des Départements* 6 (1873): 236–49.

Meysman, Stefan. "Virilitas in tijden van verandering: religieuze en profane mannelijkheden in de Nederlanden, ca. 1050–1300." PhD diss., University of Ghent, 2016.

Mews, Constant. "Debating the Authority of Pseudo-Augustine's *De spiritu et anima.*" *Przeglad Tomistyczny* 24 (2018): 321–48.

——. "The Diffusion of the *De spiritu et anima* and Cistercian Reflection on the Soul." *Viator* 49.3 (2018): 297–330.

Miller, Tanya Stabler. *Beguines of Medieval Paris: Gender, Patronage, and Spiritual Authority.* Philadelphia: University of Pennsylvania Press, 2014.

Milner, Matthew. "The Physics of Holy Oats: Vernacular Knowledge, Qualities, and Remedy in Fifteenth-Century England." *Journal of Medieval and Early Modern Studies* 43.2 (2013): 219–45.

Mitchell, W. J. T. *Iconology: Image, Text, Ideology.* Chicago: University of Chicago Press, 1987.

Moens, Sara. "Beatrice's World: The Rise of Cistercian Nunneries in the Bishoprics of Liège and Cambrai." *Ons Geestelijk Erf* 89.3–4 (2020): 225–74.

Mollat, Michel. *The Poor in the Middle Ages: An Essay in Social History.* Translated by Arthur Goldhammer. New Haven: Yale University Press, 1986.

Mols, Roger. *Introduction à la démographie historique des villes du Europe du XIVe au XVIIIe siècle.* Gembloux: Duculot, 1954.

Mooney, Catherine. *Clare of Assisi and the Thirteenth-Century Church: Religious Women, Rules, and Resistance.* Philadelphia: University of Pennsylvania Press, 2016.

——. "The 'Lesser Sisters' in Jacques de Vitry's 1216 Letter." *Franciscan Studies* 69 (2011): 1–29.

Mora-Dieu, Guillaume. "Liège/Liège: Évaluation archéologique sur le site de l'ancien hôpital Tirebourse." *Chronique de l'Archéologie Wallonne* 15 (2008): 132–34.

More, Alison. "Convergence, Conversion, and Transformation: Gender and Sanctity in Thirteenth-Century Liège." In *Representing Medieval Genders and Sexualities: Construction, Transformation, and Subversion, 600–1530,* edited by Elizabeth L'Estrange, 33–48. Surrey: Ashgate, 2011.

——. "Dynamics of Regulation, Innovation, and Invention." In *Observant Reform in the Late Middle Ages and Beyond,* edited by James D. Mixon and Bert Roest, 85–110. Leiden: Brill, 2015.

——. *Fictive Orders and Feminine Religious Identities, 1200–1600.* Oxford: Oxford University Press, 2019.

Moreau, Édouard de. *L'abbaye de Villers en Brabant aux XIIe et XIIIe siècles: Étude d'histoire religieuse et économique, suivie d'une notice archéologique par le chanoine R. Maere.* Brussels: Dewit, 1909.

Moreton-Robinson, Aileen, ed. *Sovereign Subjects: Indigenous Sovereignty Matters.* Crows Nest, Australia: Allen & Unwin, 2008.

Morse, Mary. "Seeing and Hearing: Margery Kempe and the Mis-en-Page." *Studia Mystica* 20 (1999): 15–42.

——. "'Thys moche more ys oure Lady Mary longe': Takamiya MS 56 and the English Birth Girdle Tradition." In *Middle English Texts in Transition: A Festschrift Dedicated to Toshiyuki Takamiya on His 70th Birthday,* edited by Simon Horobin and Linne Mooney, 199–219. Woodbridge: York Medieval Press, 2014.

Moulinier, Laurence. "Élisabeth, Ursule et les Onze mille Vierges: Un cas d'invention de reliques à Cologne au XIIe siècle." *Médiévales* 22–23 (1992): 173–86.

Mt. Pleasant, Alyssa, Caroline Wigginton, and Kelly Wisecup. "Materials and Methods in Native American and Indigenous Studies: Completing the Turn." *William and Mary Quarterly* 75 (April 2018): 207–36.

Muessig, Carolyn. *The Faces of Women in the Sermons of Jacques de Vitry.* Toronto: Peregrina Press, 1999.

Mulder-Bakker, Anneke, ed. *The Invention of Saintliness.* London: Routledge, 2002.

——. *Lives of the Anchoresses: The Rise of the Urban Recluse.* Philadelphia: University of Pennsylvania Press, 2005.

——, ed. *Living Saints of the Thirteenth Century.* Turnhout: Brepols, 2011.

——, ed. *Mary of Oignies: Mother of Salvation.* Turnhout: Brepols, 2006.

Munkoff, Richelle. "Poor Women and Parish Public Health." *Renaissance Studies* 28.4 (2014): 579–96.

Neel, Carol. "The Origins of the Beguines." *Signs* 14.2 (1989): 321–41.

Newman, Martha. "Crucified by the Virtues: Monks, Laybrothers, and Women in Thirteenth-Century Cistercian Saints' Lives." In *Gender and Difference in the Middle Ages,* edited by Sharon Farmer and Carol Braun Pasternack, 182–209. Minneapolis: University of Minnesota Press, 2003.

Nichols, Ann Eljenholm. "The Footprints of Christ as Arma Christi: The Evidence of Morgan B.54." In *The Arma Christi in Medieval and Early Modern Material*

Culture, edited by Lisa Cooper and Andrea Denny-Brown, 113–42. Aldershot: Ashgate, 2014.

Nicoud, Marilyn. *Les régimes de santé au Moyen Âge: Naissance et diffusion d'une écriture médicale (XIIIe–XVe siècles)*. Rome: École française, 2007.

Nie, Giselle de. *"Mutatio Sensus*: Poetics of Holiness and Healing in Paulinus of Périgueux's *Life of Saint Martin*." In *Studies on Medieval Empathies*, edited by Karl Morrison and Rudolph Bell, 61–89. Turnhout: Brepols, 2013.

——. *Poetics of Wonder: Testimonies of the New Christian Miracles in the Late Antique Latin World*. Leiden: Brill, 2011.

Niebyl, P. H. "The Non-Naturals." *Bulletin of the History of Medicine* 45.5 (1971): 486–92.

Nieus, Jean-François. "La route, les pauvres et le prince: L'hôpital rural de Grand-Vaux à Balâtre/Boignée; Approche historique (XIIIe–XVIe siècles)." In *Voyageurs, En Route! Au detour du chemin, trouver le vivre et le couvert*, edited by Aurélie Stuckens, 91–109. Bouvignes-Dinant: Maison du patrimonie médiéval mosan, 2019.

Noell, Brian. "Expectation and Unrest among Cistercian Laybrothers in the Twelfth and Thirteenth Centuries." *Journal of Medieval History* 32 (2006): 253–74.

Norpoth, Leo. *Der pseudo-augustinische Traktat "De Spiritu et anima."* Würzburg: Institut für Geschichte de Medizin, 1971.

Nutton, Vivian. *Galen: On Problematical Movements*. Cambridge: Cambridge University Press, 2011.

——. "God, Galen, and the Depaganization of Ancient Religion." In *Religion and Medicine in the Middle Ages*, edited by Peter Biller and Joseph Ziegler, 15–32. York: York Medieval Press, 2001.

——. "Medicine in Medieval Western Europe, 1000–1500." In *The Western Medical Tradition, 800 BC to 1800 AD*, edited by W. F. Bynum, 139–206. Cambridge: Cambridge University Press, 1995.

Nuyttens, M. "Abbaye de Zwijveke à Termonde." In *Monasticon Belge* VII: *Province de Flandre Orientale*, edited by U. Berlière, 473–75. Liège: Revue Belge de Philologie et d'Histoire, 1980.

Oberste, Judith. "Zeit und Ewigkeit: 128 Tage in St. Marienstern." In *Neues Archiv für sächsische Geschichte*, edited by K. Blaschke, 361–62. Stuttgart: Verlag Hermann Böhlaus, 1999.

O'Brien, Jean M., and Robert Warrior. "Building a Professional Infrastructure for Critical Indigenous Studies: A(n Intellectual) History of and Prospectus for the Native American and Indigenous Studies Association." In *Critical Indigenous Studies: Engagements in First World Locations*, edited by Aileen Moreton-Robinson, 33–48. Tucson: University of Arizona Press, 2016.

Oliver, Judith. "Devotional Psalters and the Study of Beguine Spirituality." *Vox Benedictina* 9.2 (1992): 199–225.

——. *Gothic Manuscript Illumination in the Diocese of Liège, 1250–1350*. 2 vols. Leuven: Peeters, 1988.

——. "Je pecherise renc grasces a vos: Some French Devotional Texts in Beguine Psalters." In *Medieval Codicology, Iconography, Literature, and Translation: Studies for Keith Val Sinclair*, edited by Peter Rolfe Monks, 248–62. Leiden: Brill, 1994.

———. "Reflections on Beguines and Psalters." *Ons Geestelijk Erf* 66.4 (1992): 249–56.

Olsan, Lea. "Charms and Prayers in Medieval Medical Theory and Practice." *Social History of Medicine* 16.3 (2003): 343–66.

———. "Latin Charms of Medieval England: Verbal Healing in a Christian Oral Tradition." *Oral Tradition* 7.1 (1992): 116–42.

———. "The Three Good Brothers Charm: Some Historical Points." *Incantatio* 1 (2011): 48–78.

Olson, Glending. *Literature as Recreation in the Middle Ages.* Ithaca: Cornell University Press, 1982.

Orlemanski, Julie. *Symptomatic Subjects: Bodies, Medicine, and Causation in the Literature of Late Medieval England.* Philadelphia: Pennsylvania University Press, 2019.

Orsi, Robert. "Abundant History: Marian Apparitions as Alternative Modernity." *Historically Speaking* 9.7 (2008): 12–16.

———. *History and Presence.* Cambridge, MA: Harvard University Press, 2016.

Otter, Monika. "Entrances and Exits: Performing the Psalms in Goscelin's *Liber confortatorius.*" *Speculum* 83 (2008): 283–302.

Page, Christopher. "Music and Medicine in the Thirteenth Century." In *Music as Medicine: The History of Music Therapy since Antiquity,* edited by Peregrine Horden, 109–19. Aldershot: Ashgate, 2000.

Palazzo, Eric. *A History of Liturgical Books from the Beginning to the Thirteenth Century.* Collegeville, MN: Liturgical Press, 1998.

Palmer, James. *Virtues of Economy: Governance, Power, and Piety in Late Medieval Rome.* Ithaca: Cornell University Press, 2019.

Park, Katherine. *Doctors and Medicine in Early Renaissance Florence.* Princeton: Princeton University Press, 1985.

Parnell, Suzanne, and Lea Olsan. "Index of Charms: Purpose, Design, and Implementation." *Literary and Linguistic Computing* 6.1 (1991): 59–63.

Paschetto, Eugenia. *Pietro d'Abano, medico e filosofo.* Florence: E. Vallecchi, 1984.

Pasnau, Robert. "Scholastic Qualities, Primary and Secondary." In *Primary and Secondary Qualities: The Historical and Ongoing Debate,* edited by Lawrence Nolan, 41–61. Oxford: Oxford Scholarship Online, 2011.

Paul, Nicholas. *To Follow in Their Footsteps: Crusades and Family Memory in the High Middle Ages.* Ithaca: Cornell University Press, 2012.

Paxton, Frederick. *Christianizing Death: The Creation of a Ritual Process in Early Medieval Europe.* Ithaca: Cornell University Press, 1990.

Pelikan, Jaroslav. *The Growth of Medieval Theology, 600–1300.* Chicago: University of Chicago Press, 1978.

Pelling, Margaret. "Thoroughly Resented? Older Women and the Medical Role in Early Modern London." In *Women, Science, and Medicine, 1500–1700,* edited by Lynette Hunter and Sarah Hutton, 63–88. Gloucestershire: Sutton, 1997.

Pelling, Margaret, and Charles Webster. "Medical Practitioners." In *Health, Medicine, and Mortality in the Sixteenth Century,* edited by Charles Webster, 165–235. Cambridge: Cambridge University Press, 1979.

Peterson, Janine. *Suspect Saints and Holy Heretics: Disputed Sanctity and Communal Identity in Late Medieval Italy.* Ithaca: Cornell University Press, 2019.

Peyroux, Catherine. "The Leper's Kiss." In *Monks, Nuns, Saints, and Outcasts: Religion in Medieval Society; Essays in Honor of Lester K. Little*, edited by Sharon Farmer and Barbara Rosenwein, 172–88. Ithaca: Cornell University Press, 2000.

Pfister, Manfred. *Theory and Analysis of Drama*. Cambridge: Cambridge University Press, 1988.

Pingree, David. *From Astral Omens to Astrology: From Babylon to Bīkāner*. Rome: Italian Institute for Africa and the Orient, 1997.

Pirenne, Henri. "Les dénombrements de la population d'Ypres au XVe siècle (1412–1506): Contribution à la statistique sociale du Moyen Âge." *Vierteljahrschrift für Sozial und Wirtschaftsgeschichte* 1 (1903): 1–32.

Pissart, Madeleine. "*Tirebourse et Florichamps*: Histoire d'un hôpital reserve aux beguines (Tirebourse) et d'une léproserie (Florichamps)." *Annuaire d'Histoire Liégeoise* 3 (1950): 301–44.

Pomata, Gianna. "Practicing between Earth and Heaven: Women Healers in Seventeenth-Century Bologna." *Dynamis* 19 (1999): 119–43.

Pormann, Peter, and Emilie Savage-Smith. *Medieval Islamic Medicine*. Washington, DC: Georgetown University Press, 2007.

Porter, Roy. *The Greatest Benefit to Mankind: A Medical History of Humanity from Antiquity to the Present*. New York: Norton, 1999.

Power, Eileen. "Some Women Practitioners of Medicine in the Middle Ages." *Proceedings of the Royal Society of Medicine* 15.6 (1922): 20–23.

Pratt, Karen. "*De vetula*: The Figure of the Old Woman in Medieval French Literature." In *Old Age in the Middle Ages and the Renaissance: Interdisciplinary Approaches to a Neglected Topic*, edited by Albrecht Classen, 321–42. Berlin: De Gruyter, 2007.

Raciti, Gaetano. "L'autore del *De spiritu et anima*." *Rivista di Filosofia Neo Scolastica* 53 (1961): 385–401.

Ragab, Ahmed. *Medieval Islamic Hospital: Medicine, Religion, and Charity*. Cambridge: Cambridge University Press, 2018.

Rankin, Alicia. *Panaceia's Daughters: Noblewomen as Healers in Early Modern Germany*. Chicago: University of Chicago Press, 2013.

Rappaport, Roy. *Ritual and Religion in the Making of Humanity*. Cambridge: Cambridge University Press, 1999.

Rather, L. J. "The Six Things Non Natural: A Note on the Origin and Fate of a Doctrine and a Phrase." *Clio Medica* 3 (1968): 337–47.

Rawcliffe, Carole. "Hospital Nurses and Their Work." In *Daily Life in the Late Middle Ages*, edited by R. H. Britnell, 42–64. London: Stroud, 1998.

———. "Learning to Love the Leper: Aspects of Institutional Charity in Anglo Norman England." *Anglo-Norman Studies* 23 (2001): 231–50.

———. *Leprosy in Medieval England*. Woodbridge: Boydell, 2006.

———. *Medicine for the Soul: The Life, Death, and Resurrection of an English Medieval Hospital; St. Giles's Norwich, 1249–1550*. Stroud: Sutton, 1999.

———. "Women, Childbirth, and Religion in Later Medieval England." In *Women and Religion in Medieval England*, edited by Diana Wood, 91–117. Oxford: Oxbow Books, 2003.

Ray, Anthony. "Brothers and Sisters in Christ, Brothers and Sisters Indeed: Two Thirteenth-Century Letters of Thomas, Cantor of Villers, to His Sister Alice,

Nun of Parc-les-Dames." In *Partners in Spirit: Women, Men, and Religious Life in Germany, 1100–1500*, edited by Fiona Griffiths and Julie Hotchin, 213–36. Turnhout: Brepols, 2014.

Reddy, William. *The Navigation of Feeling: A Framework for the History of Emotion.* Cambridge: Cambridge University Press, 2001.

Reinberg, Virginia. *French Books of Hours: Making an Archive of Prayer, 1400–1600.* Cambridge: Cambridge University Press, 2012.

——. "Prayer and the Book of Hours." In *Time Sanctified: The Book of Hours in Medieval Art*, edited by Roger Wieck, 39–44. Baltimore: Walters Art Gallery, 2001.

Rembry, Ernest. *Saint Gilles: Sa vie, ses reliques, son culte en Belgique et dans le nord de la France.* Bruges: Gailliard, 1881–82.

Resnick, Irven. *Marks of Distinction: Christian Perception of Jews in the High Middle Ages.* Washington, DC: Catholic University of America Press, 2012.

Reverby, Susan. *Ordered to Care: The Dilemma of American Nursing, 1850–1945.* Cambridge: Cambridge University Press, 1987.

Richardson, Kristina. "Blue and Green Eyes in the Islamicate Middle Ages." *Annales Islamologiques* 48.1 (2014): 13–30.

Ritchey, Sara, and Sharon Strocchia, eds. *Gender, Health, and Healing, 1250–1550.* Amsterdam: Amsterdam University Press, 2020.

Rivard, Derek. *Blessing the World: Ritual and Lay Piety in Medieval Religion.* Washington, DC: Catholic University of America Press, 2008.

Roisin, Simone. *L'hagiographie cistercienne dans le diocèse de Liège au XIIIe siècle.* Louvain: Bibliothèque de l'Université, 1947.

Rosenwein, Barbara. *Emotional Communities in the Early Middle Ages.* Ithaca: Cornell University Press, 2006.

Rosier-Catach, Irène. *La parole efficace: Signe, rituel, sacré.* Paris: Éditions du Seuil, 2004.

Rowell, Geoffrey. *The Liturgy of Christian Burial: An Introductory Survey of the Historical Development of Christian Burial Rites.* London: Alcuin Club, 1977.

Rubin, Miri. *Charity and Community in Medieval Cambridge.* Cambridge: Cambridge University Press, 2002.

——. *Corpus Christi: The Eucharist in Late Medieval Culture.* Cambridge: Cambridge University Press, 1991.

Rudy, Kathryn. *Rubrics, Images, and Indulgences in Late Medieval Netherlandish Manuscripts.* Leiden: Brill, 2016.

——. *Virtual Pilgrimages in the Convent: Imagining Jerusalem in the Late Middle Ages.* Turnhout: Brepols, 2011.

Ruhrberg, Christine. *Der literarische Körper der Heiligen Leben und Viten der Christina Stommeln.* Tubingen: Bibliotecha Germanica, 1995.

Saint-Denis, Alain. *L'hôtel-Dieu de Laon, 1150–1300.* Nancy: Presses Universitaires de Nancy, 1983.

Salmón, Fernando. "The Physician as Cure." In *Ritual Healing: Magic, Ritual, and Medical Therapy from Antiquity until the Early Modern Period*, edited by Ildikó Csepregi and Charles Burnett, 193–216. Florence: SISMEL, 2012.

——. "The Pleasures and Joys of the Humoral Body in Medieval Medicine." In *Pleasure in the Middle Ages*, edited by Naama Cohen-Hanegbi and Piroska Nagy, 39–58. Turnhout: Brepols, 2018.

Salmón, Fernando, and Montserrat Cabré. "Fascinating Women: The Evil Eye in Medical Scholasticism." In *Medicine from the Black Death to the French Disease*, edited by Roger French, 53–84. Aldershot: Ashgate, 1998.

Sargent, Carolyn. *The Cultural Context of Therapeutic Choice: Obstetrical Care Decisions among the Beriba of Benin*. Dordrecht: D. Reidel, 1982.

Saucier, Catherine. *A Paradise of Priests: Singing the Civic and Episcopal Hagiography of Liège*. Rochester: University of Rochester Press, 2014.

——. "Sacrament and Sacrifice: Conflating Corpus Christi and Martyrdom in Medieval Liège." *Speculum* 87 (2012): 682–723.

Scheepsma, Wybren. *The Limburg Sermons: Preaching in the Medieval Low Countries at the Turn of the Fourteenth Century*. Leuven: Brill, 2008.

Scheutz, Martin, et al., eds. *Europäisches Spitalwesen: Institutionelle Fürsorge in Mittelalter und Früher Neuzeit/Hospitals and Institutional Care in Medieval and Early Modern Europe*. Vienna: Oldenbourg Verlag, 2008.

Schmitt, Jean-Claude. *Ghosts in the Middle Ages: The Living and the Dead in Medieval Society*. Chicago: University of Chicago Press, 1998.

——. *Mort d'une hérésie: L'Église et les clercs face aux béguines et aux béghards du Rhin supérieur du XIVe au XVe siècle*. Paris: Mouton, 1978.

Searle, John, and Daniel Vanderveken. *Foundations of Illocutionary Logic*. Cambridge: Cambridge University Press, 1985.

Shyovitz, David. *A Remembrance of His Wonders: Nature and the Supernatural in Medieval Ashkenaz*. Philadelphia: University of Pennsylvania Press, 2017.

Simons, Walter. "Beginnings: Naming Beguines in the Southern Low Countries, 1200–50." In *Labels and Libels: Naming Beguines in Northern Medieval Europe*, edited by Letha Böhringer, Jennifer Kolpacoff Deane, and Hildo van Engen, 9–52. Turnhout: Brepols, 2014.

——. "The Beguine Movement in the Southern Low Countries: A Reassessment." *Bulletin de l'Institut Historique Belge de Rome* 59 (1989): 63–105.

——. *Cities of Ladies: Beguine Communities in the Medieval Low Countries, 1200–1565*. Philadelphia: University of Pennsylvania Press, 2001.

——. "Reading a Saint's Body: Rapture and Bodily Movement in the *Vitae* of Thirteenth-Century Beguines." In *Framing Medieval Bodies*, edited by Sarah Kay and Miri Rubin, 10–23. Manchester: Manchester University Press, 1994.

——. "Staining the Speech of Things Divine: The Uses of Literacy in Medieval Beguine Communities." In *The Voice of Silence: Women's Literacy in a Men's Church*, edited by Thérèse de Hemptinne and María Eugenia Góngora, 85–110. Turnhout: Brepols, 2004.

Sinclair, Keith. "Les manuscrits du psautier de Lambert le Bègue." *Romania* 86 (1965): 22–47.

Siraisi, Nancy. *Medieval and Early Renaissance Medicine: An Introduction to Knowledge and Practice*. Chicago: University of Chicago Press, 1990.

——. "The Music of the Pulse in the Writings of Italian Academic Physicians (Fourteenth and Fifteenth Centuries)." *Speculum* 50 (1975): 689–710.

Skemer, Don. *Binding Words: Textual Amulets in the Middle Ages*. University Park: Pennsylvania State University Press, 2006.

Smith, Jonathan Z. "Religion, Religions, Religious." In *Critical Terms for Religious Studies*, edited by Mark Taylor, 269–84. Chicago: University of Chicago Press, 1988.

Smith, Julia. "Oral and Written: Saints, Miracles, and Relics in Britany, *c.* 850–1250." *Speculum* 65 (1990): 309–43.

Smith, Pamela H. *The Body of the Artisan: Art and Experience in the Scientific Revolution.* Chicago: University of Chicago Press, 2004.

Smith, Rachel. *Excessive Saints: Gender, Narrative, and Theological Invention in Thomas of Cantimpré's Mystical Hagiographies.* New York: Columbia University Press, 2019.

——. "Language, Literacy, and the Saintly Body: Cistercian Reading Practices and the Life of Lutgard of Aywières." *Harvard Theological Review* 109.4 (2016): 586–610.

Solomon, Michael. *Fictions of Well-Being: Sickly Readers and Vernacular Medical Writing in Late Medieval and Early Modern Spain.* Philadelphia: University of Pennsylvania Press, 2010.

Sotres, Pedro Gil. "The Regimens of Health." In *Western Medical Thought from Antiquity to the Middle Ages,* edited by Mirko Grmek, 291–318. Cambridge, MA: Harvard University Press, 2002.

Southern, Richard. *Saint Anselm and His Biographer.* Cambridge: Cambridge University Press, 1963.

Spiegeler, Pierre de. "La léproserie de Cornillon et la cité de Liège (xiie–xve)." *Annales de la Société Belge d'Histoire des Hôpitaux* 18 (1980): 5–16.

——. *Les hôpitaux et l'assistance à Liège: Aspects institutionnels et sociaux.* Paris: Les Belles Lettres, 1987.

Spillers, Hortense. "Mamas Baby, Papas Maybe: An American Grammar Book." *Diacritics* 17 (1987): 64–81.

Spivak, Gayatri Chakravorty. *The Post-Colonial Critic: Interviews, Strategies, Dialogues.* New York: Routledge, 1990.

Stabel, Peter. *Dwarfs among Giants: The Flemish Urban Network in the Late Middle Ages.* Louvain: Garant, 1997.

Stanton, Anne Rudloff. *Queen Mary Psalter: A Study of Affect and Audience.* Philadelphia: American Philosophical Society, 2011.

Stemmle, Jennifer. "From Cure to Care: Indignation, Assistance, and Leprosy in the High Middle Ages." In *Experiences of Charity, 1250–1650,* edited by Anne Scott, 43–62. Farnham: Ashgate, 2015.

Stewart, Kathleen. *Ordinary Affects.* Durham: Duke University Press, 2007.

Stock, Brian. *The Implications of Literacy: Written Language and Models of Interpretation in the 11th and 12th Centuries.* Princeton: Princeton University Press, 1987.

——. *The Integrated Self: Augustine, the Bible, and Ancient Thought.* Philadelphia: University of Pennsylvania Press, 2017.

Stoller, Ann Laura. *Along the Archival Grain: Epistemic Anxieties and Colonial Common Sense.* Princeton: Princeton University Press, 2009.

Stracke, D. A. "Arnulf van Leuven, O. Cist. versus gelukz. Hermann Jozef, O. Praem." *Ons Geestelijk Erf* 24 (1950): 27–50.

Strengers, Jean. *Les juifs dans les Pays-Bas au Moyen Âge.* Brussels: Palais des Académies, 1950.

Stuart, Heather. "A Ninth-Century Account of Diets and Dies Aegyptiaci." *Scriptorium* 33 (1979): 237–44.

Sutherland, Annie. "Performing the Penitential Psalms in the Middle Ages." In *Aspects of the Performative in Medieval Culture*, edited by Almut Suerbam and Manuele Gragnolati, 15–37. Berlin: De Gruyter, 2010.

Suydam, Mary. "Visionaries in the Public Eye: Beguine Literature as Performance." In *The Texture of Society: Medieval Women in the Southern Low Countries*, edited by Ellen Kittell and Mary Suydam, 131–52. New York: Palgrave, 2004.

——. "Women's Texts and Performances in the Medieval Southern Low Countries." In *Visualizing Medieval Performance: Perspectives, Histories, Contexts*, edited by Elina Gertsman, 143–59. Aldershot: Ashgate, 2008.

Tarlier, Jules. *Geographie et histoire des communes Belges: Province de Brabant*. Brussels: Decq, 1865.

Tasiaux, Michelle. "L'hospice Terarken, à Bruxelles des origins à 1386." *Annales de la Société Royale d'Archéologie de Bruxelles* 57 (1980): 3–37.

Taylor, Diana. *The Archive and the Repertoire: Performing Cultural Memory in the Americas*. Durham: Duke University Press, 2003.

——. "Remapping Genre through Performance: From 'American' to 'Hemispheric' Studies." *PMLA* 122 (2007): 1416–30.

Thorndike, Lynn. *A History of Magic and Experimental Science*. New York: Columbia University Press, 1923.

Tierney, Brian. "The Decretists and the 'Deserving Poor.'" *Comparative Studies in Society and History* 1.4 (1959): 360–73.

Touati, François-Olivier. *Maladie et société au Moyen Âge: La lèpre, les lèpreux, et les lèpro-saries dans la province ecclésiastique de Sens jusqu'au milieu du XIV siècle*. Paris: De Boeck, 1998.

Trouillot, Michel-Rolph. *Silencing the Past: Power and the Production of History*. New York: Beacon, 1997.

Valdman, Albert, et al., eds. *Dictionary of Louisiana French: As Spoken in Cajun, Creole, and American Indian Communities*. Jackson: University of Mississippi Press, 2009.

Van Dam, Raymond. *Saints and Their Miracles in Late Antique Gaul*. Princeton: Princeton University Press, 1993.

Van Der Elst, Emmanuel. *L'Hôpital Saint-Jean de Bruges de 1188 à 1500*. Bruges: Vercruysse-Vanhove, 1975.

Van Der Lugt, Maaike. "The Learned Physician as Charismatic Healer: Urso of Salerno on Incantations in Medicine, Magic, and Religion." *Bulletin of the History of Medicine* 87.3 (2013): 307–46.

Vanderputten, Steven, Tjamke Snijders, and Jay Diehl. *Medieval Liège at the Crossroads of Europe: Monastic Society and Culture, 1000–1300*. Turnhout: Brill, 2017.

Van der Wee, Herman, ed. *The Rise and Decline of the Urban Industries in Italy and the Low Countries*. Leuven: Leuven University Press, 1988.

Van Gerven, Jan. "Vrouwen, arbeid en sociale positie: Een voorlopig onderzoek naar de economische rol en maatschappelijke positie van vrouwen in de Brabantse steden in de late Middeleeuwen." *Revue Belge de Philologie et d'Histoire* 73 (1995): 947–66.

Van Puyvelde, Leopold. *Un hôpital du Moyen Âge et une abbaye y annexée: La Biloke de Gand; Étude archéologique*. Ghent: University of Ghent, 1925.

Vauchez, André. *La spiritualité du Moyen Âge occidental (VIIIe-XIIIe siècle)*. Paris: Seuil, 1994.

——. *Sainthood in the Later Middle Ages*. Cambridge: Cambridge University Press, 1997.

Wallis, Faith. "Medicine in Medieval Calendar Manuscripts." In *Manuscript Sources of Medieval Medicine*, ed. Margaret Schleissner, 105–44. New York: Garland, 1995.

Walters, Barbara, Vincent Corrigan, and Peter Ricketts, eds. *The Feast of Corpus Christi*. University Park: Pennsylvania State University Press, 2006.

Walters, Jozef. *Geschiedenis der Zusters der Bijloke te Gent*. Ghent: Veritas, 1929–30.

Ward, Benedicta. *Miracles and the Medieval Mind: Theory, Record, and Event, 1000–1215*. Philadelphia: University of Pennsylvania Press, 1987.

Weinryb, Ittai, ed. *Ex Voto: Votive Giving across Cultures*. New York: Bard Graduate Center, 2015.

Wharton, Amy. "The Sociology of Emotional Labor." *American Review of Sociology* 35 (2009): 147–65.

Wieck, Roger. *Painted Prayers: The Book of Hours in Medieval and Renaissance Art*. New York: George Braziller, 1997.

——. *Time Sanctified: The Book of Hours in Medieval Art and Life*. New York: George Braziller, 1988.

Wilcox, Judith, and John Riddle. "Qūsta Ibn Lūqā's *Physical Ligatures* and the Recognition of the Placebo Effect: With an Edition and Translation." *Medieval Encounters* 1.1 (1995): 1–25.

Williams, Patricia. *Seeing a Colorblind Future: The Paradox of Race (the Reith Lectures, 1997)*. New York: Farrar, Straus and Giroux, 1998.

Wogan-Browne, Jocelyn. "The Apple's Message: Some Post-Conquest Hagiographic Accounts of Textual Transmission." In *Late Medieval Religious Texts and Their Transmission*, edited by Alistair Minnis, 39–53. Cambridge: D.S. Brewer, 1993.

——. "Clerc u lai, muïne u dame: Women and Anglo-Norman Hagiography in the Twelfth and Thirteenth Centuries." In *Women and Literature in Britain, 1150–1500*, edited by Carole Meale, 61–85. Cambridge: Cambridge University Press, 2009.

Wolf, Kenneth. *The Life and Afterlife of St. Elizabeth of Hungary*. Oxford: Oxford University Press, 2010.

Yarrow, Simon. *Saints and Their Communities: Miracle Stories in Twelfth-Century England*. Oxford: Clarendon Press, 2006.

——. "Twelfth-Century Miracle Narratives." In *Contextualizing Medieval Miracles in the Christian West*, edited by Matthew Mesley and Louise Wilson, 41–62. Oxford: Medium Aevum, 2014.

Yoshikawa, Naoë Kukita. "Holy Medicine and Diseases of the Soul: Henry of Lancaster and *Le livre de seyntz medicines*." *Medical History* 53 (2009): 397–414.

——. "The Virgin in the Hortus conclusus: Healing the Body and Healing the Soul." *Medieval Feminist Forum* 50.1 (2014): 11–32.

Zarri, Gabriella. *Le sante vive: Cultura e religiosità femminile nella prima età moderna*. Turin: Rosenberg & Sellier, 1990.

Ziegler, Joanna. *The Sculpture of Compassion: The Pietà and the Beguines in the Southern Low Countries, 1300–1600*. Brussels: Institut Historique Belge de Rome, 1992.

Ziegler, Joseph. *Medicine and Religion, c. 1300: The Case of Arnau de Vilanova*. Oxford: Clarendon Press, 1998.

——. "Ut dicunt medici: Medical Knowledge and Theological Debates in the Second Half of the Thirteenth Century." *Bulletin of the History of Medicine* 73 (1999): 208–37.

Ziegler, Tiffany. "The Hospital of St. John: Exploring Charitable Distribution in High Medieval Brussels." *Ëa: Journal of Medical Humanities and Social Studies of Science & Technology* 3 (2011): 1–32.

INDEX

Page numbers in *italics* indicate illustrations. Authored texts are located under the author's name. Manuscripts are listed by location and institution under the entry, "manuscripts," and by their commonly used names. Institutions such as hospitals usually are listed by location.

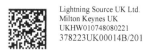
Lightning Source UK Ltd.
Milton Keynes UK
UKHW010748080221
378223UK00014B/201

9 781501 758324